The Digestive System

SYSTEMS OF THE BODY

The Digestive System

BASIC SCIENCE AND CLINICAL CONDITIONS

THIRD EDITION

Richard Horniblow MSci, PhD, PGCHE, FHEA
Lecturer of Biomedical Science
School of Biomedical Sciences
College of Medical and Dental Sciences
University of Birmingham
Birmingham, UK

Chris Tselepis BSc, PhD, FRSB, PFHEA
Professor of Biomedical Science
School of Biomedical Sciences
College of Medical and Dental Sciences
University of Birmingham
Birmingham, UK

Mohammed Nabil Quraishi

PhD, MRCP, FEBGH
Consultant Gastroenterologist
Honorary Senior Clinical Lecturer
University Hospitals Birmingham
NHS Foundation Trust
University of Birmingham
Birmingham, UK

1st and 2nd edition authors:

Margaret Smith
Dion Morton

Series Editor

Stephen Hughes BSc, MSc, MBBS, FRCSEd, FRCEM, FHEA
Consultant in Emergency Medicine, Broomfield Hospital
Senior Lecturer in Medicine, School of Medicine, Anglia Ruskin University
Chelmsford, UK

For additional online content visit ExpertConsult.com

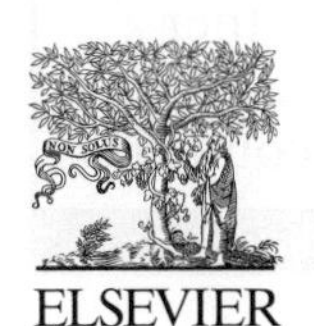

ELSEVIER

First edition 2003
Second edition 2010

Notices

Practitioners and researchers must always rely on their own experience and knowledge in evaluating and using any information, methods, compounds or experiments described herein. Because of rapid advances in the medical sciences, in particular, independent verification of diagnoses and drug dosages should be made. To the fullest extent of the law, no responsibility is assumed by Elsevier, authors, editors or contributors for any injury and/or damage to persons or property as a matter of products liability, negligence or otherwise, or from any use or operation of any methods, products, instructions, or ideas contained in the material herein.

ISBN: 978-0-7020-8376-1

Publisher: Jeremy Bowes
Content Project Manager: Fariha Nadeem
Design: Margaret Reid
Illustration Manager: Anitha Rajarathnam
Marketing Manager: Deborah Watkins

Copyedited by Editage, a unit of Cactus Communications Services Pte. Ltd.
Typeset by TNQ Technologies Pvt. Ltd.
Printed in Scotland

Last digit is the print number: 9 8 7 6 5 4 3 2 1

SERIES EDITOR FOREWORD

Most students now study medicine through a form of integrated curriculum. These courses blend basic science with exposure to clinical medicine from an early stage. These students have the good fortune to be left in no doubt, from the outset, why they are studying medicine. I teach in a medical school that delivers a fully integrated curriculum and I can compare it with the traditional model according to which I received my early medical education. That comparison is very favourable.

Unlike many other texts, the *Systems of the Body* series has been designed very specifically to support an integrated approach to learning medicine. Our carefully selected panel of authors drawn from across the English-speaking world have combined basic science with clinical application. Links to clinical skills, clinical investigation and therapeutics are made clear throughout.

The aim is to offer highly accessible guidance for all student types and stages. It will be invaluable to those who are approaching the subject for the first time or who may have found a topic challenging when using other more traditionally configured resources – as well as greatly assist all students wishing to excel as their course progresses. The clear layout and writing style, together with detail that informs without overwhelming, go a long way to supporting students. It may also provide welcome reminders to postgraduates facing their own examinations.

Whatever curriculum you follow, wherever you are in the world, and whichever stage you are at, we know that the Systems of the Body volumes will serve as great places to start when learning something new and enable you to effectively piece together the essential components of each major body system, in a modern clinical context.

Good luck!

Stephen Hughes, MSc MBBS FRCSEd FRCEM FHEA
Senior Lecturer in Medicine
Anglia Ruskin University
Chelmsford, UK
and
Consultant, Emergency Medicine
Broomfield Hospital
Chelmsford, UK

The field of gastroenterology is a dynamic and exciting area of clinical medicine and biomedical science. The evolution of this system, enabling us to extract nutrients from our diet, has allowed us to thrive. What appears to the uninformed to be a simple hollow tract traversing our body is, in reality, a complex, multi-compartmental system, vital for human life. However, students studying the subject can often feel somewhat overwhelmed with this complexity, particularly as the gastrointestinal tract is commonly dissected into many individual functioning parts. Consequently, this third edition of *The Digestive System* has focussed the subject content in addition to streamlining the learning outcomes. Furthermore, there is now an opportunity for self-assessment at the end of each chapter which allows for reflection and assessing understanding of the subject. Similarly, many years teaching both preclinical and biomedical scientists on the subject has highlighted a continued disconnect between the descriptive physiology of the gastrointestinal tract and clinical manifestations. Thus, in this edition, there is increased integration between the basic science and clinical cases of common diseases presenting in healthcare settings, enabling the reader to easily grasp the underpinning physiological changes associated with disease. Furthermore, gastrointestinal pathologies and treatment pathways are now described within their respective chapters to better compartmentalise information. Finally, this edition now includes a chapter on the intestinal microbiome, a subject which has come to the fore in the last decade, becoming incredibly important to gastrointestinal biology and is now implicated in many intestinal and extra-intestinal diseases and processes.

We are grateful for the help given by various academics and clinicians in the preparation of this new edition of *The Digestive System*. This edit builds on the successful previous editions of the book and, as such, we wish to thank all contributing individuals acknowledged in the previous editions. Furthermore, we wish to thank Prof. Margaret Smith and Prof. Dion Morton who established the basis of the previous editions and for providing us with the opportunity to develop this new edition. Key individuals who provided guidance and support for this update include Dr Revers Donga and Dr Robert Stephenson for their contributions to anatomical sections and Dr Praveen Sharma from the School of Dentistry, University of Birmingham.

DIGESTION FROM THE START: THE MOUTH, SALIVARY GLANDS AND OESOPHAGUS 1

THE STOMACH: BASIC FUNCTIONS AND CONTROL MECHANISMS 25

EXOCRINE FUNCTIONS OF THE PANCREAS 45

LIVER AND BILIARY SYSTEM 59

THE SMALL INTESTINE 79

DIGESTION AND ABSORPTION 97

THE ABSORPTIVE AND POST-ABSORPTIVE STATES 117

THE COLON 131

THE INTESTINAL MICROBIOME 145

DIGESTION FROM THE START: THE MOUTH, SALIVARY GLANDS AND OESOPHAGUS

1

Chapter objectives and clinical presentations

After reading this chapter, review your learning by considering the following:

1. Can you describe the role of the mouth and tongue in digestion?
2. Are you able to describe how saliva is secreted, its composition and its function?
3. Do you understand the phases of swallowing and the structure of the oesophagus?

Also, you should be familiar with the following clinical presentations:

- Xerostomia
- Gastro-oesophageal reflux disorder (GORD)
- Barrett's metaplasia/oesophagus
- Oesophageal cancer
- Achalasia
- Loss of swallowing function following stroke
- Eosinophilic oesophagus

Clinical outlook

The most common presentations relevant to the mouth, salivary glands and oesophagus are heartburn and difficulty swallowing. Common diagnoses in patients presenting with these symptoms include gastro-oesophageal reflux disease (GORD), Barrett's oesophagus, conditions associated with oesophageal dysmotility such as achalasia, eosinophilic oesophagitis, oropharyngeal dysphagia due to cerebrovascular accidents and oesophageal malignancies. Problems with salivary gland functions are often seen in relation to rheumatological conditions such as Sjögren's syndrome.

Introduction

The mouth represents the start of the gastrointestinal (GI) tract which has multiple functions including speech, digestion and protection of the body from ingestion of harmful foods. Additionally, the mouth is important for:

- Mastication
- Taste
- Swallowing
- Lubrication
- Digestion
- Speech
- Signalling of thirst
- Protection of the body from harmful ingested substances

The performance of all of these functions depends on the presence of saliva. In this chapter, the functional importance of saliva is illustrated by the problems encountered in individuals with xerostomia (dry mouth), a condition characterised by pathological changes in the salivary and mucous glands that result in impaired secretion. In addition, swallowing function can be impaired in stroke patients. Both of these clinical cases are presented in Cases 1.1 and 1.2, respectively. In Case 1.3, the common clinical progression from GORD to oesophageal cancer is detailed. Finally, the most common clinical presentation of eosinophilic oesophagus is given in Case 1.4.

The mouth

Anatomical features of the mouth

The mouth is concerned primarily with the ingestion and mastication of food (which is mainly the function of the teeth). The oral cavity (mouth) is closed by the apposition of the lips. Within the cavity, the palate forms the roof of the mouth, which separates the oral and nasal cavities; the floor of the mouth is occupied by the tongue. Three pairs of major salivary glands open into the mouth: the parotid, submandibular and sublingual salivary glands. The lips and the cheeks form the anterior and lateral boundaries and are composed mainly of skeletal muscle embedded in elastic fibro-connective tissue (Fig. 1.1).

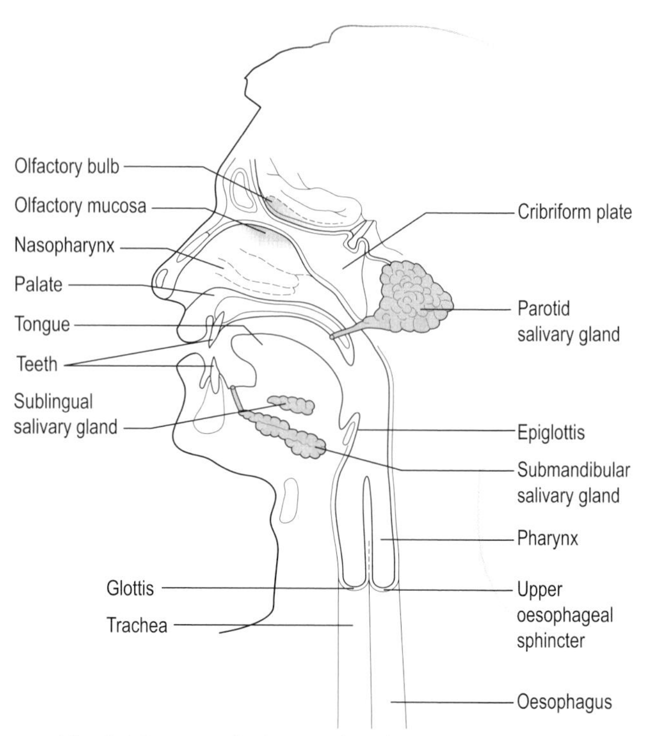

Fig. 1.1 Structures in the mouth and associated structures.

Oral mucosa

The oral cavity has been described as a 'mirror of health', reflecting the wellbeing of an individual. Alterations in the oral mucosal lining are commonly observed in several systemic conditions (including diabetes and nutrient deficiency) and the local effects of chronic tobacco or alcohol use. The mucosa of the mouth and oesophagus differs from the rest of the intestinal mucosa of the continuous GI tract in that they are covered by a stratifying squamous epithelium. Of note, regions of epithelium become keratinocyte-like (skin-epidermis like) when subject to mechanical forces experienced in the cavity due to mastication.

Innervation

The innervation of many structures associated with the mouth is via the four branches of the mandibular division of the trigeminal nerve (Fig. 1.2). These are as follows:

1. The anterior division, which provides motor innervation to the lateral pterygoid, temporalis and

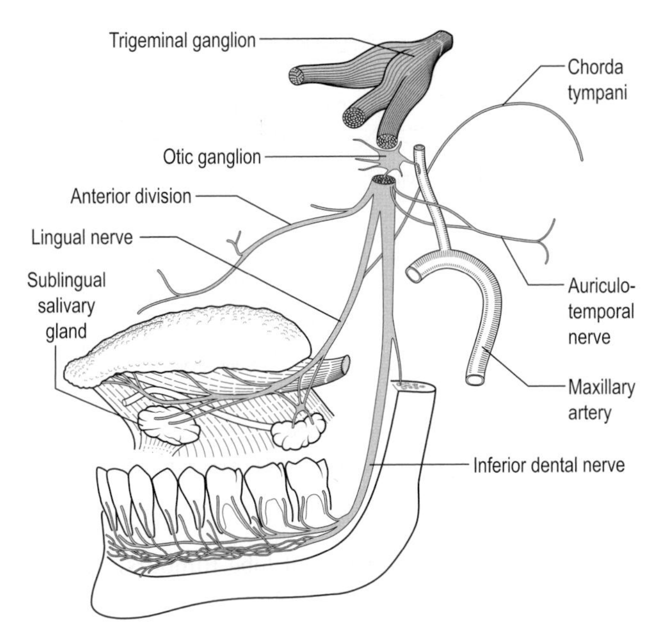

Fig. 1.2 The mandibular division of the trigeminal nerve. The lingual nerve innervates the anterior two-thirds of the tongue and the sublingual and submandibular salivary glands. The inferior dental nerve innervates the tooth pulp, periodontal ligaments and gums. The anterior division innervates the muscles of mastication (not shown). The auriculotemporal nerve innervates structures of the ear (not shown).

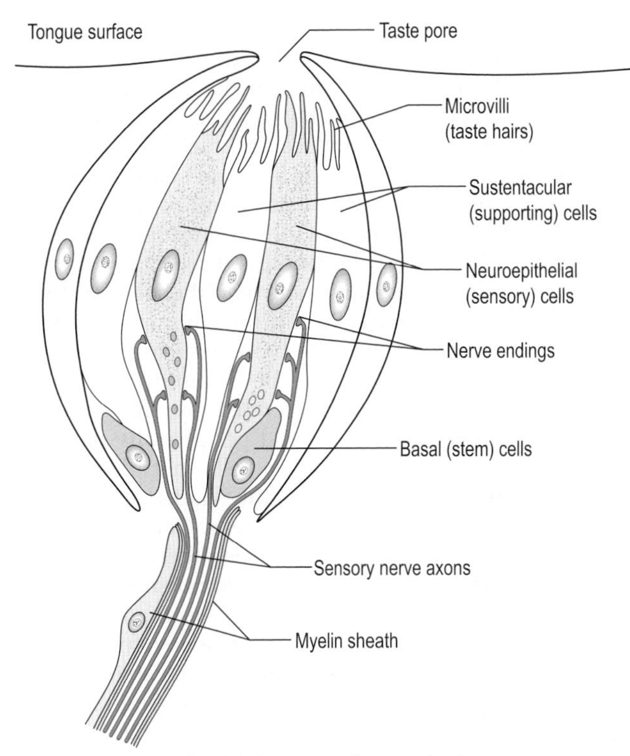

Fig. 1.3 Structure of a taste bud.

masseter muscles which are involved in mastication (see below);
2. The auriculotemporal nerve, which innervates structures of the ear;
3. The inferior dental or alveolar nerve, which provides sensory innervation to the lower lip, chin and mandibular teeth and gums;
4. The lingual nerve, which provides sensory innervation to the anterior two-thirds of the tongue, the floor of the mouth and the gum on the lingual side of the lower teeth.

The lingual nerve is joined by the chorda tympani that run through the lateral pterygoid muscle. The chorda tympani carry sensory taste fibres from the lingual nerve to the facial nerve and secretomotor (parasympathetic) fibres from the facial nerve to the lingual nerve. These fibres innervate the submandibular and sublingual salivary glands. Nerve damage is an uncommon but serious complication following certain dental procedures.

Anatomy and histology of the tongue

The tongue has a freely moveable portion known as the body, and a root portion that is attached to the floor of the oral cavity and forms part of the anterior wall of the pharynx. It is divided into anterior and posterior regions by the sulcus terminalis, a V-shaped groove with the apex of the V directed posteriorly. The glands in the base of the tongue are mainly mucous-producing and their ducts open behind the sulcus terminalis. In the body of the tongue, the glands are mainly serous (enzyme-producing) and their ducts open anterior to the sulcus. The glands are mixed near the tip and their ducts open onto the inferior surface of the tongue.

On the dorsal surface of the tongue are numerous small protuberances, or papillae, which give the tongue its roughened appearance. The papillae have different distributions on the tongue; fungiform (mushroom-like) papillae are the smallest and most common, and filiform (thread-like) papillae occur evenly spaced between the anterior and lateral surface. Circumvallate papillae are on the base of the tongue, the largest of all papillae with only 8–12 of them found on human tongues. Papillae contain numerous nerve endings that sense touch and most have associated taste buds (see below). Lymphatic nodules (the lingual tonsil) protrude from the surface of the posterior one-third of the tongue and give it a nodular, irregular appearance. Between the nodules are crypts where the epithelium is infiltrated with numerous lymphocytes. The ventral surface of the tongue is smooth with an underlying submucosa.

Taste

Taste buds

There are several thousand taste buds on the human tongue. Fig. 1.3 details the structure of an individual taste bud.

Each circumvallate papilla contains several hundred taste buds. The taste buds contain the gustatory (taste) receptor cells. They are located in the oral epithelium, mainly in association with the papillae, but can be situated elsewhere in the oral cavity such as the palate and the epiglottis. They have a barrel-shaped appearance with a depression (the taste pore) on the surface. This is an aperture that provides communication with the exterior. The taste bud contains three types of cells: supporting (sustentacular), neuro-epithelial taste and basal. Both the sensory cells and the support cells have long apical microvilli, or taste hairs, which project into the taste pore. The taste hairs lie in amorphous polysaccharide material that is secreted by the supporting cells. The basal cell is located peripherally near the basal lamina. These are the stem cells that give rise to all other cell types. There are club-shaped endings of sensory nerves lying between the cells. Chemical (taste) stimuli are received by the neuroepithelial cells and transmitted via the release of neurotransmitters from the cells to the nerve endings. The secretions of the serous glands of the papillae wash away food material and permit new taste stimuli to be received by the receptors. Papillae additionally create a rough surface on the tongue which is important for cleaning the tooth surfaces.

Taste sensation

The solubilisation of food constituents by saliva enables the sense of taste to be experienced. Thus taste depends on the detection of chemicals that are dissolved in the saliva and for this reason, taste is compromised in a condition called xerostomia (see Case 1.1) where saliva production is diminished. Historically, four submodalities (tastes) were recognised: salt, sour (acid), sweet and bitter. A fifth distinct taste is now recognised: umami, elicited by L-glutamate, a chemical found in foods such as seafood, cured meats and mushrooms. Further research is potentially identifying more submodalities, including receptors for fats. Dissolved substances with these properties stimulate the receptors (the taste buds) on the tongue. Acid is the most potent stimulus; in humans, sucking a lemon can lead to the maximum rate of secretion, which elicits 7–8 mL of saliva production per minute. Whilst a taste bud is most sensitive to one particular taste, it can also respond to most submodalities if in high enough concentration. The nerves from the taste buds in the anterior of the tongue pass in the chorda tympani (a branch of the facial nerve) and those from the taste buds in the posterior third travel in the glossopharyngeal nerve. These nerves project to the tractus solitarius (Fig. 1.4). The sensory nerves from the taste buds in the palate and epiglottis ascend in the vagus nerve.

Taste (and smell) sensations often become lost in many disease states, including upper respiratory tract infections (as seen with severe acute respiratory coronavirus 2 [SARS-CoV-2]) and neurological conditions such as multiple sclerosis and frontal lobe tumours, in addition to chemotherapy and antibiotics.

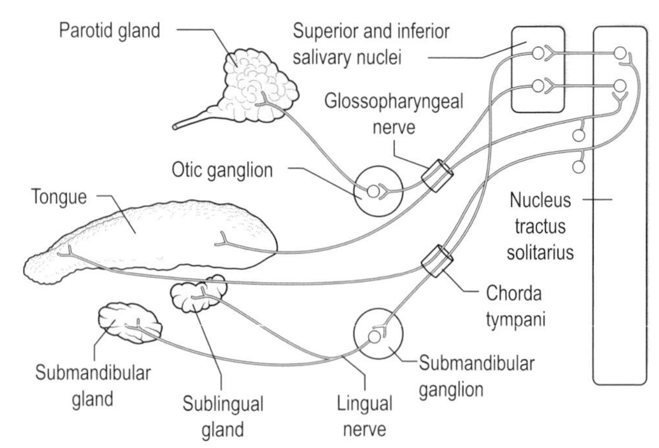

Fig. 1.4 Reflex pathway for the secretion of saliva in response to the stimulation of taste bud receptors.

Causes, diagnosis and treatment

Causes

Xerostomia is a sensation of a dry mouth condition usually due to hyposalivation. It primarily affects older adults and can have a significant negative effect on quality of life. More women than men tend to be affected by it with incidence increasing with age. It frequently occurs in conjunction with dryness of eyes as seen in Sjögren's syndrome. The major causes are as follows:

- Medication, especially tricyclic antidepressants and sympathomimetic drugs,
- Head and neck irradiation and
- Autoimmune inflammatory diseases such as Sjögren's syndrome, which targets exocrine glands in general.

Sjögren's syndrome

Sjögren syndrome is the most commonly recognised autoimmune disease associated with xerostomia. In this condition, the salivary glands are infiltrated by the immune cells specifically macrophages, B cells, T cells, mast cells and plasma cells. The plasma cells produce autoantibodies anti-Ro and anti-La, which target the muscarinic 3 receptor, leading to atrophy of the glands. Measurement of these antibodies are often used to help diagnose this condition (Fig. 1.6).

A histological section of a minor salivary gland in a patient with Sjögren's syndrome, in which focal aggregates of lymphocytes can be seen in Fig. 1.7. In non-autoimmune inflammatory disease, the infiltration by lymphocytes is more diffuse. Atrophy of the

Case 1.1 **Xerostomia**

A 60-year-old woman visited her general practitioner and complained of a persistent dry mouth, difficulties in chewing and swallowing and the feeling of sore and gritty eyes. She also said that her food seemed tasteless. The doctor examined the patient's mouth. Her gums and teeth appeared inflamed and infected, and her tongue appeared lobulated. The patient was sent for investigation of salivary function. The most frequent cause of dry mouth (xerostomia) is hypofunction of the salivary glands (which is often accompanied by hypofunction of the lacrimal glands). Fig. 1.5 shows the appearance of the tongue in a patient with xerostomia.

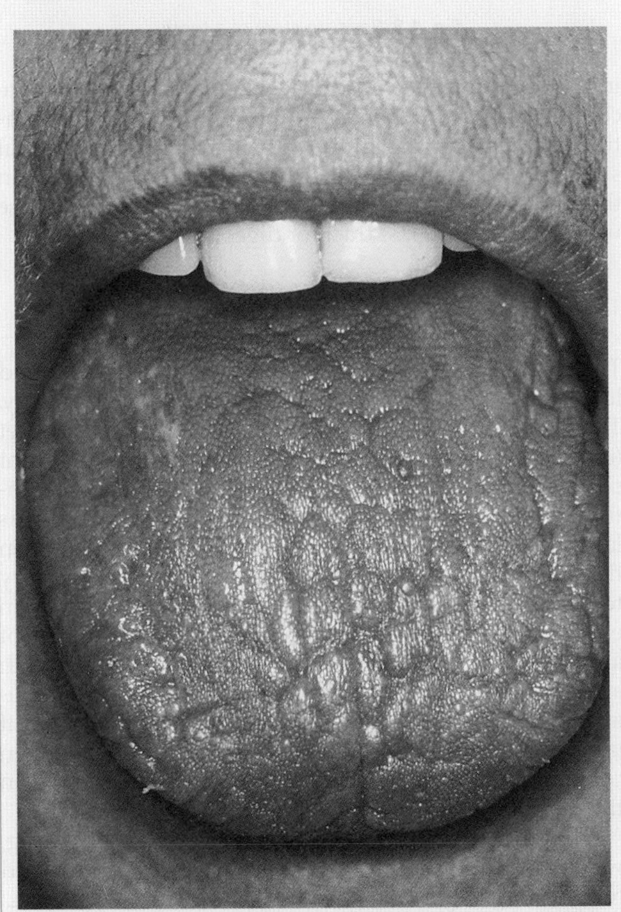

Fig. 1.5 The tongue of a patient with xerostomia, showing a characteristic grooved appearance. (Courtesy Mr J. Hamburger, Dental School, University of Birmingham.)

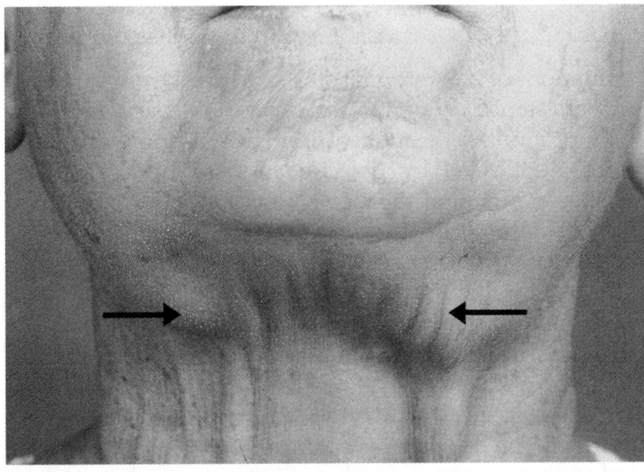

Fig. 1.6 Swollen submandibular glands (*arrows*) in a patient with Sjögren's syndrome. The inflammatory process can cause the ducts to become blocked with mucoid saliva. The ducts may also be narrowed (stenosis). As a consequence, the glands swell. (Courtesy Mr J. Hamburger, Dental School, University of Birmingham.)

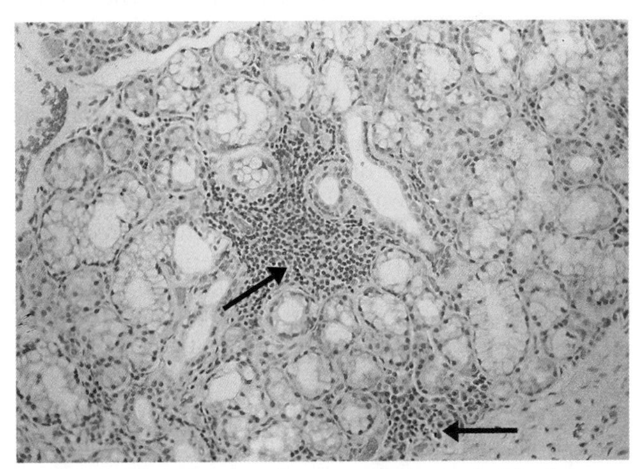

Fig. 1.7 Histological section of a minor salivary gland of the lip in a patient with Sjögren's syndrome. Focal infiltrates of lymphocytes are indicated by arrows. (Courtesy Mr J. Hamburger, Dental School, University of Birmingham.)

mucous glands in the buccal mucosa may also be present. Primary Sjögren's syndrome is characterised by dry mouth and eyes, but a secondary form exists in which these symptoms are accompanied by connective tissue disease, usually rheumatoid arthritis or lupus erythematosus, primary biliary cirrhosis, polymyositis and a number of other conditions. In some patients infected with HIV, the condition resembles Sjögren's syndrome. Diabetes can also cause symptoms of xerostomia as these conditions are accompanied by dehydration resulting from copious urine flow.

Symptomatic xerostomia

The perception of oral dryness in the absence of actual oral dryness, termed 'symptomatic xerostomia', can be the result of sensory or cognitive disorder. In addition, altered perception of oral sensation (oral dysaesthesia) is a feature of anxiety, although acute anxiety can actually cause clinical symptoms and signs of xerostomia.

Diagnosis

Evaluation of xerostomia starts with enquiring about the persistence of symptoms on a daily basis for three or more months through validated questions. This may then be followed by objective assessment of salivary gland hypofunction through salivary gland scintigraphy or measurement of rate of saliva production by whole sialometry. However, these tests are rarely done in a clinical setting and often may form part of clinical studies. Imaging of salivary glands may be done through a cross-sectional imaging (computed tomography [CT] or magnetic resonance imaging [MRI]) or ultrasonography in order to identify structural abnormalities. Finally, tests specific to the underlying autoimmune conditions associated with xerostomia (such as Sjögren's syndrome) may be performed.

Treatment and side-effects

The treatment of xerostomia depends on whether the patient can secrete saliva in response to a stimulus, i.e., whether he or she is a 'responder' who has functioning salivary gland epithelium or a 'non-responder' who does not. Artificial saliva can be used in non-responders, but this is not wholly satisfactory. Low doses of pilocarpine or cevimeline are often used to treat the condition in individuals with residual salivary function. This drug is a partial agonist of muscarinic acetylcholine receptors. These drugs, known as sialagogues, mimic the effect of stimulation of the parasympathetic nerves, causing the acinar cells to secrete saliva and kallikreins, which in turn cause vasodilatation via bradykinin and hence increased secretion.

Smell

Activation of olfactory receptors, in conjunction with central nervous system processing of their responses, enables many different types of odours or flavours to be distinguished. Smell has more primary qualities than taste. These include floral, ethereal, musky, camphor, putrid and pungent submodalities. Blockage of the nose by the common cold or olfactory nerve lesions renders taste discrimination crude as it then relies only on the taste buds. The sense of smell, like that of taste, is an important stimulant of appetite and digestion. The olfactory mucosa that detects the odours is located in the upper nasopharynx (see Fig. 1.1). Odorant molecules are borne to the olfactory mucosa via the inspired air, or air in the oral cavity during feeding. Chemical odours are detected by receptors in bipolar cells present in the mucosa. There are about 10 million chemoreceptor cells in the human olfactory mucosa. Immobile cilia on the surface of the cells detect odorants dissolved in the mucous layer that overlies the mucosa. The chemical odorants depolarise receptor cells, triggering a discharge

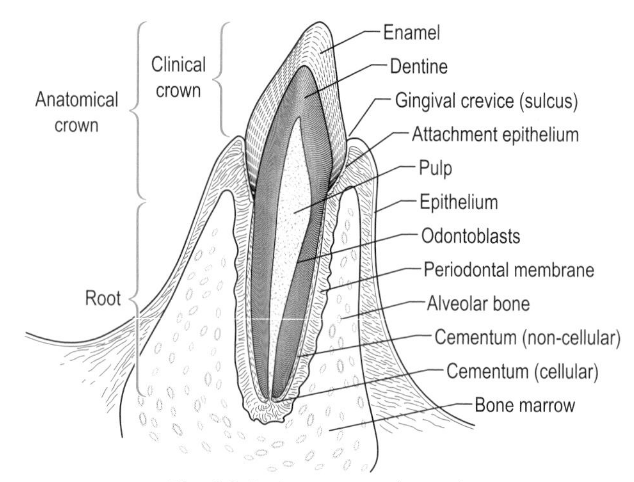

Fig. 1.8 Basic structure of a tooth.

in the sensory nerve. Coding for a particular smell, like coding for taste, depends on the response of a population of receptors. The information is integrated in cortical structures. The smell of food is an important trigger in the cephalic phase of digestion. This is the initial phase which prepares the GI tract for digestion.

Teeth

The teeth are suspended in the bone of the upper and lower jaws, or the maxilla and mandible, respectively. The periodontal membrane holds the tooth in its socket (alveolus). This arrangement of a peg-and-socket joint permits slight movement of the teeth during mastication. They are arranged in two arches. The upper arch is larger than the lower arch and this commonly results in the mandibular teeth being overlapped by the maxillary teeth. In humans, there are 10 primary (milk) teeth in each half jaw (20 in total) that erupt between the ages of approximately 6 months and 2 years of age. These teeth are shed between 6 and 13 years of age and are gradually replaced by 16 permanent adult teeth in each half jaw (32 in total). Of these, the 4 wisdom teeth are often congenitally missing or unerupted/partially erupted in the mouth.

The sharp incisor teeth are specialised for biting, while the larger, more flattened molars are specialised for grinding. Fig. 1.8 shows the basic structure of a tooth.

Each tooth has a basic similar structure with a visible crown projecting above the gingiva (gum) and a root that is buried in the alveolus of the maxilla or the mandible. The neck is at the junction between the crown and the root. In the centre of each tooth is the pulp cavity that contains nervous and vascular tissues. The pulp communicates via small openings (apical foramina) with the surrounding tissue. The following are the hard tissues of the pulp:

- Dentine: a calcified tissue similar to bone, which surrounds the pulp cavity and forms the bulk of the tooth. This is 70% inorganic and 30% organic.

- Enamel: the hardest material which is mainly composed of apatite crystals and covers the dentine of the crown. This is more than 95% inorganic.
- Cementum: which is similar to dentine and covers the dentine of the root.

Mastication (chewing)

The sight, smell and thought of food elicit the secretion of saliva before food enters the mouth. However, the palatability of food also depends on orally sensed properties after food has been taken into the mouth, such as taste, texture and temperature. Once present in the mouth, the food is chewed, a process known as mastication. This involves movements of the mandible and the tongue. It is controlled by sensations from touch and pressure receptors located in the oral mucosa and the periodontium (area around the teeth), as well as from stretch and other receptors in the masticatory muscles, temporomandibular joints and periosteum.

Mastication, the mechanical breakdown of solid foods, prepares the food-bolus for swallowing. The vertical (up and down) movements of the mandibles result in biting by the incisor teeth. After a piece of food has been taken into the mouth, both vertical movements and horizontal (side to side) movements enable the molars to crush and break the food into fragments of a size suitable for swallowing. Chewing food breaks it down into smaller fragments for easier swallowing and increases the surface area exposed to digestive enzymes present in saliva (see later). Chewing additionally releases chemicals from food contributing to the taste and smell. The process of mastication encourages the development and maintenance of the jaw bones and associated muscles, which is important as the biting forces exerted by the muscles and the incisors and molars are 110–250 N and 390–900 N, respectively. The efficiency of mastication is reduced in those who wear dentures, and they often tend to eat foods that are not difficult to chew; the toughness of the foods chosen seems to be related to the biting force that can be exerted on the dentures. Mastication stops at a specific moment (although the neurophysiological mechanism underpinning this moment is poorly understood) and swallowing follows. The swallowing reflex is a complex neuromotor reflex involving more than 25 muscles and 5 different cranial nerves.

Control of mastication

The muscles of mastication are the lateral pterygoids that are responsible for jaw opening and the masseters, the temporalis and the medial pterygoid muscles that are responsible for jaw closing (Fig. 1.9). The control is exerted by neural mechanisms. Two important aspects of the control are as follows:

1. the generation of movements, and
2. the regulation of bite.

Case 1.2 Stroke–loss of swallowing function

A 78-year-old female presented to A&E with right upper and lower limb weakness along with slurring of speech. She underwent a CT scan of her brain which reveals a cerebral infarction. She is commenced on medications; however, she reported difficulty in swallowing, often coughing while eating or drinking. A swallow assessment revealed abnormal initiation of swallowing as a consequence of the stroke. As her swallow function failed to improve, a percutaneous endoscopic gastrostomy (PEG) tube was inserted to help her with her nutrition.

The patient described problems with initiation of swallowing and coughing while eating, suggestive of oropharyngeal dysphagia. Patients with oropharyngeal dysphagia report difficulty with transferring food from the mouth to their oropharynx and may describe a feeling of an obstruction in the throat. They may present with coughing and choking and have a history of chest infections due to aspiration of food and fluid. Videofluoroscopy is the gold standard for the evaluation of oropharyngeal dysphagia as it allows dynamic functional evaluation of the swallowing process. Oropharyngeal dysphagia can be caused by neuromuscular diseases or acutely by a cerebrovascular accident involving the region of the brain that controls swallowing. Management may involve dietary modification: for example, by thickening of fluids and increasing bolus viscosity and enteral feeding in those at high risk of aspiration.

Generation of movements

Chewing is a programmed pattern of movements organised in the central nervous system, which can become a conditioned reflex. Recent functional MRI (fMRI) studies have revealed that the generation of chewing movements in humans is highly complex, involving multiple brain regions.

Regulation of the bite

As the jaws close, the teeth come into contact with food or the opposing set of teeth.

Stimulation of mechanoreceptors associated with the teeth is important. Many sensory receptors are present in the tooth pulp and the periodontal ligaments. Stimulation of receptors in the periodontal ligament sends impulses along fibres in the lingual nerve (see Fig. 1.2). Activation of the receptors causes information to be transmitted to the brainstem, to inhibit jaw closing when the biting force rises, and therefore to regulate the force applied. When these receptors are stimulated, the amplitude of the jaw movement bursting responses changes and activity in the masseter jaw closing muscles increases. These inputs therefore modify the activity of the pattern generator and contribute to the control of the chewing force. The texture

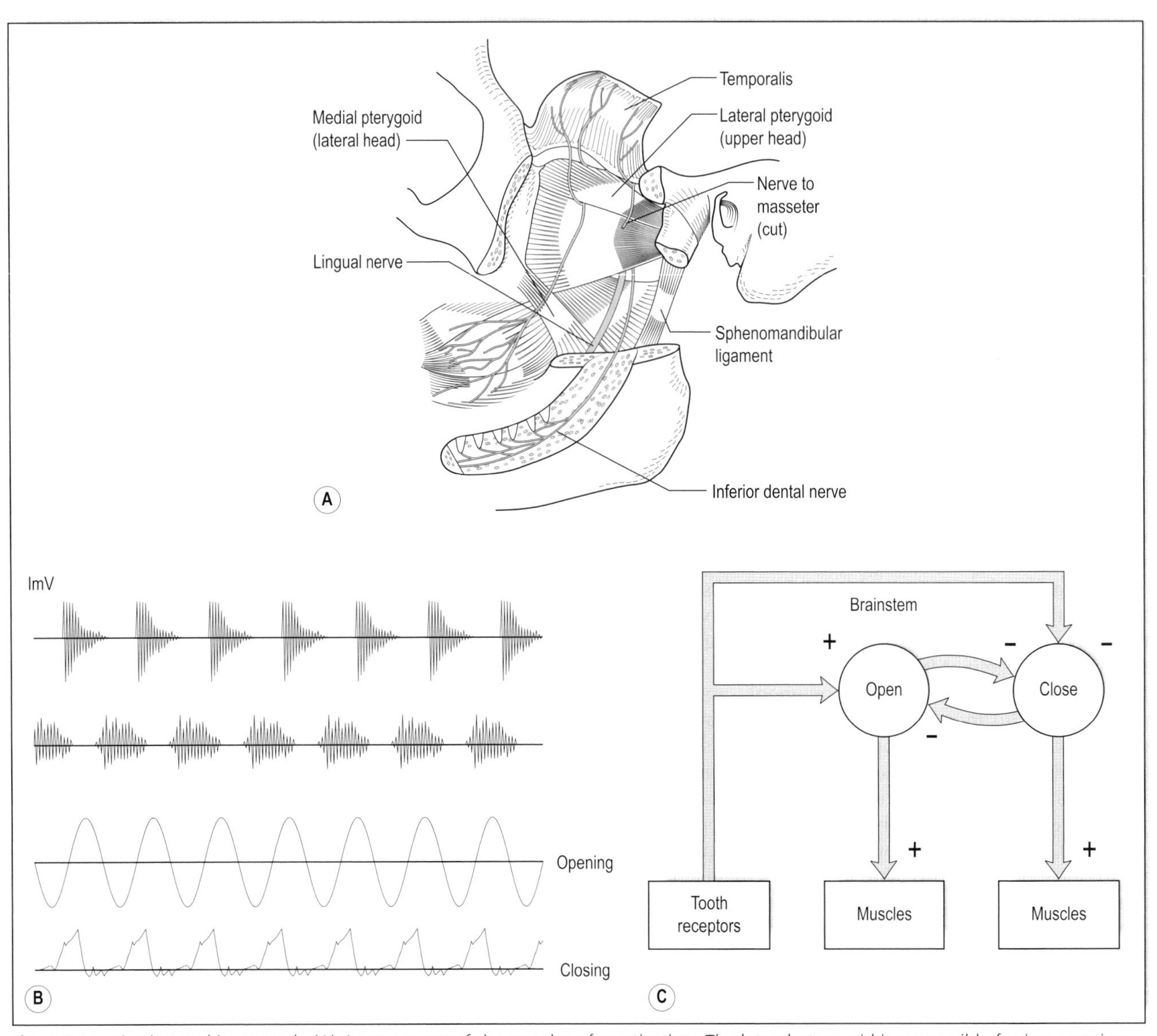

Fig. 1.9 Mastication and its control. (A) Arrangement of the muscles of mastication. The lateral pterygoid is responsible for jaw opening, and the medial pterygoid, the masseters and the temporalis are responsible for jaw closing. (B) The pattern of electrical activity (EMG) in the muscles of opening and closing. (C) Simplified representation of a pattern generator that could control the opening and closing of jaws.

of food is perceived during chewing by excitation of mechanoreceptors in the periodontal ligaments. Slight displacement of a tooth during chewing, causes the periodontal ligaments to be stretched and this deforms and excites the receptors. Each afferent responds maximally to one particular direction of applied force. The pressure stimulus threshold for perception of a stimulus applied to a tooth is 10 mN and is higher for the molars than for the incisors or canines. The threshold level depends on the velocity of application of the force. Nevertheless, people who have lost all their teeth can control masticatory force, indicating that tactile sensation in the periodontal ligaments is not the only input controlling the biting force. Muscle spindles in the masticatory muscles, temporomandibular joints and periosteum may also contribute.

Role of tongue movements in mastication

The density of mechanoreceptors is high in the front of the oral cavity and low in the posterior part. The tip of the tongue has the highest density. Two-point discrimination on the tip of the tongue can be less than 1 mm. Tactile information from the oral cavity and the tongue is transmitted to the brain via the trigeminal nerve. The tongue is a sophisticated motor organ that moves rhythmically in concert with the lower jaw (usually without being bitten) during chewing. The tongue can perform these movements because of the arrangement of its musculature. The extrinsic muscles enable it to change its overall position. These, together with the intrinsic muscles that terminate on the mucosa or on other muscles of the tongue, enable it to both alter its shape and perform rapid movements. The nerve endings in the papillae transmit the senses of touch, pressure, temperature and pain. There are also proprioreceptors within the muscles and abundant muscle spindles in the human tongue, and these are also important for the intricate movements involved in chewing. The tongue mixes saliva with the crushed food by alternations from one side to the other, coating it with mucus.

Saliva

In humans the paired major salivary glands (parotid, submandibular and sublingual) and many small, minor submucosal glands constantly secrete saliva at a basal rate. This resting secretion soon becomes stimulated in response to the taste and smell of food and whilst chewing. The parotid glands are the largest of the glands. Each parotid is located below and anterior to the ear. Its main duct (Stensen's duct) passes forward to penetrate the cheek and opens into the mouth opposite the upper first/second adult molar tooth. The submandibular gland lies in the floor of the mouth beneath the body of the mandible, extending below its lower border into the side of the neck. It has a duct (Wharton's duct) that opens on the ventral surface of the tongue where it attaches to the floor of the mouth. Autoimmune conditions like Sjögren's syndrome affect the salivary glands, impairing their ability to produce saliva which manifest as a dry mouth or xerostomia. Autoimmune destruction can affect all salivary glands and can lead to obstruction and swelling.

The sublingual gland is actually a collection of glands that lie the duct of the submandibular gland beneath the mucous membrane of the floor of the mouth. Each of these sublingual glands has a separate duct that opens beneath the tongue. The three pairs of glands differ with respect to the type of acini present, and they secrete saliva that differs in composition with respect to the mucus content. The parotids have acini that contain only serous cells. They produce a watery secretion that has a high content of α-amylase but very little mucus. Most acini of the submandibular glands are serous, but some are mucous, and some are mixed and contain mucous cells with serous crescents (demilunes) (Fig. 1.10).

The saliva secreted by these glands has a weak α-amylase activity but contains lysozyme that is secreted by the serous demilunes. The sublingual glands contain mainly mucous acini but some of these have serous demilunes. Very few pure serous acini are present in the sublingual gland. Consequently, they produce a particularly thick mucous secretion.

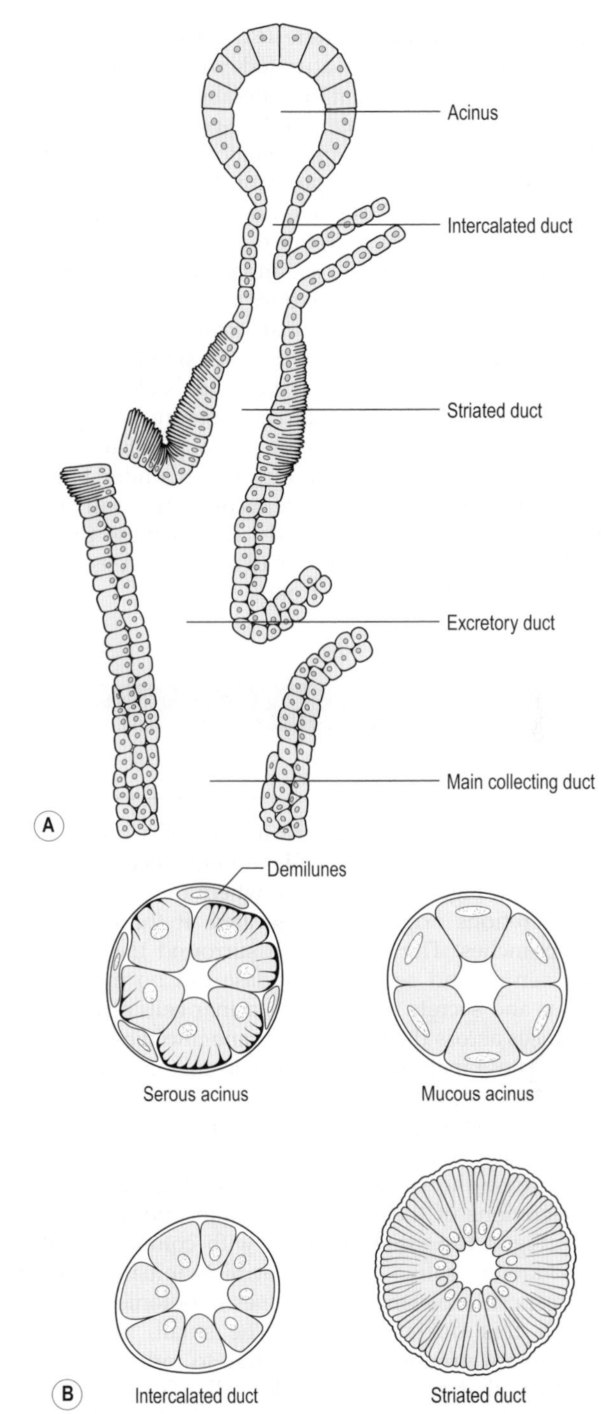

Fig. 1.10 (A) Regions of a salivary gland. (B) Cell types present in different regions.

Composition of saliva

Whole saliva is composed of water, peptides and proteins, hormones, sugars, lipids and electrolytes. Saliva in the mouth is a mixture of secretions from all the glands present. Human saliva consists of 99% water. Additionally, saliva contains a variety of electrolytes including sodium (Na^+), potassium (K^+), calcium (Ca^{2+}), magnesium (Mg^{2+}), phosphate (PO_4^{3-}) and bicarbonate (HCO_3^-). Saliva is supersaturated with calcium phosphates that help to prevent demineralisation of the teeth. Specific phosphoproteins (proline-rich proteins and statherin) that inhibit the precipitation of calcium phosphate crystals from the supersaturated saliva onto the teeth are also present. The alkalinity or acidity of saliva depends on the rate of flow, but the pH is usually within the range of 6.2–8.0. There are more than 2000 different proteins in saliva, the major ones being the enzyme α-amylase. In addition, there are an array of glycoproteins including mucins. Those present in smaller amounts include the enzymes lysozyme and sialoperoxidase (see below), as well as lactoferrin, histatins and various immunoglobulins, all of which have protective functions in the mouth. Interestingly, as our understanding and characterisation of the proteins present in saliva continues, it is estimated that nearly 40% of these proteins could be candidate markers for diseases such as cancer, cardiovascular disease and stroke.

Salivary glands

Structure and histology

Fig. 1.10A shows the structure of part of a mixed salivary gland. The salivary glands are branched structures as shown in Fig. 1.10. The acini, where the primary salivary secretions originate, are located at the termini of these branches. The cells which surround the acini are either serous and secrete α-amylase but no mucins, or mucous and secrete mucins. The acinar cells also secrete substances across the basal membrane into the interstitial spaces. These include the proteolytic enzymes known as kallikreins, which have a role in controlling the regional blood flow to the glands (Fig. 1.13). The basal membrane of the serous acinar cell has thin finger-like projections that increase the surface area for secretion (Fig. 1.10B). The secretions of the acinar cells drain into intercalated ducts (Fig. 1.10A) that are lined with columnar epithelium. Flowing saliva from the acini is initially isotonic with respect to plasma yet becomes hypotonic as it runs through this ductal network. The small, intercalated ducts from a number of acini merge to form larger striated ducts that are lined by taller cells. The basal membranes of these cells have numerous infoldings. Between the infoldings are rows of mitochondria that impart a striated appearance to the cells. These striated ducts drain into larger, excretory ducts, which in turn drain into a large collecting duct that opens into the mouth. The cells lining the striated ducts and the excretory ducts modify the secretion as it flows past them. Somewhat sparsely distributed myoepithelial cells are present around the ducts and the acini of a salivary gland. These cells support the glandular elements and contract when the glands are stimulated, to assist the extrusion of the saliva from the ducts.

Functions of saliva

Taste

The hypotonicity of saliva provides an ideal medium for the dissolution of substances from food within the mouth and, as such, allows the taste buds to perceive the different flavours.

Lubrication

The lubricant property of saliva depends on its mucin content. These carbohydrate-rich proteins are gel-like and coat the food-bolus, making it more easily moved in the mouth. This lubricant property of saliva enables chewing and swallowing to be performed. Additionally, lubrication is important for protection against dehydration and in the process of speech. With respect to antimicrobial protection and the control of bacterial colonisation, mucins modulate the adhesion of microorganisms to the oral surfaces.

Digestion

α-Amylase is the major digestive enzyme in saliva and is responsible for the initial digestion of starches. It hydrolyses α-1,4 glycosidic linkages in starch. The efficiency of mastication is important for salivary amylase to penetrate the food bolus. Despite the short exposure of saliva in the mouth, the salivary digestion of starch is important because it continues after the food has reached the stomach. Gastric acid in the stomach inactivates α-amylase, but as the bolus of food takes time to disintegrate in the stomach, salivary digestion can continue within it for as long as half an hour. When the acid has completely penetrated the food, the enzyme is inactivated.

Protective functions of saliva

Saliva has many properties that enable it to promote oral and dental health:

- The large volume of the fluid produced enables the buccal cavity to be continually rinsed, thereby removing ingested substances and particles from it.
- It contains mucins that impart a slippery property to the secretion. It coats the mouth, thereby protecting it against abrasion by sharp pieces of food.
- The alkaline pH of the saliva produced when a meal is being eaten buffers acids present in the food. The copious secretion of saliva prior to vomiting protects the mouth from gastric acid in the vomit by virtue of its mucus content and its pH. Buffering of the acids in food prevents the erosion of tooth enamel.
- It is bacteriostatic because it contains an antimicrobial substance, thiocyanate, and an enzyme, sialoperoxidase, which catalyses the reaction of

metabolic products of bacteria, such as that of hydrogen peroxide with salivary thiocyanate:

$$\underset{\substack{\text{Hydrogen}\\\text{peroxide}\\\text{(bacterial}\\\text{activity)}}}{H_2O_2} + \underset{\substack{\text{thiocyanate}\\\text{(saliva)}}}{CNS^-} \xrightarrow{\text{Sialoperoxidase}} \underset{\substack{\text{e.g. } OSCN^-\\\text{hypothiocyanate}\\\text{(toxic to bacteria)}}}{\text{oxidation products,}}$$

The oxidised derivatives produced in this reaction are highly toxic to bacteria. There are many other antibacterial properties of saliva (i.e., immunoglobin A, lysozymes and lactoferrin). Infections in the mouth are rare, even after oral or dental surgery when aseptic precautions are difficult to maintain, because of the potent bacteriostatic properties of saliva.

- It has a tissue repair function as the bleeding time of oral tissues appears to be shorter than other tissues; this is attributed to epidermal growth factor found within saliva.

Control of water intake

Thirst is the desire for increased water intake, and it is perceived as a dry mouth. When we become dehydrated, saliva production reduces to almost zero to conserve water; the reverse is observed during hyperhydration. Changes in blood osmolarity are detected by the subfornical organ and organum vasculosum of the lamina terminalis in the forebrain (two of the sensory circumventricular organs of the brain). The two structures are located outside the blood-brain barrier and therefore have enhanced access to the circulation and greater detection of blood osmolarity. There is a delay of around 10 minutes between drinking water and subsequent effects on blood solute concentration after absorption. However, the thirst-quenching sensation is signalled in seconds after ingesting water; as such, thirst cannot be quenched by the reverse of the process that generates it. The mechanisms involved are still poorly understood, but sensory cues from the oropharynx and upper GI tract inhibit the same thirst neurones that respond to blood osmolarity. These cues may include temperature receptors (decreases in oropharynx temperature decrease activity of thirst neurones), somatosensory receptors (detecting the sensation of water in the oral cavity) and stretch receptors (volume of the liquid in the upper GI tract stretches the intestine). The desire to drink is completely satisfied only when the plasma osmolarity, volume and pressure are adjusted to within the normal range.

Absorption in the mouth

Absorption of low-molecular-weight molecules can occur, to some extent, directly from the oral cavity. This route of absorption can be useful for absorption of certain drugs, especially when a rapid treatment response is required. Such drugs are usually placed under the tongue. One example is glyceryl trinitrate, which is used to treat an angina attack. It can also be a useful route for drugs which are unstable at the pH of the stomach, or which are rapidly metabolised by the liver. Drugs that are absorbed from the oral cavity enter the systemic circulation directly and therefore escape the 'first-pass' metabolism that occurs in the liver, unlike substances that are absorbed into the portal system. An example of a drug that is rapidly inactivated in the liver is isoprenaline, which is sometimes used to treat heart block. This drug can be effective if given sublingually. High-molecular-weight substances are not well-absorbed from the mouth.

Mechanisms of secretion

The basal rate of secretion of saliva is very low during sleep: approximately 0.05 mL/min. In the resting or awake state, it increases to about 0.5 mL/min, which is just enough to keep the mouth moist. During the course of the day, 1–2 L of saliva are secreted. Most of it is swallowed. The proteins in saliva are broken down in the GI tract by digestive enzymes. The amino acids and peptides produced, together with the water and ions, are reabsorbed across the walls of the intestines.

A simplified representation of a salivary secretory unit (a salivon), consisting of an acinus and a duct, is given in Fig. 1.11. The blood flows first past the duct and then past the acinus. The blood supply constitutes a portal system because substances reabsorbed from the duct cells into the blood capillaries surrounding the duct are transported to the capillaries surrounding the acinus via an efferent arteriole prior to being returned to the heart via the veins. The acinar cells secrete the primary saliva that passes down the ducts. The primary secretion consists of an ultrafiltrate of plasma to which some components synthesised by the acinar cells (such as α-amylase and mucins) have been added. It is therefore almost isotonic with plasma. The rates of secretion of the primary juice and the α-amylase concentration vary with the type of stimulation, but the ionic composition of the primary juice is fairly constant.

As the primary juice flows past the duct cells, it undergoes secondary modification via transport systems in the membranes of the secretory and striated duct cells. Certain substances are produced by the duct cells and secreted into the saliva and others are extracted from the saliva by the cells. Sodium ions and chloride are extracted from the saliva and potassium is added. In fact, Na^+ and K^+ are exchanged by an active mechanism in the duct cells. However, more Na^+ is extracted than K^+ is added by this mechanism, and the duct epithelium has a very low permeability to water. Consequently, secondary saliva becomes more hypotonic as it flows down the ducts; in humans, saliva is always hypotonic compared to plasma.

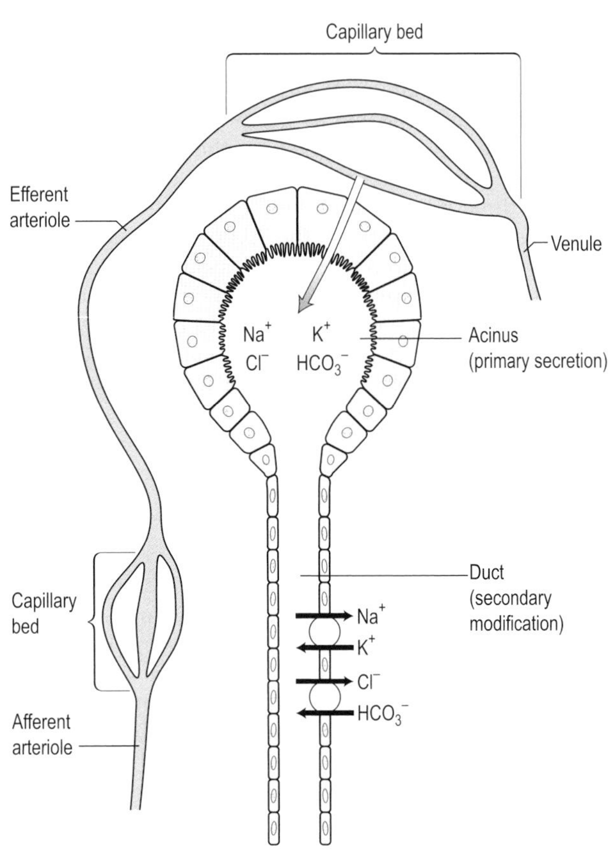

Fig. 1.11 Secretion of primary saliva in the acinus of a salivary gland and secondary modification in the duct.

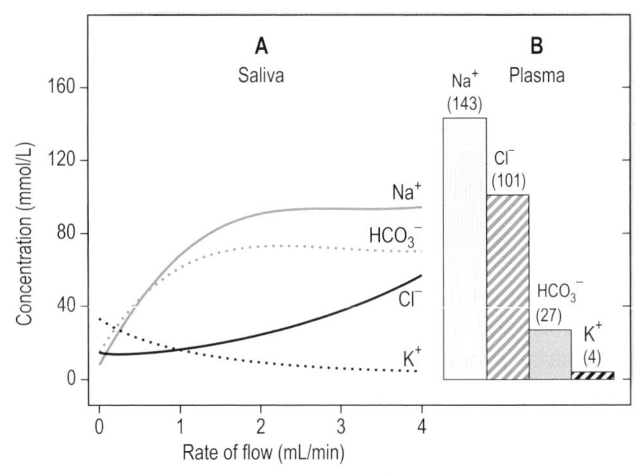

Fig. 1.12 (A) Changes in concentration of some ions in saliva with rate of flow. (B) Concentrations of the same ions in blood plasma.

Bicarbonate ions in saliva are produced from CO_2 and water in the duct cells via the reactions:

$$CO_2 + H_2O \xleftrightarrow{\text{carbonic anhydrase}} H_2CO_3 \longleftrightarrow H^+ + HCO_3^-$$

Duct cells are rich in carbonic anhydrase, an enzyme which catalyses the formation of carbonic acid from CO_2 and water. Bicarbonate is secreted across the membranes into the ducts in exchange for Cl^- (Fig. 1.11).

The composition of saliva changes with the rate of flow because, at fast flow rates, there is less time for the exchange processes occurring in the ducts to modify the composition. Thus the composition at high flow rates approaches that of the primary juice. Fig. 1.12 shows the changes in the concentration of some ions in the saliva flowing from the ducts, with the rate of flow, and compares them with the concentration of those ions in the plasma.

The concentrations of Na^+ ions and bicarbonate ions increase with the rate of flow until a plateau is reached, whilst the concentration of K^+ ions decreases and plateaus at low flow rates. Sodium ions are exchanged for K^+, but the Na:K exchange ratio is 3:1. It is only at low flow rates that the active transport processes for these ions in the ducts make a measurable difference to their concentrations in the saliva. At maximum rates of flow, the tonicity of human saliva is approximately 70% of that of plasma. The ducts extract more ions than they deliver to the saliva, and the osmotic gradient is therefore in the direction of the plasma, but the ducts are relatively impermeable to water and so the saliva is always hypotonic to plasma. Table 1.1 compares the ionic composition of primary saliva produced in the acinus, secondary saliva produced at a low flow rate (unstimulated), and secondary saliva produced at a high flow rate (stimulated).

Saliva has a normal pH range of 6.2–7.6 with an average pH of 6.7. It becomes more alkaline with increasing rate of flow as the concentration of HCO_3^- ions increases; bicarbonate is an important component of saliva since it plays a major role in buffering salivary pH near neutrality.

Control of secretion

In humans, the secretion of saliva is exclusively controlled by both sympathetic and parasympathetic innervations. Hormonal control of salivary production has also been demonstrated. The postganglionic sympathetic nerve fibres have their cell bodies in the superior cervical ganglion. The preganglionic parasympathetic nerve fibres travel in branches of the facial (cranial nerve VII) and the glossopharyngeal (cranial nerve XI) nerves. These synapse with postganglionic fibres in or near the glands. There is a parasympathetic innervation of all acini and most usually also have a sympathetic innervation. Several nerve fibres supply each acinus but not every cell is innervated. However, the acinar cells are electrically coupled so that the membrane depolarisation brought about by nerve impulses in the innervated cells is transmitted to the neighbouring cells. Myoepithelial cells in the vicinity of the acini are innervated by the same nerve fibres. The duct cells, myoepithelial cells and arterioles of the gland are also innervated by both parasympathetic and sympathetic nerves.

Nerve stimulation induces changes in both the composition and the volume of the secretion. The parasympathetic nerve is mainly responsible for the secretion of water and electrolytes, whereas secretion of proteins is

Table 1.1 Concentrations of some important constituents in primary and secondary saliva

Ions (mmol/L)	*Primary saliva*	*Secondary saliva*	
		Unstimulated	*Stimulated*
Na^+	145	2	85
K^+	4	25	18
Cl^-	100	23	55
HCO_3^-	24	4	40
α-Amylase (g/L)		0.1	1.0
Flow rate (mL/min)		0.5	3.5

The ionic composition of the primary juice is similar to that of blood plasma. The differences in ionic compositions of the primary and secondary saliva are due to the modifications that take place as the saliva flows down the ducts. Thus Na^+ is extracted and K^+ is added in the ducts. HCO_3^- secretion is stimulated at high rates of flow. The fate of Cl^- is complex; it is exchanged for HCO_3^- and is transported down the electrical gradient created by the transport of Na^+. In stimulated saliva, there is less time for such modifications to take place, as the flow rate is faster. The composition of the stimulated secondary juice is therefore intermediate between that of the primary juice and the unstimulated secondary juice. The concentration of α-amylase is higher at high flow rates as its secretion from the acinar cells is stimulated.

under sympathetic control. Simulation of either the parasympathetic nerves or the sympathetic nerves increases the rate of secretion. However, the parasympathetic nerves provide a stronger and longer lasting stimulus. The parasympathetic nerves release acetylcholine, substance P and vasoactive intestinal peptide (VIP), while the sympathetic nerves release noradrenaline.

The processes stimulated by parasympathetic nerve activity include the flow of saliva, the release of α-amylase and mucins from the acinar cells, transport events in the duct cells, the extrusion of saliva from the ducts, blood flow and the metabolism and growth of the acinar and duct cells. Stimulation of the sympathetic nerves is a transient effect causing the release of saliva rich in α-amylase, mucins, HCO_3^- and K^+ and the contraction of the myoepithelial cells. It also causes vasoconstriction that reduces the blood flow to the glands. This effect may be exaggerated when an individual is frightened and may explain why some people experience a dry mouth when they are afraid. Circulating catecholamines reinforce the effect of sympathetic nerve stimulation. Acinar cell membranes have both α- and β-adrenergic receptors. Other hormones are not a major influence in the control of secretion of saliva, although both vasopressin and aldosterone can stimulate Na^+/K^+ exchange in the duct dells.

Cellular mechanisms of control

The acinar cells of resting glands contain granules. Within these granules, the zymogen precursor of α-amylase is stored. If the gland is stimulated, the number of granules diminishes as the enzyme is released. Enzyme production occurs rapidly in the acinar cell after stimulation, although it is the release by exocytosis, not the synthesis, that is directly stimulated by the transmitter.

The second messengers involved in the actions of the neurotransmitters on acinar cells are intracellular cAMP and Ca^{2+}. Activation of either β-adrenergic receptors or VIP receptors causes an increase in intracellular cAMP, while activation of α-adrenergic receptors, muscarinic acetylcholine receptors, or substance P receptors results in increased Ca^{2+} influx into the cell. Substances that increase intracellular cAMP tend to produce a secretion that is richer in α-amylase than those that increase intracellular Ca^{2+} concentration, whilst those that increase intracellular Ca^{2+} concentration tend to produce a greater increase in the volume of acinar cell secretion. Mucins are also released by exocytosis as a consequence of influx of Ca^{2+} into the cell.

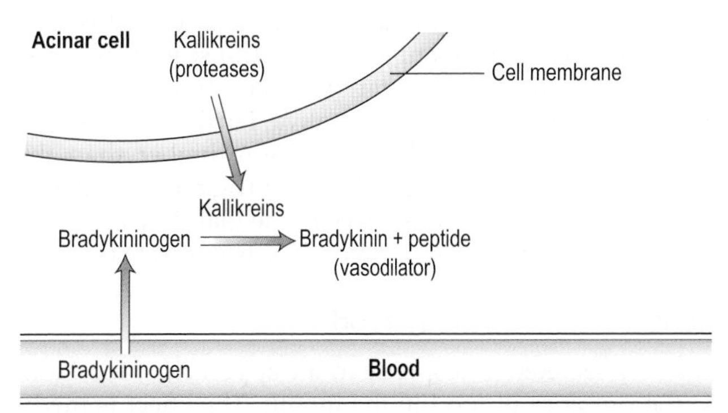

Fig. 1.13 Mechanism of vasodilation during stimulation of salivary secretion.

Blood flow

When the parasympathetic nerves are stimulated, there is a rapid vasodilatation that can result in up to a five-fold increase in blood flow. This is followed by a slower vasodilatory effect. The immediate effect is probably due to a direct action of the transmitters acetylcholine and VIP released from parasympathetic nerve fibres that terminate on the arterioles in the glandular tissue. Stimulation of the sympathetic nerves causes vasoconstriction via the release of noradrenaline that acts on α-adrenergic receptors on the arteriolar smooth muscle.

The slower vasodilatory effect is an indirect consequence of stimulation of the parasympathetics. It is due to the formation of vasodilator metabolites, mainly bradykinin, by processes occurring following stimulation of the acinar cells that results in the release of proteolytic enzymes known as kallikreins into the interstitial fluid. These enzymes catalyse the conversion of a precursor, bradykininogen to bradykinin, the active vasodilator (see Fig. 1.13).

Bradykinin acts on the arteriolar smooth muscle to cause vasodilatation. When the arterioles dilate, the pressure drop across them diminishes and the pressure is transferred to the capillaries. The increased hydrostatic pressure and consequent increased transcapillary pressure result in increased filtration in the gland. The consequence is an increased flow of saliva. Furthermore, saliva can actually be secreted at a pressure higher than the arterial pressure to the gland, as the triggering of active processes at the luminal surface of the gland by the parasympathetic nerves causes secondary water transport.

Control of secretion by food

Saliva is secreted in response to the approach of food and to the presence of food in the mouth. The effect is mediated via the parasympathetic nerves. Up to 50% of the secretion during a meal comes from the parotid glands. Two reflexes are involved: a conditioned reflex and an unconditioned reflex.

The conditioned reflex is due mainly to the sight and smell of food, although other sensory inputs such as sounds can trigger it. The reflex was first studied in dogs by Ivan Pavlov, a Russian physiologist who worked in St Petersburg. He usually fed the dogs at a time when the bells of the cathedral chimed. He discovered that they salivated when the bells chimed even on occasions when they were not being fed, presumably in anticipation. Thus the conditioned reflex is a learned response because the first time the stimulus is presented, it does not elicit a secretion.

The unconditioned reflex is due to the presence of food in the mouth. It occurs in response to activation of touch or taste receptors. Stimulation by food of taste receptors on the tongue, or pressure receptors in the mouth, results in impulses being set up in the afferent nerves to the brainstem. Fig. 1.4 shows the arrangement of the neural pathways of the secretory reflex that occurs following stimulation of the taste buds. This involves afferent pathways from the tongue to the superior and inferior salivary nuclei. The afferent nerve fibres run in the chorda tympani and the glossopharyngeal nerves (see above). The efferent preganglionic parasympathetic nerves to the salivary glands also run in these nerves (see Fig 1.4). The preganglionic fibres in the glossopharyngeal nerve synapse with postganglionic fibres in the otic ganglion and the postganglionic fibres innervate the parotid glands. The preganglionic fibres in the chorda tympani synapse with postganglionic fibres in the submandibular ganglion and the postganglionic fibres innervate the submandibular and sublingual glands.

Oesophagus

Anatomical arrangements of the oesophagus

The primary function of the oesophagus is to connect the pharynx to the stomach. The arrangement of the smooth muscle in the wall of the oesophagus is similar to that of the rest of the GI tract in that there is an inner circular layer and an outer longitudinal layer. However, only the lower two-thirds of the oesophagus contain smooth muscle. The top one-third contains skeletal muscle. The muscle tissue in an area in the middle of the oesophagus consists of a mixture of skeletal muscle and smooth muscle fibres, with the skeletal muscle gradually being replaced by smooth muscle in the caudal direction. Whilst skeletal and smooth muscle fibres are under the control of the vagus nerve, skeletal muscle is innervated directly by somatic motor neurones from the nucleus ambiguus, and the smooth muscle is innervated indirectly by neurones in the vagus nerve that synapse with neurones in the myenteric plexus; the myenteric plexus is a part of the enteric nervous system. The intrinsic nerves are, in effect, postganglionic autonomic nerves. Preganglionic parasympathetic neurones in the vagus nerve from the dorsal motor nucleus synapse with the cell bodies of these neurones.

The upper oesophageal sphincter (the hypopharyngeal sphincter or cricopharyngeus muscle) is composed of skeletal muscle. It is a thickening of the circular muscle layer. The lower sphincter comprises the last 1–2 cm of the oesophagus. It is not anatomically distinguishable as a discrete sphincter, but the pressure is normally greater in this region than in the stomach to aid transit of the food bolus.

Oesophageal varices

Oesophageal varices are due to portal hypertension. This is a common complication of cirrhosis of the liver which causes obstruction to the portal blood flow. The portosystemic anastomoses at the lower end of the oesophagus become unusually dilated in response to the raised venous pressure. These veins are thin-walled and bleed easily. Bleeding can be life-threatening. The associated liver disease can complicate the situation because of impaired coagulation. Optimal management requires occlusion of the veins by beta blockade, endoscopic ligation, or sclerotherapy.

Swallowing (deglutition)

The arrangement of the structures associated with swallowing is shown in Fig. 1.1. The events involved are represented in Fig. 1.14.

The whole process lasts only a few seconds. It is initiated voluntarily but once initiated it cannot be stopped voluntarily. The process can be divided into three phases: voluntary, pharyngeal and oesophageal.

Phases of swallowing

Voluntary phase

In the voluntary phase, the tongue separates the food into a bolus and then moves it backwards and upwards

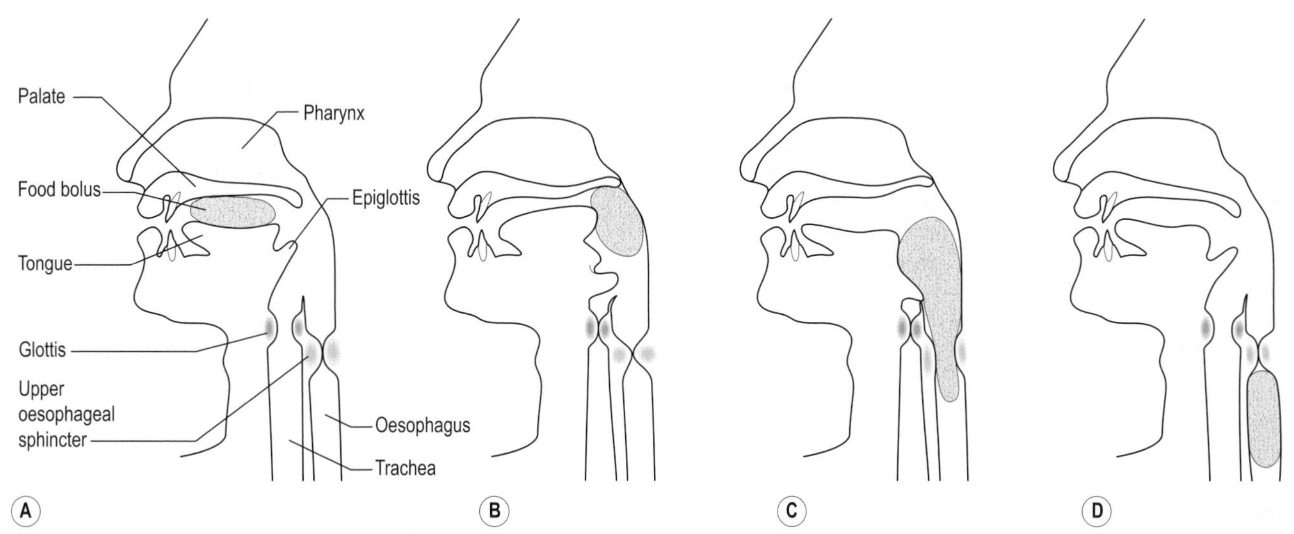

Fig. 1.14 (A–D) Sequential events involved in swallowing.

towards the back of the mouth. The lubricating properties of saliva are important for swallowing, and individuals suffering from xerostomia have difficulty in swallowing.

Pharyngeal phase

As the bolus of food moves into the pharynx, it activates pressure receptors in the palate and anterior pharynx. This results in impulses in the trigeminal and glossopharyngeal nerves being transmitted to the swallowing centre in the brainstem. Each impulse serves as a trigger for the swallowing reflex. This causes the elevation of the soft palate that seals the nasal cavity and prevents food from entering it. The swallowing centre inhibits respiration, raises the larynx and closes the glottis (the opening between the vocal cords). This prevents food from getting into the trachea. As the tongue forces the food further back into the pharynx, the bolus tilts the epiglottis backwards to cover the closed glottis. However, it is closure of the glottis, not the tilting of the epiglottis, that is mainly responsible for preventing food from entering the trachea.

The upper oesophageal sphincter is closed at rest. It opens during swallowing, allowing the bolus of food to pass into the oesophagus. Immediately after the bolus has passed, it closes again, resealing the junction. The glottis then opens and breathing resumes. The skeletal muscle fibres of the upper oesophageal sphincter are so arranged that they contract when the sphincter opens and relax when it closes. This pharyngeal phase of swallowing lasts approximately 1 s. The relationship between the oesophagus and other thoracic structures is shown in Fig. 1.15.

Oesophageal phase

The food is moved along the oesophagus by peristalsis. A peristaltic wave consists of a wave of contraction of the circular muscle, followed by a wave of relaxation. The wave of contraction passes along the walls of the oesophagus and moves the food towards the stomach.

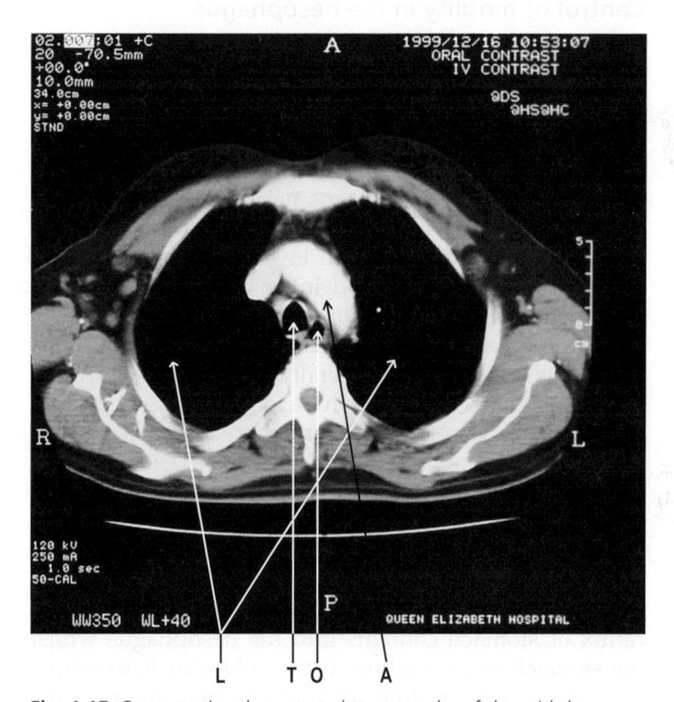

Fig. 1.15 Cross-sectional computed tomography of the mid-thorax showing the anatomical relationship of the lungs (L), aortic arch (A), overlying the trachea (T) and the oesophagus (O).

The wave of contraction takes about 9 s to travel the length of the oesophagus. The progression of the wave is controlled by autonomic nerves and is coordinated by the swallowing centre in the medulla. Thus it is not primarily gravity, but peristalsis that causes the food to move towards the stomach, although gravity assists the process. The importance of peristalsis to the process compared to that of gravity is seen by the fact that food can be swallowed and will reach the stomach even in someone who is upside down. It is noteworthy that, in other parts of the GI tract, the peristaltic waves are coordinated largely by the internal nerve plexi and the extrinsic nerves are less important and can be sectioned without GI function being dramatically affected.

As the peristaltic waves reach the lower oesophageal sphincter, the sphincter relaxes and opens, allowing the food bolus to enter the stomach. The sphincter muscle then contracts and reseals the junction. It remains closed in the absence of peristalsis, preventing reflux of the stomach's contents.

Control of swallowing

Swallowing is coordinated by the 'swallowing centre' in the medulla oblongata. It involves efferent impulses from the medulla to 25 different skeletal muscles of the pharynx, the larynx and the early oesophagus and the smooth muscles in the lower oesophagus.

Control of motility in the oesophagus

Swallowed food is propelled along the oesophagus to the stomach by the coordinated contraction of the muscle in the body of the oesophagus. This wave of contraction is due to a sequential activation of the muscles in the pharynx and oesophagus by neural impulses in the segmental efferent neurones of the vagus nerve that utilise acetylcholine as the neurotransmitter (Fig. 1.16).

The smooth muscle of the lower sphincter is innervated by both extrinsic and intrinsic nerves. Impulses in the cholinergic nerve fibres in the vagus are partly responsible for the maintained contraction of the muscle, or its tone, when peristaltic activity is absent in the oesophagus. Stimulation of noradrenergic sympathetic nerves also causes contraction via activation of α-adrenergic receptors. However, if the extrinsic nerves are cut, there is still some tone, indicating that the intrinsic nerves are also important. An increase in the blood concentration of gastrin that is released from the stomach can also increase the tone of the sphincter muscle. This mechanism may be important in preventing reflux of stomach contents into the oesophagus whilst the stomach is contracting. If the sphincter is incompetent, the reflux of stomach contents may damage the mucosa.

Relaxation of the lower oesophageal sphincter is caused by impulses in inhibitory nerve fibres that innervate the circular smooth muscle. The transmitters involved may be VIP and nitric oxide. A decrease in cholinergic impulses also promotes relaxation of the sphincter.

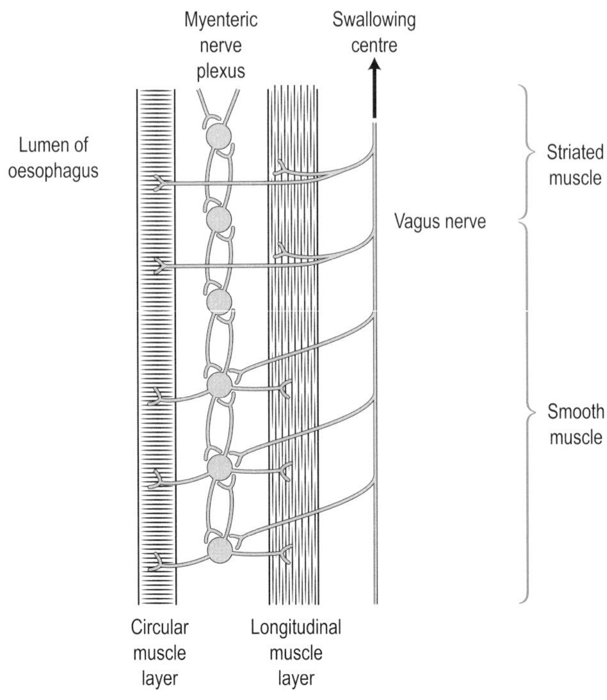

Fig. 1.16 Segmental innervation of the skeletal and smooth muscle of the oesophagus. Somatic motor neurones in the vagus nerve innervate the skeletal muscle directly. Autonomic nerve fibres in the vagus innervate the smooth muscle indirectly via the intrinsic nerves in the myenteric plexus. *Note*: The transition from skeletal muscle to smooth muscle in a region approximately one-third of the way down the oesophagus is gradual.

Gastro-oesophageal reflux disease

Gastro-oesophageal reflux disease (GORD) is defined by symptoms or complications resulting from the reflux of gastric contents into the oesophagus. The most common symptoms of GORD are heartburn, regurgitation and chest pain. However, it is important to make the distinction between individuals who occasionally suffer with symptoms of heartburn (it is predicted that up to one-third of the adult population have experienced heartburn at some time in their lifetime) and individuals with GORD. To be described as having GORD, one would experience symptoms of GORD over a chronic period of time with relatively mild symptoms at least twice a week or severe symptoms at least once a week. More alarmingly, GORD can lead to oesophageal inflammation (oesophagitis) and the premalignant condition, Barrett's metaplasia, which can lead to an increased risk of developing oesophageal adenocarcinoma. GORD is highly prevalent with approximately 10% of the adult population having had GORD at some stage in the lifetime. The common clinical presentation of GORD is described in Case 1.3.

Risk factors of GORD

- Hiatal hernias can increase the likelihood of GORD due to mechanical and motility factors associated with the condition.
- Obesity is associated with GORD, but the underlying mechanisms by which obesity is associated with GORD remain unclear. It is likely to be attributed to

enhanced intragastric pressure, which can lead to an increased risk of reflux. Obesity might promote GORD through various other mechanisms, including hormonal mechanisms involving oestrogen.

- Other factors include pregnancy, Zollinger-Ellison syndrome, and drugs such as alpha-blockers, anticholinergics, benzodiazepines, beta-blockers, bisphosphonates, calcium-channel blockers, corticosteroids, non-steroidal anti-inflammatory drugs (NSAIDs), nitrates, theophyllines and tricyclic antidepressants.

Diagnosis of GORD

A diagnosis of GORD can be made by assessing the presenting symptoms (which include chronic heartburn, regurgitation, chest pain or discomfort, chronic cough, sore throat and/or hoarseness, sleep apnoea and nausea) and the patient's response to common anti-reflux medicines, most notably proton-pump inhibitors (PPIs). However, the gold standard for diagnosing GORD is oesophageal pH monitoring. This allows for a more accurate measurement of how much of the time the oesophagus is bathed by stomach acid. If the patient presents with alarm symptoms such as anaemia and weight loss, an upper GI endoscopy is required to ensure that the oesophagus has no associated pathology including stricturing, Barrett's metaplasia and or oesophageal cancer. Importantly, not all patients with GORD present with pathology within the oesophagus, and indeed, there are patients who show no evidence of erosive effects in the oesophagus and are thus termed as having non-erosive reflux disease.

Treatment of GORD

GORD can often be remedied by simple lifestyle changes. Reflux tends to be more common after eating food and most notably at night. This is in part due to stomach acid secretion being triggered immediately before and during the consumption of food. Thus the stomach is relatively full, and reflux is more likely to occur with a relatively weak or defective gastro-oesophageal sphincter, compared with when an individual has not recently eaten and there is little stomach acid secretion. In addition, when lying down, the prevalence of acid reflux is also likely to be worse since acid is more likely to leak through the gastro-oesophageal sphincter. Thus anything which can elevate the individual's shoulders and head may help to resolve the symptoms of GORD. However, more pertinently, avoiding eating late at night will undoubtedly ameliorate symptoms of GORD. Since GORD is associated with obesity, a change in lifestyle to encourage weight loss will also have a positive effect.

Medications for GORD are also widely available, with many over-the-counter treatment options. Since the symptoms of reflux are associated with excess acid refluxing into the oesophagus, therapy can be targeted through either ablating stomach acid production (for example, with the use of PPIs), thereby preventing the acid from refluxing out of the stomach, or by neutralising the pH of acid (using alkaline ions such as calcium carbonate or sodium bicarbonate) so it is no longer erosive. The treatments include the following:

- PPIs (such as omeprazole). These are the gold standard for the treatment of GORD since the inhibitor acts on the H^+/K^+ pump itself within the parietal cells in the stomach, which are the cells responsible for the secretion of acid in the stomach. Thus PPIs will almost completely ablate stomach acid production and, consequently, reflux will not occur due to less acid in the stomach.
- H_2 receptor antagonists. Historically, H_2 receptor antagonists were utilised to suppress acid production by blocking histamine receptors. However, these drugs are not considered as effective as PPIs since acid production can still be triggered through other mechanisms independent of histamine, such as gastrin and acetylcholine.
- Physically blocking acid reflux into the oesophagus (using biopolymers like sodium alginate found in Gaviscon). The most common medications that block acid refluxing into the oesophagus are formulations based around sodium alginate. These formulations contain the antacid bicarbonate, which reacts with stomach acid to produce carbon dioxide. Alginate also reacts with calcium and polymerises into a solid material which traps the carbon dioxide produced and causes it to float on the surface of the stomach acid. This solid raft is thought to subsequently prevent the acid from refluxing into the oesophagus.
- There are various antacids which tend to be based on either aluminium hydroxide or calcium carbonate, and these tend to be the first line therapy since they are freely available and inexpensive. They act by directly neutralising the acid; however, there is limited evidence that they are effective for the treatment of GORD.
- For patients with GORD attributed to the presence of a hiatus hernia, surgical intervention to repair the hernia will in most cases resolve the symptoms of GORD. In addition, in patients with GORD that do not respond to drugs, surgery is also an option, of which Nissen fundoplication is the most common surgical procedure performed. The procedure involves the upper part of the stomach being wrapped around the gastro-oesophageal sphincter, thereby strengthening the sphincter and suppressing the likelihood of subsequent reflux episodes.

Barrett's metaplasia

Barrett's metaplasia is defined as an oesophagus in which any portion of the normal distal squamous epithelial lining has been replaced by columnar epithelium. This typically can be visualised endoscopically and is localised immediately above the gastro-oesophageal junction. It is associated with GORD, with approximately 10% of patients with GORD developing Barrett's metaplasia. Whilst the erosive effect of the stomach juice leads to the development of Barrett's metaplasia, it is still unknown how the acid-mediated damage to the oesophagus leads to this metaplastic event. However, whilst the resulting columnar mucosa is now able to withstand the reflux, it increases the risk of developing oesophageal adenocarcinoma, a cancer which has a 5-year survival of approximately 17%. Estimates suggest that approximately 1% of the adult population have Barrett's metaplasia, although many are asymptomatic; hence, this could potentially be an underestimate. In addition, it is a disease which is skewed by sex with males being approximately 10 times more likely to have the disease. Approximately 3–13% of individuals with Barrett's metaplasia will develop oesophageal adenocarcinoma in their lifetime.

Symptoms of Barrett's metaplasia

Since Barrett's metaplasia is associated with GORD, it is unsurprising that frequent and longstanding heartburn, dysphagia, regurgitation of food and retrosternal pain are known presenting symptoms. Other symptoms include hematemesis and unintentional weight loss attributed to pain when eating (odynophagia).

Risk factors

The most common risk factors for Barrett's metaplasia include being a male, old age, a family history of the disease, long-standing GORD, smoking, obesity (as determined by the waist-to-hip ratio) and White race. Of note, the presence of *Helicobacter pylori* has been shown to be inversely associated with the condition in several studies, presumably through the resulting hypochlorhydria (low stomach acid concentration) which is commonly observed in patients infected with *H. pylori*.

Diagnosis

Confirmation of Barrett's metaplasia requires endoscopy, where it is commonly found that patients have an oesophagus that is salmon-pink in colour, distinct to the off-white colouration of the native oesophagus, and is seen extending up the oesophagus from the gastro-oesophageal sphincter (Fig. 1.17A). The length of Barrett's metaplasia varies between individuals;

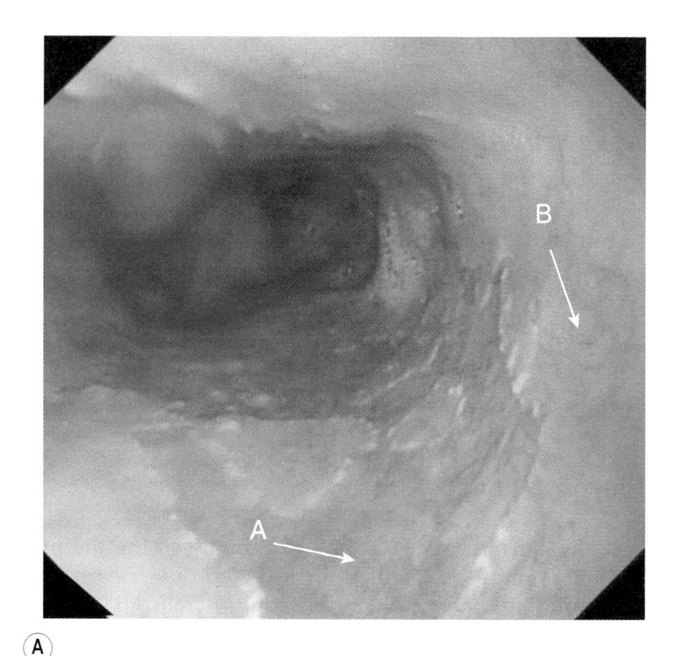

(A)

Fig. 1.17A Endoscopic image depicting the salmon-pink tissue associated with Barrett's metaplasia (A) in comparison to the adjacent healthy oesophagus (B).

however, in nearly all cases, it is confined to the distal third of the oesophagus where acid reflux is more likely to occur. Biopsies are taken of the suspected region of Barrett's metaplasia and histology confirming the presence of columnar epithelia with goblet cells in the lower oesophagus confirms a diagnosis of Barrett's metaplasia.

Treatment

Treatment of Barrett's metaplasia depends on the presence or absence of dysplasia which indicates its malignant risk. Treatment of Barrett's metaplasia with no evidence of dysplasia (which suggests that the patient is at low risk of developing adenocarcinoma of the oesophagus) is centred around the treatment of any associated symptoms rather than to attempt to remove the Barrett's metaplasia. The most commonly used medications in the treatment of Barrett's metaplasia are PPIs aimed at ameliorating any symptoms associated with reflux. More recently, a randomised control trial indicated that the use of a high-dose PPI with aspirin may confer a chemopreventative effect by protecting patients with Barrett's metaplasia from developing oesophageal adenocarcinoma. In addition, as with patients with GORD, patients with Barrett's metaplasia should avoid medications and food which exacerbate reflux, make changes to their lifestyle and consider surgery for a hiatus hernia and or Nissen fundoplication, especially if anti-reflux medicines and lifestyle changes have little impact on quality of life.

Historically, patients with evidence of dysplasia within their Barrett's metaplasia were either monitored intensely or referred for oesophagectomy, a procedure which many elderly and unfit patients are unsuitable for. However, more recently, minimally invasive procedures have been adopted which are designed to endoscopically remove the area of dysplasia. Such endoscopic procedures have radically transformed how patients are managed and their subsequent outcomes. The two main platforms are endoscopic mucosal resection (EMR) and radiofrequency ablation (RFA). EMR affords the endoscopist the ability to remove, in essence, much larger areas of tissues than can be removed with a simple biopsy. By removing the areas of dysplastic Barrett's metaplasia, it is presumed that the risk of developing oesophageal adenocarcinoma is equally reduced. This is in part achieved by initially injecting fluid into the area of dysplastic Barrett's metaplasia and then removing the tissue by suction via an endoscope. RFA is a technique which can mediate local coagulation necrosis through the induction of an electric circuit and by directing varying radiofrequency currents to the selected tissues. This platform allows for the entire circumference of the involved oesophagus to be treated and has been approved by NICE for both low- and high-grade dysplastic Barrett's.

Surveillance

Barrett's metaplasia is associated with an increased risk of developing oesophageal adenocarcinoma and has a 0.5% annual conversion rate. Since many individuals with Barrett's metaplasia are elderly and have other co-morbidities, there is still debate as to whether patients with non-dysplastic Barrett's metaplasia should be subject to surveillance. This is further questioned in the background of a conservative estimate of 1% of the adult population having Barrett's metaplasia, which would make surveillance of any large population onerous. However, although randomised clinical trial data are lacking, the evidence from published studies suggests that surveillance correlates with an improved outcome and is therefore recommended. Of note, surveillance regimens consider the extent of the metaplasia as judged by the length of the Barrett's segment. Patients with Barrett's oesophagus shorter than 3 cm with intestinal metaplasia receive endoscopic surveillance every 3–5 years, whilst patients with segments of 3 cm or longer receive surveillance every 2–3 years. Much research is currently focussed on understanding the underpinning mechanisms of Barrett's progression to adenocarcinoma and to identify biomarkers which will allow for risk stratification, which will guide more focussed surveillance of high-risk groups.

Oesophageal cancer

Oesophageal cancer is considered the 14th most common cancer in the UK, accounting for 3% of all new cancer cases and is the 7th most common cause of cancer death, accounting for 5% of all cancer deaths. The relatively poor 10-year survival figure of approximately 12% is largely attributed to advanced disease on presentation. Oesophageal cancer encompasses predominantly two types of disease: squamous cell carcinomas, which are derived from the native squamous epithelium and consequently tend to occur in the proximal and middle third of the oesophagus, and adenocarcinomas, which are derived from Barrett's metaplasia and thus tend to be localised in the distal oesophagus close to the gastro-oesophageal junction. Squamous cell cancers of the oesophagus account for over 80% of all cases of oesophageal cancers worldwide and is the predominant type of oesophageal cancer in less-developed regions. Whilst oesophageal adenocarcinoma has seen an unprecedented increase in incidence in the Western world, its incidence has surpassed that of squamous cell cancers of the oesophagus.

Case 1.3 Part 1: Achalasia, GORD, Barrett's metaplasia and cancer

A 54-year-old male presented to his general practitioner with a 5-month history of worsening dysphagia, which he noticed more when ingesting liquids than solids. He had no problems with initiating swallowing but finds that food gets stuck in the lower part of his chest. He reported some weight loss but denied early satiety. He denied heartburn and haematemesis (vomiting blood). He did not have any significant past medical or drug history and denied any allergies. He reported that his mother was diagnosed with gastric cancer in her 60s. He works as a software engineer. He smokes 20 cigarettes a day and has a 25-pack year history. He consumes 22 units of alcohol a week. On examination, his body mass index (BMI) was 38 with a blood pressure of 125/78. There were no significant clinical findings on an abdominal examination. His clinical examination was normal, and routine blood tests did not reveal any significant abnormality.

Dysphagia is an alarm symptom that needs urgent evaluation to understand the exact cause and facilitate initiation of appropriate therapy. This may be due to an anatomical or structural problem or an abnormality with the processes involved with motility associated with the passage of solids and liquids from the oral cavity into the stomach. Patients usually complain of difficulty swallowing liquids or solids, with the symptoms being acute onset or progressive in nature. The first step in evaluating patients with dysphagia is to understand if the symptoms are due to an oropharyngeal

Continued

Case 1.3 Part 1: Achalasia, GORD, Barrett's metaplasia and cancer—cont'd

or oesophageal abnormality. In oropharyngeal dysphagia, patients may report difficulty with initiating swallowing or may cough or choke while eating or drinking. With oesophageal dysphagia, patients report difficulty in swallowing several seconds after initiating a swallow and describe a sensation of food or fluids being stuck in their chest. Dysphagia needs to be characterised by determining the types of food that cause the symptoms (liquids, solids, or both); if is it progressive, intermittent, or acute onset; and if there are any other associated symptoms such as weight loss, heartburn and anaemia. The patient here reports a progressive worsening dysphagia that is oesophageal in nature and appears to be primarily associated with liquids and not solids. In addition, he has lost weight but denies symptoms suggestive of GORD.

The patient underwent an upper GI endoscopy, which revealed a dilated fluid-filled oesophagus, and a subsequent barium swallow demonstrated a dilated oesophagus with a 'bird's beak' (Fig. 1.17B). He underwent oesophageal manometry which showed absent relaxation of the lower oesophageal sphincter with high resting pressures suggestive of achalasia. Dilatation of his oesophagus only provided minimal relief. He underwent a surgical myotomy which resulted in excellent resolution of his dysphagia.

Evaluation of patients with oesophageal dysphagia includes a direct examination of the oesophagus with an endoscope or an imaging test such as contrast swallow (i.e., a barium swallow). This can help diagnose structural problems with the oesophagus such as a stricture (narrowing) from a cancer of the oesophagus or as a result of chronic inflammation of the oesophagus from acid reflux. If no specific structural abnormalities are seen on these investigations, the function and contractility of the oesophagus can be measured by performing a procedure called oesophageal manometry to assess abnormalities of the motility of the oesophagus, such as oesophageal spasm or achalasia. The patient was diagnosed with a condition called achalasia in which there is normal peristalsis and contractility of the distal oesophagus but a failure of relaxation of the lower oesophageal sphincter with swallowing. Patients usually report dysphagia to solids and liquids and often vomit undigested food and saliva. Achalasia can be treated by mechanical disruption of the lower oesophageal sphincter by cutting through the muscle fibres (surgical myotomy or endoscopic myotomy) or by stretching or tearing the muscle fibres (pneumatic dilatation). Alternatively, pharmacological therapies with injection of botulinum toxin or use of oral nitrates may be effective.

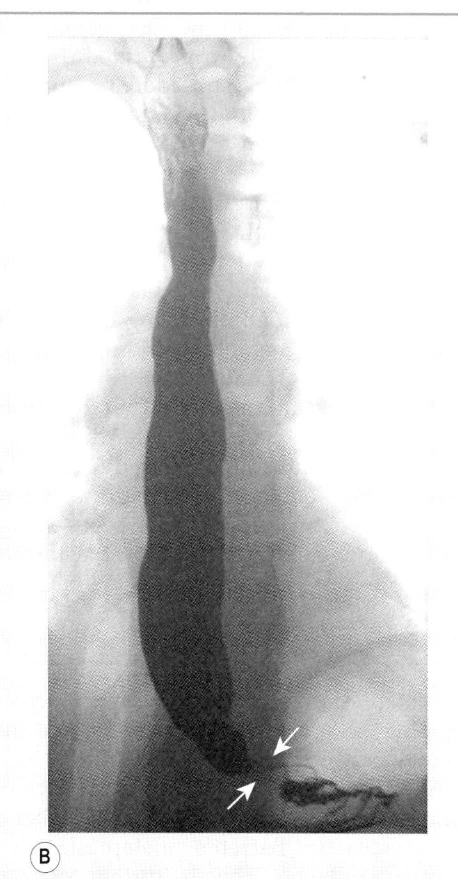

Fig. 1.17B Radiographic images depicting the characteristic bird's beak found in achalasia. Arrows highlight the unrelaxed gastro-oesophageal sphincter.

Five years later, the patient returned to his general practitioner with heartburn. His symptoms were worse at night and especially when he went to bed. He reported some relief with over-the-counter antacid medications. He underwent blood tests, which were normal. He subsequently had an upper GI endoscopy which revealed reflux oesophagitis on the background of Barrett's oesophagus along with a slight narrowing of the lumen in his lower oesophagus consistent with a peptic stricture. He was commenced on high-dose PPI therapy with significant improvement in his reflux symptoms and dysphagia.

Symptoms

Whilst the risk factors differ for these two cancer types, the presenting symptoms are broadly similar. The most common symptoms are dysphagia, which initially tends to be experienced with solid foods. Pain is also experienced in the retrosternal chest and also upon swallowing. The presence of an oesophageal tumour can also impact the motility of the oesophagus, which can lead to nausea, vomiting and regurgitation of food and coughing. Unexplained weight loss is a common presenting alarm symptom.

Risk factors of oesophageal cancers

The predominant risk factors of squamous cell cancers are socioeconomic status, tobacco smoking and the consumption of alcoholic beverages.

Socioeconomic status

Lower socioeconomic status has been shown to be associated with an increased risk in both developing and developed countries.

Tobacco smoking

Tobacco smoking is a major risk factor for oesophageal squamous cell cancers. Recent studies indicate an approximately 3- to 5-fold increased risk of oesophageal squamous cell cancers in current smokers compared with non-smokers. Data suggests that over 50% of all oesophageal squamous cell cancer cases could be attributed to tobacco smoking in some countries.

Alcohol overconsumption

Excessive use of alcohol is strongly associated with an increased risk of oesophageal squamous cell cancer, with studies from the United States indicating that overconsumption of alcohol is associated with up to a 9-fold increased risk and may account for over 70% of all oesophageal squamous cell cancer cases. Of note, the association seems to be stronger in lower-incidence Western countries than in higher-incidence Asian countries

The predominant risk factors of oesophageal adenocarcinomas are GORD, Barrett's metaplasia, obesity, tobacco smoking and *H. pylori* infection.

GORD and Barrett's metaplasia

Unsurprisingly, GORD and Barrett's metaplasia are both strong risk factors for the development of oesophageal adenocarcinoma. A number of studies have suggested an approximate 6-fold increased risk of adenocarcinoma in patients with a long-standing history of GORD. As anticipated, effective anti-reflux therapies likely prevent the development of oesophageal adenocarcinoma. The presence of Barrett's metaplasia increases the risk of developing oesophageal adenocarcinoma and equates to an approximately 0.5% annual conversion rate. Of note, 95% of oesophageal adenocarcinomas arise in individuals without a prior diagnosis of Barrett's oesophagus, hence the debate of over the value of surveillance programmes.

Obesity

A higher BMI is strongly associated with an increased risk of oesophageal adenocarcinoma. Studies indicate a 2.4-fold increased risk of oesophageal adenocarcinoma associated with a BMI of 30–34.9, 2.8-fold with a BMI of 35–39.9, and 4.8-fold with a BMI of 40 or above. The preventive potential of weight loss against the development of oesophageal adenocarcinoma remains to be evaluated

Tobacco smoking

Tobacco smoking is associated with an increased risk of oesophageal adenocarcinoma, albeit weaker than the associations with oesophageal squamous cell cancers. A number of studies have indicated an approximate 2-fold increased oesophageal adenocarcinoma risk in ever-smokers compared with non-smokers.

Helicobacter pylori

Infection with the gastric bacterium *H. pylori* has been associated with a reduced risk of oesophageal adenocarcinoma, likely attributed to the reduction in stomach acid and which consequently suppresses GORD, a recognised risk factor of oesophageal adenocarcinoma development.

Management of oesophageal cancer

Management of oesophageal cancer is very much dependent on characteristics of the patient, particularly if they are fit enough to undergo surgery if deemed necessary and the tumour itself as predominantly assessed by its Tumour-Node-Metastasis (TNM) staging. For example, relatively small early-stage tumours may be suitable for endoscopic removal, whereas more locally advanced cancers are commonly treated with chemotherapy, chemoradiotherapy, surgical resection, or combinations thereof. Patients with oesophageal cancers which are not suitable for operative management are commonly treated with palliative chemotherapy.

Surgical resection

Major surgical resection of the oesophagus is undertaken for oesophageal carcinoma when the disease is localised. Although this operation is rarely curative, it provides remarkably good symptomatic relief from pain and obstruction, allowing the patient to return to a largely normal diet. Most tumours of the oesophagus involve the lower two-thirds. Removal of this portion of the oesophagus is possible. Restoration of continuity can be achieved by mobilisation of the stomach, which is brought into the chest and connected to the remaining oesophagus in the upper thorax. This is possible because the blood supply of the stomach is so plentiful that the right gastric vessels can be divided and the blood supply sustained on the left gastric artery. If a more radical resection of the oesophagus is required, then a length of small bowel can be placed in the chest to join the throat to the stomach. This requires re-anastomosis of the arterial supply and venous drainage, as the superior mesenteric vessels (supplying the small

Case 1.3 **Part 2: Achalasia, GORD, Barrett's metaplasia and cancer**

Four years later, the patient presented with dysphagia over a 4-month period which had progressed from solids to liquids. He reported significant weight loss of 3 stones and episodes of vomiting over this period, which can be blood-stained. His blood tests revealed significant anaemia. He underwent an urgent upper GI endoscopy which revealed a circumferential tumour in his lower oesophagus, which resulted in significant narrowing of his oesophagus. Histology from biopsies taken from the tumour revealed an adenocarcinoma. He underwent an urgent staging CT scan, following which he started neoadjuvant chemotherapy and underwent oesophagectomy.

bowel) are insufficiently long to reach into the upper thorax.

Replacement of the oesophagus will result in loss of normal peristalsis, and so the patient will need to sit upright when eating. In addition, there will be impairment of motility and the storage capacity of the stomach because of division of the vagal nerves. This requires the patient to eat smaller and more frequent meals to sustain their nutrition. This minor lifestyle adaptation is usually all that is required.

Achalasia

Achalasia is a relatively rare oesophageal motility disorder characterised by oesophageal aperistalsis and a failure of the gastro-oesophageal sphincter to relax during swallowing. The overall prevalence is approximately 10 in every 100,000 people. Patients tend to present with dysphagia to solids and liquids, heartburn, chest pain, regurgitation and weight loss or nutritional deficiencies; hence there is a need to carefully distinguish it from GORD, Barrett's metaplasia and oesophageal adenocarcinoma. Patients with suspected achalasia tend to undergo an upper GI endoscopy. The current gold standard for the diagnosis of achalasia is with high-resolution manometry, and it is now generally recognised that achalasia can be categorised into three distinct types based on manometric profiles. Therapy (pharmacologic, endoscopic and surgical methods) can be subtly tailored to the subtype of achalasia.

Symptoms

Classically, achalasia presents as progressive dysphagia to solids and liquids. Heartburn is a relatively common symptom and thus patients can be misdiagnosed with GORD. Dysphagia and regurgitation are common among all ages, but younger patients are more likely to present with chest pain and heartburn whilst obese patients have more frequent choking or vomiting symptoms. Weight loss is also a common presenting symptom.

Causes

The primary aetiology of achalasia is thought to be loss of inhibitory neurones in the myenteric plexus of the distal oesophagus and lower oesophageal sphincter, resulting in a neuronal imbalance of excitatory and inhibitory activity. It is postulated that a localised decrease of VIP and nitric oxide along with unopposed excitatory activity causes failure of lower oesophageal sphincter relaxation and loss of oesophageal peristalsis. Several studies have also alluded to an association with infections, with patients with achalasia reported to have a greater prevalence of viral antibodies to herpes simplex virus, human papilloma virus and measles virus compared to control patients. There is also evidence that achalasia may be considered an autoimmune inflammatory disorder. In support of this, patients with achalasia are 3–4 times more likely to have other autoimmune diseases.

Diagnosis

A definitive diagnosis of achalasia utilises upper GI endoscopy, use of a barium swallow and high-resolution manometry:

- Endoscopy is essential to predominantly rule out pseudoachalasia from infiltrating malignancy or stricturing. Classic visual findings of achalasia include a dilated oesophageal body with a puckered lower oesophageal sphincter and proximally retained food and saliva (Fig. 1.17C).
- Barium swallow is a non-invasive radiologic procedure that allows for the evaluation of the morphology of the oesophagus and classically shows a dilated oesophagus with a narrowed lower oesophageal sphincter and 'bird's beak' appearance (see Fig. 1.17B).
- High-resolution manometry is the gold standard test for the diagnosis of achalasia. with manometry tracings in patients with achalasia showing the absence of oesophageal peristalsis and incomplete lower oesophageal sphincter relaxation.

Management of achalasia

There is currently no curative treatment for achalasia. All treatment options are targeted at symptom relief by improving the functioning of the lower oesophageal

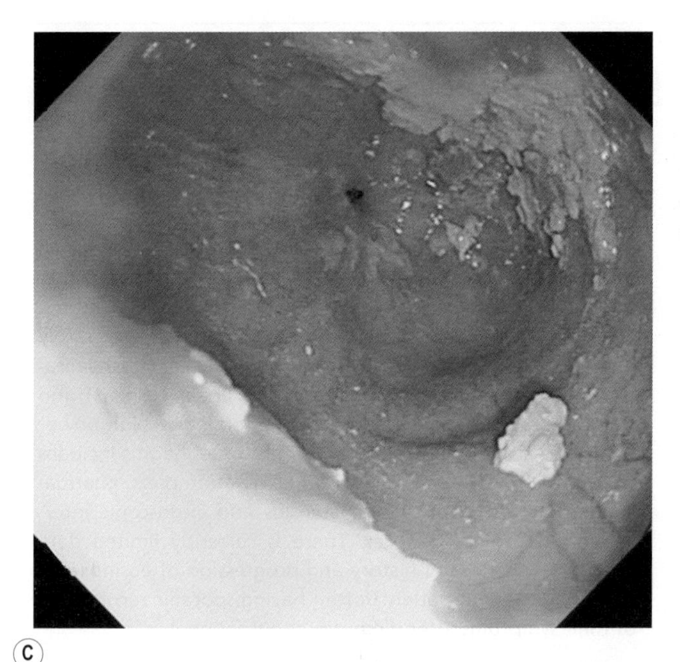

C

Fig. 1.17C Endoscopic image of a patient displaying achalasia. Puckered appearance of the gastro-oesophageal sphincter along with a dilated oesophageal and residual food adhering to the oesophageal lining.

sphincter. This includes the use of drugs, therapeutic endoscopy and surgical procedures.

- The most commonly utilised drugs are sublingually delivered calcium-channel blockers (e.g. nifedipine) and nitrates. Calcium-channel blockers act by decreasing the resting pressure of the lower oesophageal sphincter while nitrates liberate nitric oxide, which elicits relaxation of the lower oesophageal sphincter.
- Botulinum toxin injection for achalasia is an effective short-term therapy. Botulinum toxin injection into the lower oesophageal sphincter locally inhibits the release of acetylcholine, causing relaxation of the smooth muscle. Of note, approximately half of all patients have a relapse of their symptoms within a one-year period.
- Pneumatic dilatation involves the endoscopic dilatation of a balloon with the resulting radial force disrupting the muscularis propria of the lower oesophageal sphincter, resulting in the decrease of muscle tone.
- Laparoscopic Heller myotomy is a highly effective treatment for achalasia, with symptom relief for approximately 90% of patients lasting in many beyond a decade. The procedure involves fibres of the outer longitudinal muscle layer of muscle being dissected to expose the circular muscle fibres. These inner fibres are then gently lifted away from the underlying mucosa and divided. The myotomy is extended 5–6 cm proximal to the gastro-oesophageal junction and across the junction and onto the stomach for 1–2 cm. This procedure has more recently been coupled with a fundoplication so as to prevent any resulting reflux, which was a previously commonly reported side effect post-myotomy.

Case 1.4 Eosinophilic Oesophagus

A 32-year-old man presented to A&E with sudden-onset dysphagia and a sensation of food stuck in his chest while he was eating a steak. He reported a similar episode 3 months earlier which appeared to spontaneously resolve after drinking water. He suffers from asthma and eczema but is otherwise fit and well. An upper GI endoscopy was performed which revealed a food bolus obstruction and was retrieved with an endoscopic basket. Examination of the oesophagus revealed stacked circular rings and some narrowing as seen in Fig. 1.17D. Histological examination of biopsies taken from multiple segments of the oesophagus revealed at least 15 eosinophils per high-power field. A diagnosis of eosinophilic oesophagitis was made. He continued to have intermittent episodes of dysphagia after failing to respond to an initial treatment trial with a PPI and a six-food elimination diet (i.e., milk, egg, soy, wheat, peanuts and fish). He was subsequently commenced on orodispersible steroids which resulted in significant improvement of his symptoms. Repeat histological examination of biopsies taken during endoscopy after completing a 3-month course of this treatment revealed near-complete resolution of eosinophilia.

Continued

Case 1.4

Eosinophilic Oesophagus—cont'd

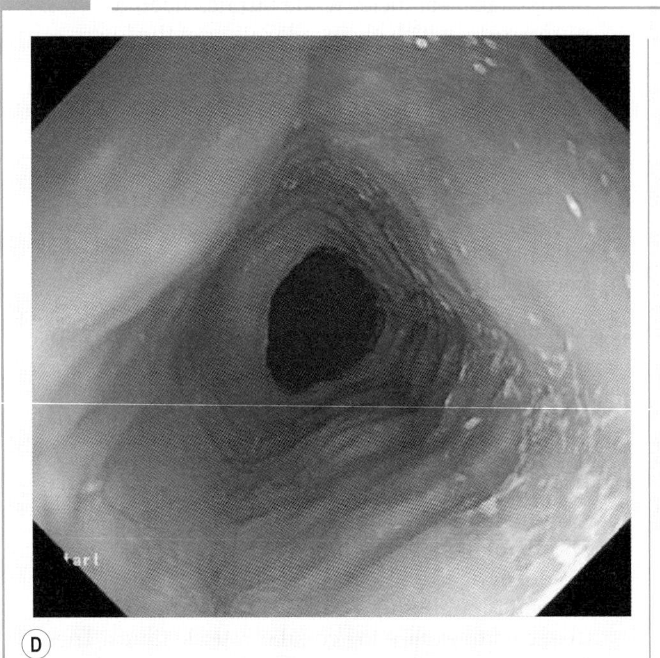

D

Fig. 1.17D Endoscopic image of oesophageal trachealisation demonstrated as furrowing or ring-like appearances.

Eosinophilic oesophagitis is an increasingly recognised cause of dysphagia and possibly heartburn that is unresponsive to PPI therapies. This condition commonly affects individuals in their 20s or 30s who frequently present with dysphagia and food impaction. There is a strong association of eosinophilic oesophagitis with allergic and atopic conditions such as asthma, atopic dermatitis and food allergies. The diagnosis is based upon symptoms (intermittent or rarely persistent dysphagia), endoscopic appearance (trachealisation of the oesophagus, strictures and linear furrows) and histological findings (at least 15 eosinophils per high-power field). The management of eosinophilic oesophagitis includes dietary exclusions such as six-food elimination diets, pharmacologic therapy with PPIs or steroids and endoscopic interventions to treat strictures. There is currently limited data regarding the natural history and progression of eosinophilic oesophagitis, with patients often having sporadic recurrences of their symptoms after discontinuing treatment.

THE STOMACH: BASIC FUNCTIONS AND CONTROL MECHANISMS

2

Chapter objectives and clinical presentations

After reading this chapter, review your learning by considering the following:

1. Can you describe the function of the following cell types found within the stomach: parietal cells, enterochromaffin-like cells, G cells, chief cells and D cells?
2. Can you recognise the different triggers of stomach acid production and the interplay between the different cell types that control acid secretion?
3. What are the different therapeutic options available to suppress stomach acid secretion?
4. Do you understand the important roles the stomach plays in the absorption of nutrients (particularly iron and vitamin B_{12})?
5. Are you familiar with the various roles of motility in stomach function?
6. Can you describe how the cephalic, gastric and intestinal phases are initiated and how these impact stomach acid secretion and motility?

Also, you should be familiar with the following clinical presentations:

- Gastritis
- Peptic ulcer disease
- Gastric cancer
- Gastroparesis

Clinical outlook

The most common presenting complaints associated with disorders of the stomach are dyspepsia (pain in upper abdomen), early satiety and vomiting. Common diagnoses in these patients include peptic ulcer disease, gastritis, gastric cancer and gastroparesis. Patients may sometimes present acutely with an upper gastrointestinal (GI) bleed due to a gastric ulcer or may have more chronic symptoms such as weight loss and iron deficiency anaemia due to a gastric malignancy.

Introduction

The primary function of the stomach is to store ingested food and to regulate its release into the duodenum. Its other functions are to churn and mix the food with the gastric secretions, producing a thick mixture known as 'chyme'. Of note, the major component of gastric secretions is gastric acid. This chapter will discuss in detail how gastric acid is synthesised and regulated in addition to addressing how it can be therapeutically ablated as a mechanism of resolving symptoms attributed to excess acid production.

Anatomy and morphology of the stomach

The stomach is a storage sac located between the oesophagus and the duodenum. Fig. 2.1 indicates the major features of the stomach. It consists of three regions: the fundus, which is the upper region; the main body; and the antrum. Folds, known as rugae, are present on the inner surface of the empty stomach. The rugae flatten out as the stomach fills.

The wall of the stomach consists of various layers of tissue (Fig. 2.2). The inner lining is known as the mucosa. It comprises the lamina propria and the gastric glands (or pits). Beneath this lie the submucosa, the muscularis mucosae, and the serosa, which is covered by the peritoneum. The wall structure of the stomach is similar to that present throughout the rest of the GI tract, except that the stomach has an oblique muscle layer in addition to the circular and longitudinal layers in the muscularis mucosae. This facilitates distension of the stomach and the storage of food. The muscle layers are not evenly distributed over the wall of the stomach. The external circular muscle layer is relatively thin in the fundus and body, and thick in the antrum, where strong muscular contractions aid the mixing of food. In addition, it is highly developed in the pylorus where it becomes a functional sphincter that regulates stomach emptying.

The lining of the stomach is covered with a protective layer of columnar epithelial cells. These have well-developed tight junctions to protect the underlying tissue from erosion by acid. In addition, the columnar cells secrete mucus and alkaline fluid to further protect the

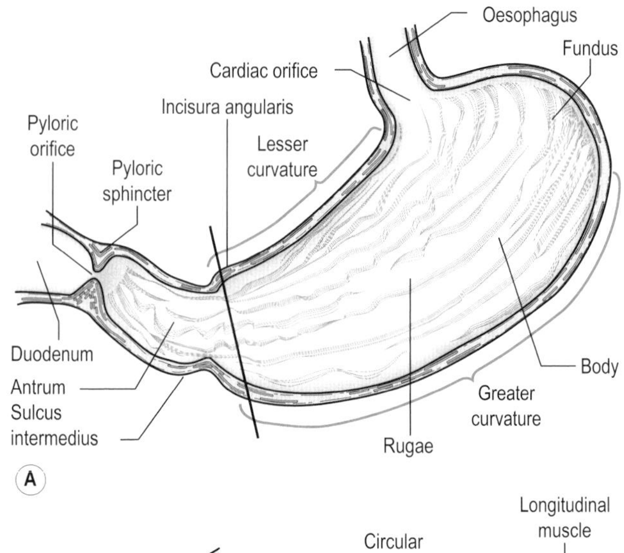

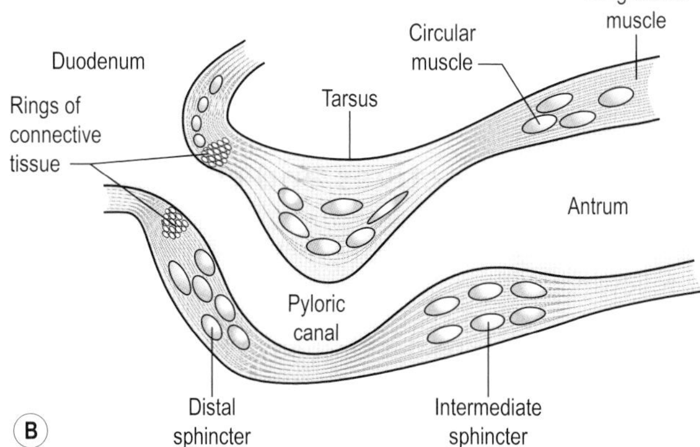

Fig. 2.1 (A) The main anatomical features of the stomach. The diagonal line shows the approximate division of the stomach into the two secretory regions: the parietal secretory area consisting of the fundus and the body, and the pyloric secretory area consisting of the pyloric antrum. (B) The structural features of the pylorus.

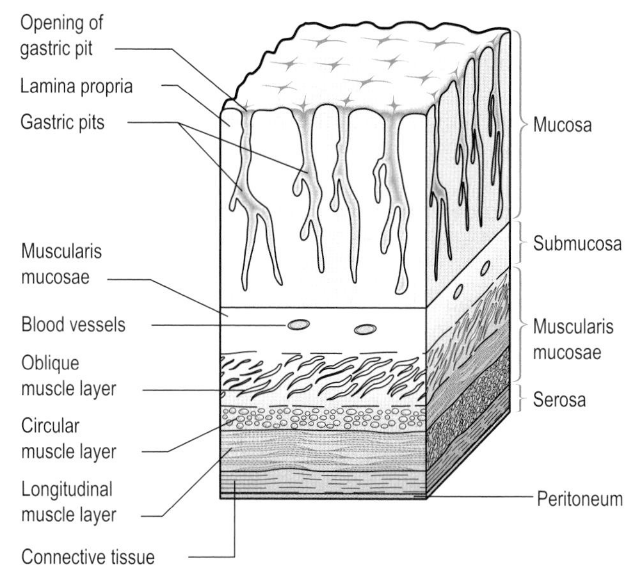

Fig. 2.2 Structure of the gastric mucosa.

gastric mucosa from injury. Numerous gastric pits (approximately 3.5 million in humans) penetrate the surface. These are short ducts into which the deeper gastric glands empty their secretions. The secretions enter the main compartment of the stomach via the necks of these ducts.

The stomach is separated from the duodenal bulb by the pyloric sphincter. Fig. 2.1B shows the main structural features of the pylorus. It is not an anatomically discrete sphincter but a development of the circular smooth muscle layer. A ring of connective tissue separates the pylorus from the duodenum, enabling the contractions of the two regions to be independent. However, the myenteric nerve plexi of the pylorus and duodenum are continuous.

Important cell types within the stomach

There are an array of different cell types within the stomach which are implicated in mediating the functions of the stomach, including acid secretion and digestion. In addition, there are also cell types which are vital in providing protection from the harsh acidic luminal environment. These cell types and their basic functions are as follows:

- Mucus-secreting cells are located in the neck region of gastric glands. They provide a protective barrier to the deeper secretory cells and ultimately to the stomach mucosal lining by secreting alkali (bicarbonate ions) and mucus.
- Parietal cells (also known as oxyntic cells) are the major acid-producing cell type. In addition, they are also responsible for producing intrinsic factor, which is essential for vitamin B_{12} absorption which occurs in the ileum.
- Enterochromaffin-like (ECL) cells are predominantly responsible for secreting histamine, which is one of the three main triggers of acid secretion by parietal cells.
- G cells are gastrin-producing cells, another major trigger for acid secretion from parietal cells. These cells, unlike the others listed, are predominantly located in the antrum of the stomach.
- Chief cells are specialised for the secretion of various digestive enzymes including pepsinogen and lipase.
- D cells are endocrine cells responsible for ultimately regulating parietal-cell acid production through the secretion of the hormone somatostatin.

Composition of gastric juice

The adult human secretes approximately 2 L of gastric juice per day. When a meal is being eaten, soluble substances in the food stimulate the secretion of gastric juice. The stomach produces two different secretions: an acid secretion known as parietal juice which is released from the parietal cells, and an alkaline juice released from the mucous cells. Gastric juice is isotonic with plasma, but the concentrations of its various constituents vary with the rate of flow: the higher the rate, the greater the acidity. Therefore, during a meal, the chyme becomes more acidic and can reach pH 2.0.

The concentration of H^+ ions increases with the rate of flow, as does that of Cl^- and K^+ ions, while the concentration of Na^+ ions decreases. These changes in composition occur because, when the stomach is stimulated during a meal, it is only the rate of acid secretion by parietal cells that increases appreciably. The secretion of alkaline fluid is mainly a passive process and so its rate is relatively unaffected. Thus, dilution of the chyme by alkaline juice is therefore less at high flow rates and the H^+ and Cl^- ion concentrations increase. Both acid and alkaline secretions are isotonic with plasma.

Parietal cells

The secretion of H^+ and Cl^- ions by the stomach are both active processes. The energy is derived from the hydrolysis of ATP and the secretion of H^+ is undertaken by the proton pump (H^+,K^+-adenosine triphosphatase [ATPase]) which must be trafficked to the surface of the cell to release H^+ ions into the lumen. H^+ ions are transported against an enormous concentration gradient: the concentration of H^+ ions in the lumen is 150,000,000 times higher than that of the blood. This requires a considerable energy expenditure and, consequently, parietal cells can contain greater than 40% mitochondria to fulfil these energy demands.

The mechanism whereby H^+ ions are generated within the cell is outlined in Fig. 2.3. Carbon dioxide diffuses into the cell from the plasma. Inside the cell, it combines with water to form carbonic acid. This reaction is catalysed by the enzyme carbonic anhydrase. The carbonic acid dissociates into H^+ and HCO_3^- ions. The HCO_3^- ions are transported into the blood, down a concentration gradient, in exchange for Cl^- ions. The secretion of

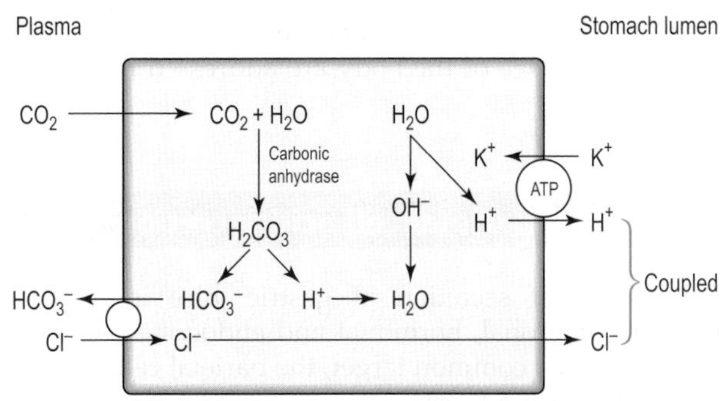

Fig. 2.3 Hydrochloric acid secretion by parietal cells.

HCO_3^- ions into the blood when the stomach is secreting acid into the lumen results in the plasma becoming transiently alkaline. This phenomenon is known as the 'alkaline tide'.

Hydrogen ion secretion across the apical surface of the parietal cell into the canaliculus is accomplished by proton pumps in the membrane of the canaliculus. The proton pump, which contains an ATPase, secretes H^+ ions in exchange for K^+ ions at a ratio of 1:1. In unstimulated cells, proton pumps are localised intracellularly in vesicles. Upon stimulation of the cell to secrete H^+ ions, the vesicles travel to the luminal membrane and the vesicle membranes become incorporated into the plasma membrane, thereby causing a substantial increase in the 'secretory' area of the membrane. Drugs that inhibit proton pumps in parietal cells are used to treat mucosal disorders such as duodenal ulcers that are potentiated by gastric acid.

Chloride ions are also secreted against a concentration gradient. The concentration of Cl^- ions in the blood is approximately 107 mM, whereas in the lumen of the stomach it can reach 170 mM. Chloride is also secreted against an electrical gradient, as the apical surface of the resting cell is electronegative (260–280 mV) with respect to the basolateral surface. Na^+/K^+ coupled pumps are present at the basolateral surface. The entry of Cl^- ions into the cell down their concentration gradient at the basolateral surface occurs in exchange for HCO_3^- ions (see above and Fig. 2.3). Cl^- ions are transported across the luminal surface via a chloride channel. This channel produces net transport of negative charges and operates without the exchange of an anion. Consequently, when the cell is stimulated to secrete, the potential difference falls (to 230–250 mV) and the apical surface becomes less electronegative. The proton and chloride pumps on the mucosal surface are coupled in secreting cells so that H^+ and Cl^- ions are secreted at a ratio of 1:1. The coupling mechanism is not yet understood.

Acid–base disturbance of the body can follow gastrectomy as the ability to secrete acid is compromised. This topic is dealt with in Case 2.2. It can also be a problem in an individual who vomits excessively. This is because a feedback mechanism operates whereby secretion is inhibited if the stomach contents become too acidic. If the stomach contents are lost, this feedback mechanism does not operate, and acid secretion is not regulated in this way. The consequences of excessive vomiting for the acid–base balance of the body are addressed in Case 2.3 below.

Triggers of parietal cell acid secretion

The control of secretion of gastric juice is complex, involving neuronal, hormonal and endocrine pathways. They share one common target, the parietal cell, which is responsible for acid section.

Hormonal control

Gastrin

Gastrin is a hormone that is secreted from the G cells in the stomach. It stimulates acid secretion and has a general role in the preparation of the GI tract for the digestion and absorption of food. Gastrin is produced mainly in the gastric antrum, although small amounts are produced in the proximal small intestine. Two major forms of gastrin exist: gastrin-34 (G34, composed of 34 amino acids) and gastrin-17 (G17, composed of 17 amino acids). In humans, over 90% of the gastrin present in the antral mucosa is the G17 form. G17 has a half-life in the circulation of approximately 6 min and G34 a half-life of approximately 36 min. Both peptides stimulate gastric acid secretion. The short half-life of G17 is consistent with its main influence being via local receptors in the stomach.

G cells and gastrin secretion

In healthy individuals, most G cells (which secrete gastrin) are found in the mucosa of the gastric antrum, although some (20%) are present in the duodenal mucosa. G cells comprise less than 1% of mucosal cells. This structural feature of the cell enables it to sample the gastric contents. Receptors present on the luminal surface membrane sense chemical substances in food, which regulate the release of gastrin (see below). Gastrin is stored in secretory granules present along the basolateral border of the cell, which lie in close proximity to the blood vessels. Gastrin is released into the circulation at the basolateral membrane in response to neural, endocrine or paracrine stimuli, and by local factors in the lumen of the stomach.

Gastrin receptors

A variety of cell types possess specific surface receptors for gastrin. Gastrin acts at cholecystokinin (CCK) receptors found on both ECL cells and parietal cells. Activation of CCK receptors on parietal cells leads to acid secretion, as does activation on ECL cells. However, this is indirect, as the binding stimulates histamine production that in turn stimulates parietal cells. This is mediated by histamine triggering H_2 receptors via a cAMP-mediated mechanism. There are two sub types of CCK receptors: the CCK-A receptor, present in the pancreas and the gall bladder, and the CCK-B receptor, present on ECL cells and parietal cells. Gastrin is more potent on the CCK-B subtype, since its predominate function is to regulate acid secretion (Fig. 2.4). Gastrin also stimulates the expression of the gene encoding the proton pump in parietal cells, thereby increasing its synthesis. Gastrin additionally has trophic actions. It controls the growth and proliferation of a variety of cell types in the gastric mucosa, including ECL cells and precursors of parietal cells. This trophic quality of gastrin may be related to potentiation of some cancers.

Neural control of gastric secretion

The functions of the stomach are controlled by intrinsic nerves in the internal nerve plexi of the enteric nervous system and by extrinsic nerve fibres in the vagus nerve and sympathetic nerves. Axons of nerve fibres (in the intramural plexi) innervate both secretory cells and smooth muscle cells. In general, activation of cholinergic fibres stimulates gastric secretion and motility. Activation of adrenergic fibres generally inhibits secretion and motility.

It should also be noted that a number of sensory nerves leave the stomach and travel in the vagus nerve and the sympathetic nerves. Sensory nerves in the stomach also provide afferent paths of intrinsic reflex arcs, which travel in the intramural plexi of the stomach. This provides some intrinsic control of smooth muscle contractions and gastric juice secretion.

Acetylcholine and gastrin-releasing peptide

Acetylcholine released from cholinergic nerve fibres in local nerves can stimulate parietal cells to release acid, or G cells to secrete gastrin. Some fibres in the vagus nerve also contain gastrin-releasing peptide (GRP), which stimulates gastrin release from the G cells (see Fig. 2.4). Interaction of the neural and gastrin control mechanisms facilitates a rapid response to food ingestion.

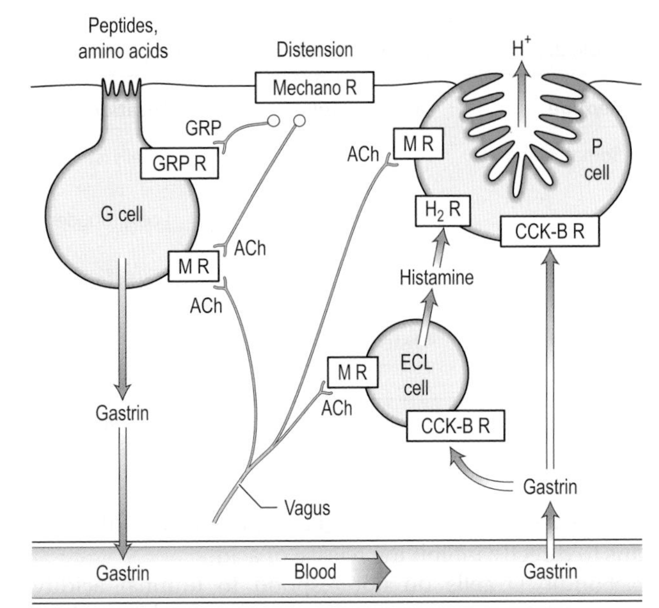

Fig. 2.4 Mechanisms of stimulation of acid secretion from the oxyntic cell by gastrin, histamine and neurotransmitters. *ACh, acetylcholine; CCK-BR, cholecystokinin B receptor; ECL, enterochromaffin-like; GRP, gastrin–releasing peptide; H2R, histamine H2 receptor; MR, muscarinic receptor; P, parietal.*

Inhibitory control of parietal cell acid secretion

Feedback control via acid concentration

Gastric acid secretion is blocked if the contents of the stomach become too acidic (pH 3.0 or lower). This is a negative feedback mechanism that prevents the gastric contents (and more importantly the duodenal contents) from becoming too acidic. When the acidity of the stomach reaches pH 2.0, it is virtually impossible to stimulate gastrin release by any means. The inhibitory action of acid on gastrin secretion is due to its ability to stimulate the release of the hormone somatostatin from D cells in the mucosa. Somatostatin is a potent inhibitor of acid secretion; it inhibits gastrin secretion from G cells and histamine secretion from ECL cells. Furthermore, D cells exhibit gastrin-binding sites, and gastrin itself can stimulate somatostatin release from these cells. However, these binding sites are probably CCK-A receptors which are more sensitive to CCK than to gastrin. Stimulation of somatostatin release via these receptors is therefore probably normally due mainly to circulating CCK (see below).

Somatostatin

The role of somatostatin here is to dampen acid secretion by parietal cells. Somatostatin exists predominantly as the 14-amino-acid peptide somatostatin-14 in D cells in the fundic and antral mucosa. It is released from cytoplasmic processes in the D cells in the antrum in the vicinity of its target cell, the G cell (Fig. 2.5). It binds to somatostatin-2 ($SSTR_2$) receptors on G cells. It acts primarily in a paracrine manner via diffusion in the intercellular spaces, but it also acts systemically through its release into the local mucosal circulation. Somatostatin also acts on ECL cells to inhibit histamine release. These interactions are outlined for the antral region in Fig. 2.5.

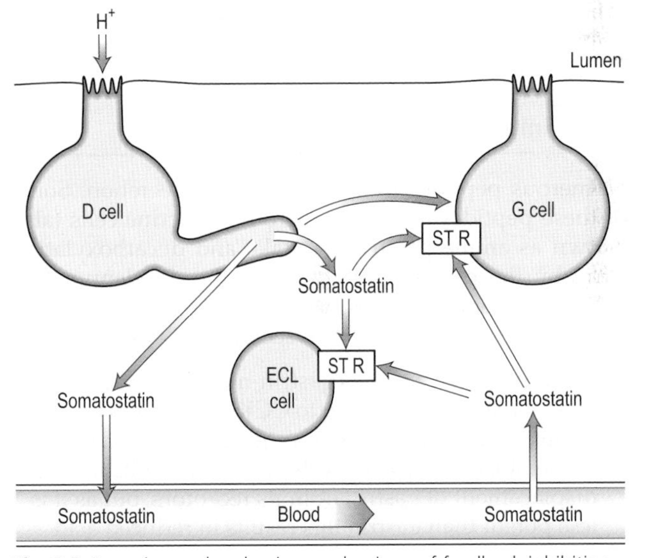

Fig. 2.5 Paracrine and endocrine mechanisms of feedback inhibition of acid secretion by somatostatin released in response to low pH in the antrum. *ECL, enterochromaffin-like; STR, somatostatin receptor.*

Table 2.1 Gastrointestinal peptides that inhibit acid production in the stomach

Peptide	*Main stimulus*	*Location*	*Mechanism of action*
Somatostatin	Acid	D cells (stomach)	Inhibition of histamine and gastrin release
CCK	Fat	I cells (duodenum)	Suppression of gastric acid secretion indirectly through somatostatin
Secretin	Acid	S cells (duodenum)	Suppression of gastric acid secretion indirectly through somatostatin
VIP	Distension of stomach	Enteric nerves	Suppression of gastric acid secretion indirectly through somatostatin

ACh, acetylcholine; CCK, cholecystokinin; VIP, vasoactive intestinal peptide.

Somatostatin also acts upon the parietal cells in the fundus to directly inhibit the release of acid.

Fundic D cells do not respond to luminal acidity. Somatostatin appears to exert a background tonic inhibition of acid release in the fundus, independent of acid concentrations. However, antral D cells respond to changes in H^+ concentration in the stomach lumen. During a meal, as the contents of the stomach become increasingly acidic, secretion from parietal cells declines due to the action of somatostatin. The release of somatostatin is inhibited when the luminal acid is neutralised.

Other inhibitory factors

Numerous peptides inhibit gastric acid secretion. Some of these peptides are released from endocrine cells (also known as amine precursor uptake and decarboxylation cells) by the presence of chyme in the duodenum (see below). Importantly, CCK, which is secreted in response to fat, causes inhibition of acid secretion in two ways:

- It competitively inhibits gastrin-mediated stimulation of acid release by binding to CCK-B receptors on parietal cells and ECL cells. A high level of CCK in the blood (if gastrin levels are high) results in displacement of gastrin from its receptors, but as it is less potent than gastrin this results in reduced acid secretion.
- It is a potent antagonist of gastrin-stimulated acid secretion by its action on CCK-B receptors on D cells to release somatostatin, which in turn inhibits acid secretion.

The duodenal hormone secretin also produces a profound inhibition of gastrin release and gastric acid secretion. It is released in response to the presence of food in the duodenum. It is a 27-amino-acid peptide which has structural similarities to the pancreatic hormone glucagon. The most potent stimulus for secretin release is acid in the duodenum. Secretin inhibits the secretion of gastrin from G cells and the secretion of acid from oxyntic cells. Other peptides which inhibit gastric acid release include gastric inhibitory peptide (GIP, a 43-amino-acid peptide), released in response to fat in the duodenum or ileum, and the 28-amino-acid peptide vasoactive intestinal peptide (VIP), which is released into the circulation from nerve endings in the enteric nerves of the submucosal and myenteric plexi. VIP and GIP have considerable sequence homology (14 amino acids) with secretin, and they act on the same receptors as secretin on parietal cells and G cells to inhibit acid release. The receptors for all these hormones are denoted as VIP receptors. Although the primary effect of these peptides is to reduce gastric juice secretion, tumours of endocrine cells, such as VIPomas, cause increased motility, and consequently diarrhoea. Table 2.1 summarises the actions of some of the endogenous peptides which inhibit acid production, their sites of release, and the likely mechanisms involved.

Finally, prostaglandins synthesised in the gastric mucosa inhibit acid secretion. They function to protect the deeper mucosal layers from damage by acid (as discussed below).

The mucosal barrier

The gastric mucosa must withstand a highly corrosive chemical environment and proteolytic enzymes. Astonishingly, the gastric mucosa is protected from the highly corrosive gastric juice by a simple columnar epithelium in addition to the following:

- Secretion of alkaline fluid to neutralise H^+ ions.
- Secretion of mucus. Surface mucous cells secrete mucous in response to chemicals, such as alcohol, and in response to contact with roughage in the food. Mucous neck cells are also stimulated by gastrin to secrete mucus. Gastric mucus is chemically complex and limits the diffusion of pepsin and hydrogen ions towards the epithelium.
- The presence of growth factors which promote the replacement of damaged cells.

Case 2.1 Gastrinomas (Zollinger–Ellison syndrome)

A 40-year-old woman who had been suffering for several years from intermittent abdominal pain and diarrhoea visited her general practitioner. She had previously been diagnosed with peptic ulcer disease by endoscopy and had been prescribed omeprazole and a short course of antibiotics, but with no long-term relief of her symptoms. Further tests were initiated to investigate the possibility that they were due to a gastrinoma. She was restarted on a high dose of omeprazole to protect against further ulceration, and arrangements were made for her to have a further endoscopy. Hypertrophy of the gastric rugae and ulceration extending into the second part of the duodenum were seen. In the light of these observations and the abnormal plasma gastrin level, a computed tomography (CT) scan of her upper abdomen was performed. This demonstrated a mass in the pancreas. A laparotomy (abdominal operation) was performed, the surgeon confirmed that a tumour was present in the pancreas, and the tumour was removed. Subsequent histological analysis of the resected specimen demonstrated that the tumour was a gastrinoma. Removal of the tumour cured the patient's symptoms and her serum gastrin concentration declined to within the normal range.

Zollinger–Ellison syndrome

Zollinger–Ellison syndrome involves excessive secretion of acid due to the high levels of circulating gastrin. Forty percent of patients with Zollinger–Ellison syndrome may have familial inheritance in an autosomal dominant fashion. The gastrinomas present may be ectopic, commonly presenting in the pancreas. In 60% of patients, the tumours are malignant. Gastrinomas secrete excessive amounts of gastrin into the portal blood stream. The high serum gastrin levels elicit massive amounts of acid secretion from parietal cells. It is the basal acid secretion (which occurs between meals) that is stimulated to the greatest extent by the high gastrin levels, which can lead to a pronounced alkaline tide. Gastrin not only stimulates acid secretion in the stomach but also stimulates the production of alkaline juices from the duct cells of the liver and pancreas. Furthermore, acid in the duodenum stimulates alkaline pancreatic juice and bile secretion via secretin, which would normally result in an 'acid tide'. However, the exaggerated alkaline tide resulting from the copious acid secretion seen in Zollinger–Ellison syndrome may overwhelm these homeostatic mechanisms. The respiratory and renal mechanisms may be inadequate to compensate for this effect, leading to metabolic alkalosis. The massive secretion of acid and pepsinogen in Zollinger–Ellison syndrome leads to widespread ulceration of the upper gastrointestinal (GI) tract. In this disease, ulcers may occur in the oesophagus, the stomach and the duodenum.

The recognised treatment for Zollinger–Ellison syndrome is to first control the overproduction of acid by treatment with a proton-pump inhibitor (PPI), such as omeprazole. This enables the ulcers to heal and controls the diarrhoea. Patients usually survive for many years with pharmacological treatment alone. When the ulcers are under control, surgery to remove a gastrinoma can be attempted to try to effect a cure.

- The more acid that is secreted by parietal cells (and enters the mucosal barrier), the more bicarbonate is automatically delivered to the epithelial surface to protect it, which is governed by simple diffusion.
- Prostaglandins maintain mucosal integrity, decrease acid secretion, increase bicarbonate and mucin production, and increase blood flow, all of which modify the local inflammatory response caused by high acidity. Gastric mucosal protection can become compromised in individuals taking non-steroidal anti-inflammatory drugs (NSAIDs) including aspirin. This is attributed to the fact that NSAIDs inhibit enzymes key to prostaglandin synthesis.

In peptic ulcer disease, the protective mechanisms are inadequate. The mechanisms of ulcer formation in the stomach and the duodenum are described in Case 2.2.

Secretions of the mucous cell

Mucus is a viscous sticky substance that contains glycoproteins known as mucins, which consist of about 80% carbohydrates, largely galactose and N-acetylglucosamine. The molecules are tetramers with a molecular weight of approximately 2,000,000 g/mol. The carbohydrate chains protect the molecule from digestion by pepsin. Gastric mucus lubricates the pieces of food (in conjunction with salivary mucus), enabling them to be moved about and churned by the contractions of the stomach. Epithelial cells secrete an opaque alkaline mucus which has a high bicarbonate content. This secretion increases when food is eaten. In addition, the mucous neck cells secrete a clear mucus in response to food. Mucus is released from the mucous neck cells and surface epithelium by exocytosis. It can also be released by desquamation of the epithelial cells from the surface.

Mucin tetramers form a dissolved gel when their concentration exceeds approximately 50 mg/mL. This gel forms a layer on the surface of the mucosa. Its stability depends on charged $SO4^-$, COO^- groups, and H^+ bonds, and dramatic changes in pH can cause precipitation of the mucus. Surface epithelial cells secrete non-parietal alkaline fluid (see above) and this fluid is entrapped in the layer of mucus. The alkaline mucus forms a barrier that lines the stomach and protects it from damage by acid and pepsin. Damage to the mucosal barrier results in the development of ulcers.

Acid reduction therapy

Several different classes of drugs can be effective in the treatment of peptic ulcer disease (a consequence of acid attacking the epithelium due to ineffective mucosal protection) and other conditions such as gastrinomas and acid reflux. The treatment of peptic ulcer disease and gastrinomas with such drugs is discussed in Case 2.2. Reduction of acid secretion by drug therapy will increase the pH of the chyme and thereby reduce the activity of pepsin, and so also protect the mucosa from its action. Acid reduction therapy also has utility in the treatment of heartburn and gastro-oesophageal reflux disease (discussed in Chapter 1).

Antacids

Antacids are weak bases that act by directly neutralising gastric acid. Raising the pH of the stomach contents results in suppression of the action of pepsin that exacerbates ulceration due to acid. Thus, antacids can be used to relieve gastric pain caused by excessive acid secretion. Compounds are commonly various salts of calcium, magnesium and aluminium as the active ingredients. Sodium bicarbonate is a fast-acting antacid, but it should not be used for long-term treatment in peptic ulcer disease as it is absorbed in the intestines and may cause metabolic alkalosis. The release of CO_2 from bicarbonate dissolved in the stomach chyme can also be a problem as it causes belching (eructation). Other potential adverse effects of antacids in general are constipation, nausea and abdominal pain.

H2 receptor antagonists

Histamine H2 receptor antagonists competitively inhibit the actions of histamine at H2 receptors on parietal cells, thereby reducing acid secretion. These drugs are usually effective in relieving the symptoms of peptic ulcer disease (Case 2.2). These drugs can inhibit acid secretion by up to 90% and promote healing of ulcers. Long-term maintenance with these drugs was widely used until effective treatment with PPIs became available. H_2 receptor antagonists are also sometimes included in a multi-drug regimen for *Helicobacter pylori* eradication. *H. pylori* is a bacterial infection of the stomach associated with peptic ulcers (discussed in detail later). Drug interactions with this class of drugs may occur since the therapeutic increase in gastric pH could alter the absorption of drugs that require low pH environments for absorption. Cimetidine is also a potent cytochrome P450 (CYP450) enzyme inhibitor.

Proton-pump inhibitors

Proton-pump inhibitors (PPIs) block the hydrogen ion pumps in oxyntic cells. They include omeprazole and lansoprazole and are the drugs of first choice for treating peptic ulcers and other conditions associated with high gastric acid. Omeprazole is among the top 10 most prescribed drugs in the United States, and some classes of PPIs are now available over the counter in the UK. These powerful drugs block the H^+/K^+ ATPase proton pump, markedly inhibiting both basal and stimulated secretion of gastric acid. Omeprazole is a weak base and is inactive at neutral pH, but it is activated in acid conditions (pH 3.0 and below). Such conditions exist only in the canaliculi of parietal cells. The action of the drug is therefore restricted to this location in the GI tract, thereby avoiding the unwanted side effects of disruption of Cl^- ion transport, which could occur in other organs such as the lungs, pancreas and skin (sweating) with use of other H^+ transport inhibitors which are active in less acid conditions.

Omeprazole has few unwanted side effects, although there remains concern about lowering acid secretion too drastically because of the resultant elevation of serum gastrin levels, which in theory could be mitogenic (and therefore tumour-promoting) because acid is a potent inhibitor of G cell proliferation. Because of this, the chronic administration of a PPI such as omeprazole results in proliferation of G cells and ECL cells.

The continued administration of PPIs also comes with a risk of infection. As the acidic environment of the stomach serves as a chemical barrier against bacterial infection, PPIs, which reduce acid concentrations, can make the stomach contents more subject to colonisation. Indeed, PPI use correlates with an increased likelihood of *Clostridium difficile* infections and other enteric foodborne infections. Interestingly, there is a potentially increased risk of community-acquired pneumonia since this can be associated with bacterial overgrowth in the stomach.

Muscarinic receptor antagonists

Anticholinergic drugs that bind to muscarinic M2 receptors on parietal cells and ECL cells can antagonise the effects of vagal nerve stimulation and reduce gastric acid secretion. Most muscarinic M2 antagonists are less effective than H2 receptor antagonists or PPIs, although they can have beneficial antispasmodic effects on gut smooth muscle. Furthermore, muscarinic receptors are present at many locations within the GI tract and outside it, and for this reason, parasympathetic side effects, including effects on the cardiovascular system, are common with these drugs.

However, the drug pirenzepine is a relatively specific M1 receptor antagonist that probably acts on postsynaptic nerves in parasympathetic ganglia to block the stimulation of oxyntic cells.

Case 2.2 Part 1 Epigastric discomfort

A 42-year-old man presented with a history of upper abdominal (epigastric) discomfort with intermittent nausea and heartburn. There was no history of weight loss or change in bowel habits. He had a history of a myocardial infarction and takes regular aspirin, statin and a beta-blocker. He was a smoker and consumed excessive alcohol. He had been taking over-the-counter antacids with some relief. On examination, he had mild tenderness in his epigastrium. He was given a course of a PPI; however, his symptoms persisted despite this. He was referred for an upper GI endoscopy and was asked to pause his PPI beforehand. His endoscopy revealed erythema (redness) of the gastric antrum with scattered superficial erosions in his stomach but no ulcers. A CLO test (urease) was done, and this was positive. He was given eradication therapy for *H. pylori* with antibiotics and PPIs.

Helicobacter pylori

H. pylori is a Gram-negative micro-aerophilic organism that has been classified by the World Health Organization as a class 1 carcinogen and which infects approximately half of the world's population. It is usually found colonising the stomach, where in 90% of individuals there are no associated symptoms. However, in the remainder, *H. pylori* can lead to chronic gastritis, peptic ulcers, and even gastric cancer.

H. pylori has adapted in a number of ways to be able to survive the noxious environment of the stomach, particularly the very low pH. Most notably, *H. pylori* expresses an enzyme called urease which converts stomach urea into ammonium ions and carbon dioxide. These react with the acid to allow the bacterium to neutralise its niche. In addition, *H. pylori* has flagella which it uses for motility. By using its flagella, it swims through the stomach juice to the mucosa. When it reaches the mucosa, it is able to express mucinases amongst other enzymes, which digest the mucin layer and allow the bacterium to migrate into the mucous layer, which is a far less acidic environment than the lumen of the stomach. It also utilises chemotaxis as a mechanism to migrate towards a less acidic environment. Once through the mucous layer, the bacterium can then adhere to the epithelial cells through the expression of various adhesion proteins. Ammonia, a product of urease, is toxic to epithelial cells. In addition, the bacterium produces proteases, vacuolating cytotoxin A (VacA), phospholipases, and cytotoxin associated gene A (CagA), which can all contribute to an inflammatory cascade and ultimately cancer. Thus, unsurprisingly, some individuals present with chronic gastritis at the site of infection: in the background of stomach acid and pepsin, the buffering capacity of the mucosa can be affected, exacerbating the inflammatory response and ultimately epithelial integrity.

H. pylori can infect any portion of the stomach. However, *H. pylori* infection of the antrum of the stomach can stimulate G cell gastrin production, resulting in excess acid, which in turn can overwhelm the buffering capacity of the small intestine, resulting in duodenal ulcers. The presence of pepsin is also implicated in acid-induced ulceration. This enzyme can digest damaged mucosa in the oesophagus, stomach and duodenum when activated by the presence of acid. Disruption of the mucosal barrier will provide the opportunity for pepsin to digest the columnar epithelium and promote ulceration. Thus, pepsin potentiates (rather than initiates) ulcer formation. Inflammatory responses at sites of infection in the stomach can result in the production of Il-1β, which is a potent acid suppressant. This ultimately causes hypochlorhydria, gastritis and gastric atrophy.

A breath, stool or blood test can be used to assess the presence of *H. pylori*. The breath test relies on the presence of urease which, if present, will convert an ingested formulation of $^{13/14}C$-labelled urea into ammonia and labelled carbon dioxide. The blood test assesses the presence of antibodies to *H. pylori*, while the stool test assesses for the direct presence of *H. pylori* proteins. If positive for *H. pylori*, a triple therapy of two antibiotics and a PPI is commonly prescribed (e.g., amoxicillin, clarithromycin and omeprazole).

The role of the stomach in nutrient absorption

Very few substances are absorbed in the stomach and the stomach is virtually impermeable to water. Aspirin and alcohol are the main substances that are absorbed at this location. Alcohol is lipid-soluble, and aspirin becomes more lipid-soluble when it meets the acidic pH present in the stomach. Despite this, the stomach has indirect actions in the absorption of two very important nutrients: vitamin B_{12} and iron.

Vitamin B_{12}

Intrinsic factor is secreted by the stomach. It is a 55,000-kDa glycoprotein which complexes with vitamin B_{12} (cobalamin) and enables its absorption in the ileum. The glycoprotein dimerises and the dimer binds two molecules of vitamin B_{12}. The complex is resistant to digestion. There are four physiologically important forms of vitamin B_{12}. These cyanocobalamins bind to protein in the food and are released from them by the action of acid and pepsin in the stomach. Vitamin B_{12} is absorbed inefficiently by passive diffusion in its free un-complexed state along the length of the intestine, but a specialised absorption mechanism exists in the distal ileum whereby vitamin B_{12} complexed to intrinsic factor can be absorbed at a relatively rapid rate. Vitamin B_{12} deficiency leads to pernicious anaemia. This condition can result from disorders of the stomach mucosa that releases intrinsic factor, or from disorders such as Crohn's disease that affect the terminal ileum where vitamin B_{12} is absorbed. The consequences of vitamin B_{12} deficiency due to lack of intrinsic factor after gastrectomy are discussed in Case 2.2.

Pernicious anaemia

After gastrectomy, pernicious anaemia can develop as a consequence of vitamin B_{12} deficiency due to lack of intrinsic factor, unless replacement therapy is instigated. However, vitamin B_{12} is stored in the liver and pernicious anaemia does not develop until the stores have become depleted (i.e., probably after several years). In pernicious anaemia, abnormal immature macrocytic (large) red cells are produced by the bone marrow. The results of the patient's blood tests would show a low red cell count and a high mean cell volume of the cells. The preferred treatment is intramuscular injections of vitamin B_{12} every 3 months.

Iron

The average adult loses approximately 1–2 mg of iron per day predominantly through the sloughing of epithelial cells (keratinocytes and enterocytes) and thus an equivalent amount of iron needs to be absorbed in the small intestine every day to ensure there is enough iron to meet the body's demands in essential processes such as erythropoiesis. The stomach has an important role in the absorption of iron as its acidic environment ensures that iron remains in a soluble and absorbable form. The acid keeps iron in its reduced ferrous state which is absorbed by enterocytes in the duodenum.

Iron-deficiency anaemia

After removal of the stomach, iron–deficiency anaemia can develop because the acid in the stomach tends to convert ferric iron (Fe^{3+}) in the diet to the ferrous form, the only form of non-haem iron that can be absorbed to any appreciable extent. Even if only the antrum of the stomach is removed, iron deficiency can develop because of the removal of the gastrin-secreting G cells, as gastrin is a major stimulus for acid secretion in the stomach. The body's iron stores are more limited than those of vitamin B_{12} and iron-deficiency anaemia can manifest within a few months of partial gastrectomy, while pernicious anaemia may not occur for 2 years or so. Iron deficiency is characterised by the presence of small red blood corpuscles (microcytosis), although after gastrectomy, this may eventually be obscured by pernicious anaemia in which the red blood corpuscles are macrocytic.

Secretions of the chief cell

Pepsin, the proteolytic enzyme of the stomach, is normally responsible for less than 20% of the protein digestion that occurs in the GI tract. It is an endopeptidase that degrades proteins to peptides. It preferentially hydrolyses peptide linkages where one of the amino acids is aromatic. Pepsin, like other protease enzymes, is formed from an inactive precursor, pepsinogen, which is stored in granules in the chief cells of the stomach and released by exocytosis. The synthesis and exocytosis of pepsinogen is essentially similar to that described for pancreatic enzymes. Pepsinogen is also secreted by mucous cells and cells in the glands of Brunner in the duodenum.

Pepsinogen is activated in the stomach lumen by hydrolysis, with the removal of a short peptide. H^+ ions are important for pepsin function because:

- Pepsinogen is initially activated by the H^+ ions. The activated enzyme then acts autocatalytically to increase the rate of formation of more pepsin.
- It provides the appropriate pH for the enzyme to act. The optimum pH for pepsin is approximately pH 3.5.
- It denatures ingested protein. Denatured protein is a better substrate for the enzyme than native protein.

Control of pepsinogen secretion

Pepsinogen, the precursor of pepsin, is released from chief cells by acetylcholine and a number of other GI hormones. Fig. 2.6 illustrates the various secretogogues and their receptors and the second messenger systems involved in their actions. Acetylcholine released upon stimulation of the vagus nerve and local nerves is probably the most potent stimulus. It acts on muscarinic receptors on the chief cell membrane. H^+ ions trigger the local cholinergic reflex that stimulates chief cells. They also enhance the effects of other stimuli on chief cells. In addition, H^+ ions stimulate the release of secretin in the duodenum (see below) and secretin also stimulates pepsinogen secretion. These effects of H^+ may account in part for the correlation between acid and pepsin secretion. Gastrin stimulates pepsinogen secretion directly via CCK receptors, but the most potent effect of gastrin on pepsinogen secretion is its indirect action via acid secretion. Pepsinogen secretion is decreased by somatostatin.

Drug therapy

A variety of different classes of drugs can be effective in the treatment of peptic ulcer disease. Currently, antacids, H_2 receptor blockers, PPIs and antibiotics all have a role to play. Long-term treatment with antacids can produce

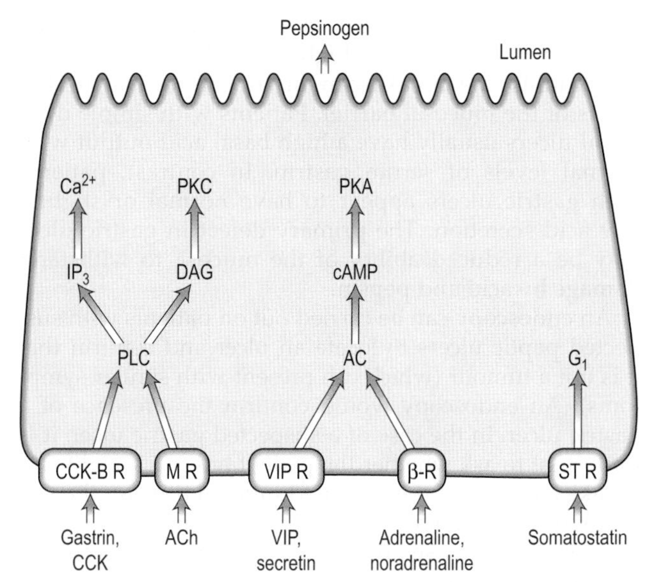

Fig. 2.6 Mechanisms of secretion of pepsinogen from the chief cell. *AC, adenyl cyclase; ACh, acetylcholine; CCK, cholecystokinin; DAG, diacylglycerol; G1, G protein; IP3, inositol trisphosphate; MR, muscarinic receptor; PKA, protein kinase A; PKC, protein kinase C; R, receptor; STR, somatostatin receptor; VIP, vasoactive intestinal peptide; β-R, β-adrenergic receptor.*

Case 2.2 **Part 2 Gastric ulcer**

One year later, the patient's epigastric pain reoccurred despite taking regular PPIs. His pain radiated to the back and was worse 6 hours after eating. His pain improved by eating a meal. On direct questioning, he also reported transient black tarry stools over a period of 4 days. His blood tests demonstrated anaemia with raised urea. He was admitted to hospital and underwent an urgent upper GI endoscopy. This demonstrated an acute gastric ulcer in the antrum which was actively oozing. The base of the ulcer was injected with adrenaline and a clip was placed across the ulcer which stopped the bleeding. He was commenced on an intravenous infusion of PPIs and a further course of *H. pylori* eradication therapy was given. He improved and was discharged home. A urease breath test was negative at 6 weeks following discharge, suggesting successful eradication of *H. pylori*. A repeat endoscopy to confirm healing of the gastric ulcer was arranged which he unfortunately did not attend.

healing of duodenal ulcers but they are ineffective for healing gastric ulcers.

Patients often self-medicate with H_2 blockers or PPIs as they are available without prescription and are effective in controlling symptoms. They are most effective if taken at night because the hypersecretion of acid from the empty stomach at night and its entry into the empty duodenum may be the most important factor in duodenal ulcer formation. When the stomach contains food, buffering of acid (by proteins, for example) and the mixing of acid in the chyme reduces the exposure of the mucosa to the acid. These drugs can inhibit acid secretion by up to 90% and promote healing of ulcers. However, if treatment is withdrawn in patients with duodenal ulcers, the ulcers are likely to reoccur.

Triple therapy

Combinations of omeprazole (see below) and antibiotics have proved to be extremely effective in the treatment and often the cure of duodenal ulcers. In practice, 'triple therapy' consisting of a PPI and the antibiotics amoxicillin and either metronidazole or clarithromycin is often instigated. *H. pylori* is generally eradicated after 2 weeks of this regimen.

Surgery

Treatment with H_2 antagonists or PPIs and antibiotics is highly effective for duodenal or gastric ulcers, but surgery is sometimes necessary. Prior to the development of effective drug treatment, surgery used to be the main treatment for chronic peptic ulcer disease. It involved either division of the vagus nerve (vagotomy), or antrectomy (resection of the stomach antrum). Vagotomy is performed to reduce vagal stimulation of acid secretion in the stomach. Unfortunately, this also results in impaired gastric motility and emptying. Bleeding is a complication of a peptic ulcer. Most bleeding ulcers require endoscopy to stop bleeding with cautery or injection. On occasions when endoscopic procedures are unable to stop the bleeding, radiological embolization of the bleeding vessel or surgery may be considered.

Peptic ulcer disease

A peptic ulcer is a defect in the gastric or duodenal mucosa and may present with epigastric pain (dyspepsia) or other GI symptoms. Patients can often initially be asymptomatic and then present with complications, such as upper GI bleeding or perforation. In a patient with gastric ulcer, the pain is poorly localised but may be perceived in the midline area. It occurs at any time but is often worse during or after a meal. Physical examination does not usually demonstrate epigastric tenderness. There is not usually nausea or vomiting and food does not ease the pain. In practice, however, the differential diagnosis between gastric and duodenal ulcer cannot be ascertained on the basis of symptoms alone. Eating provides relief because food buffers the acid. Symptoms of hypersecretion at night are supposedly more usually seen with a duodenal rather than a gastric ulcer, but in practice, there is often overlap of symptoms between the two types. In the case of a duodenal ulcer, the symptoms usually last for a few weeks followed by a period of remission.

The most common site in the stomach for ulcers to occur is the antrum, where the oxyntic mucosa meets the pyloric mucosa (i.e., the acid acts on the mucosa that does not have the same protective mechanisms as the body and fundus). The stomach normally has a low permeability to acid due to the presence of the protective mucosal barrier. The barrier is partly due to the presence of mucins, but other factors such as adequate blood flow and the presence of growth factors, which promote the replacement of damaged cells, are also important. However, it should be noted that mucus does not form a continuous layer and the protection is due to a great extent to the fact that the rate of acid production keeps pace with the buffering capacity of the food. Peptic ulcers (Fig. 2.7) form in the stomach due to the action of acid when the mucosal barrier is damaged, and the stomach is unable to protect itself and replace the damaged cells. Thus, ulcers in the stomach are not usually due to an increased rate of acid secretion but rather to a defect in the ability of the mucosa to withstand damage (which may be caused by substances such as aspirin, ethanol or bile salts).

The duodenum is the most frequent site for ulcer formation, with the duodenal cap being the most vulnerable area. Excessive secretion of acid and pepsinogen are directly implicated in chronic ulceration of the duodenum. In individuals with duodenal ulcers, there is often a higher-than-normal basal secretion of acid, and an abnormally high rate of maximum secretion in response to histamine stimulation. Individuals with duodenal ulcer may have twice the average normal number of

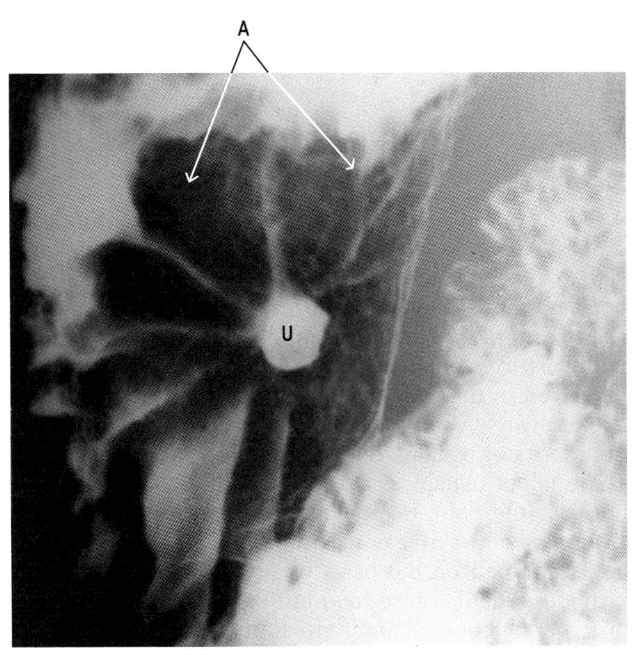

Fig. 2.7 An X-ray of the stomach taken after ingestion of barium. The normal folds of the antrum (A) have been disrupted by chronic ulceration, giving rise to linear scarring around the ulcer (U).

parietal cells in their mucosae. In addition, pepsinogen secretion is also usually high. High H^+ concentration can lead to the breakdown of the protective mechanisms of the mucosal barrier. Patients with simple duodenal ulcers usually have a high basal acid output with normal levels of serum gastrin. In contrast, patients with gastric ulcers appear to have normal or slightly low acid secretion. The primary defect in gastric ulcer may be a reduced ability of the mucosa to withstand damage by acid and pepsin.

An endoscopy can be carried out on patients with suspected peptic ulcers to locate an ulcer and confirm that it is not a tumour (which can present with similar symptoms). An endoscopy would confirm the presence of a gastric ulcer. In the case of a suspected gastric ulcer, it is important to ask whether the patient has lost weight and to take a biopsy of the ulcerated mucosa because there is a risk of malignancy, which is not seen in the case of a duodenal ulcer. A small amount of blood loss (occult) is usually associated with the ulcer, and in chronic ulcers this will result in anaemia. Occasionally, the ulceration can erode into a major vessel (commonly the gastroduodenal artery behind the first part of the duodenum) and life-threatening bleeding can occur.

Gastric cancer

Gastric cancer is the 17th most common cancer in the UK accounting for 2% of all new cancer cases, and the 14th most common cause of cancer death in the UK accounting for 3% of all cancer deaths. The 5-year survival is approximately 20%. A person's risk of developing gastric cancer depends on many factors, including age, genetics and exposure to risk factors. The major risk factors include *H. pylori* infection (41% of stomach cancer cases), smoking (15% of stomach cancer cases) and obesity or being overweight (6% of stomach cancer cases). Thus unsurprisingly, 54% of stomach cancer cases in the UK are thought to be preventable.

Surgical resection

Removal of the antrum and pylorus of the stomach can be undertaken for the complications of peptic ulcer disease and occasionally for carcinoma of the stomach. This portion of the stomach mucosa contains the majority of the gastrin-secreting G cells, and as a result, resection dramatically reduces acid secretion in the stomach. In addition, there is loss of the pyloric control of gastric emptying and reduced storage capacity. The stomach remnant can be reconnected to the proximal duodenum or the upper jejunum. This results in premature release of chyme from the stomach in advance of the release of digestive juices from the gall bladder and pancreatic duct. The main consequence of this is impaired fat absorption and sometimes osmotic diarrhoea from incomplete digestion.

Case 2.2 Part 3 Gastric cancer

Around 2 years later, the patient presented with 2 stones of weight loss, epigastric discomfort, intermittent vomiting, and fullness after eating a small meal (early satiety). His blood tests revealed iron-deficiency anaemia and elevated inflammatory markers. An endoscopy was performed which showed evidence of a large, friable, ulcerated mass in the gastric antrum. Biopsies were taken which confirmed a gastric adenocarcinoma. He underwent urgent staging of his cancer that included a CT scan which did not show spread. A partial gastrectomy was performed and a follow-up CT scan at 12 months did not show any evidence of recurrence (Fig. 2.8)

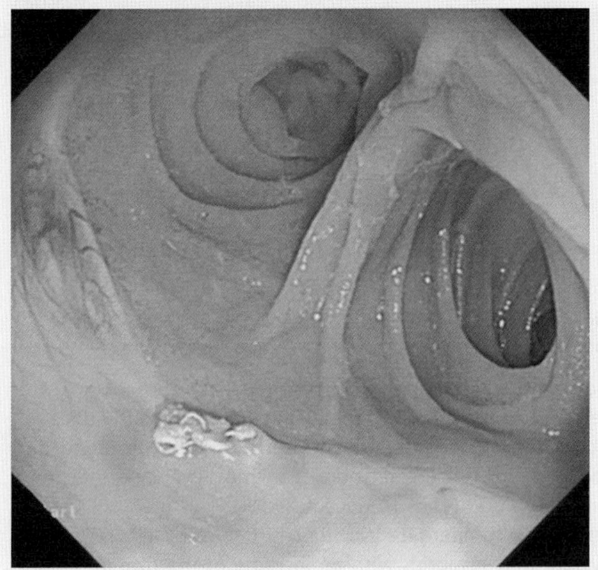

Fig. 2.8 Endoscopic appearances of the stomach following partial gastrectomy in a patient with gastric cancer. This is known as a Billroth II gastrojejunostomy where the part of the stomach that is not resected is connected to the first part of the jejunum in an end-to-end anastomosis.

Patients can usually control these symptoms by simple modification of their diet. The functional consequences of the loss of gastrin are not usually clinically apparent. An interesting but relatively rare complication of this operation is paradoxical hypoglycaemia following meals. The patient complains of symptoms of sweating and feeling faint soon after meals. This is due to inappropriate release of insulin from the pancreas in response to ingestion of food, but in advance of sufficient absorption of glucose from the GI tract to counterbalance the insulin release.

Gastric carcinoma may require total gastrectomy in an attempt to cure the disease. In this case, the jejunum is brought up to connect with the oesophagus, and the distal one-fourth of the duodenum is re-joined to the jejunum more distally. This anatomical rearrangement is necessary because the alkaline secretions from the gall bladder and pancreas would cause severe ulceration of the unprotected oesophageal mucosa if allowed to come into direct contact with it. Loss of the whole stomach does significantly impair the storage capacity of the digestive tract. As a consequence, the patients must eat more frequent and smaller meals to maintain nutrition. Loss of acid secretion, pepsinogen and gastrin all have surprisingly little effect on GI function. However, loss of intrinsic factor does require replacement therapy by subcutaneous injection of vitamin B_{12}.

Stomach motility

One of the most important functions of the stomach is its ability to regulate the rate at which material enters the small intestine, where digestion and absorption of most nutrients occurs. The stomach is responsible for churning the food and mixing it with gastric juice to produce a semi-liquid mass known as chyme. The empty stomach in the adult has a volume of approximately 50 mL. The interior surface of the stomach is highly folded into ridges. Upon being filled with food, the folds undergo 'receptive relaxation', which is a process mediated via the vagus nerve that allows the folds to relax and open out, thus expanding the accommodating volume of the stomach. Importantly, this also ensures that the intraluminal pressure does not increase whilst the stomach is being filled.

Mixing and emptying

The contractions of the stomach that are responsible for mixing the chyme and emptying it into the small intestine depend on the activity of the smooth muscle in the wall. The stomach, like the rest of the GI tract, is surrounded by layers of smooth muscle (see Fig. 2.2). The process by which chyme empties into the duodenum involves three steps: propulsion, grinding and retropropulsion. Once food enters the stomach and initiates chemical digestion, mechanical digestion is also initiated through peristaltic contractions which propel food from the proximal stomach towards the contracted pylorus. This phase is known as propulsion. Once in the antrum, the material is then ground down by forceful peristaltic contractions mediated by the thickened antral walls. This grinding action against a closed pylorus acts to reduce the particle size and matter less than 2 mm is able to pass through the contracted pylorus. This phase is known as grinding. The remaining bolus which consists of particles greater than 2 mm is propelled back into the main body of the stomach in a process known as retropropulsion. This sequence repeats until the bolus is completed ground to less than 2 mm and has emptied into the duodenum. Any matter which remains in the stomach is eventually swept through the pylorus in the fasted state through a series of strong peristaltic contractions known

Case 2.2

Part 4 Gastric cancer

Four years later, the patient presented to his general practitioner as he had started to feel tired and listless. He also complained of longstanding symptoms of dizziness, sweating and palpitations after meals. He reported that he had become forgetful and did not attend the clinic for vitamin B_{12} injections. He was advised to restart the medication and to attempt to regulate his food intake more carefully by eating smaller but more frequent meals, as his symptoms were partly due to the rapid entry of large amounts of material into the small intestine. The doctor also sent him for a blood test. The patient was found to be suffering from megaloblastic anaemia and mild metabolic acidosis. His blood vitamin B_{12} level was low, and he was found to be mildly iron-deficient.

The consequences of partial surgical resection of the stomach depend on the part being removed. Removal of the upper part of the stomach (body and fundus), as in this patient, will remove the majority of the parietal cells, whereas resection of the lower part (antrum and pylorus) will remove most of the G cells.

It can be inferred from studying the details of this case that a good quality of life can be maintained after such a partial gastrectomy if:

- The development of pernicious anaemia is prevented,
- The development of iron-deficiency anaemia is prevented, and
- Food intake is carefully regulated.

Effect of gastrectomy on acid–base balance

Secretion of acid by the stomach during a meal is accompanied by transport of HCO_3^- ions into the blood (the alkaline tide). When the food reaches the duodenum, it is mixed with the alkaline secretions from the pancreas, liver and walls of the intestines. The cellular mechanisms whereby these alkaline juices are secreted are in some ways the reverse of those whereby acid is secreted in the stomach (see Fig. 2.3). Thus, transport of HCO_3^- ions into the glandular ducts of these organs occurs simultaneously with the transport of an equal number of H^+ ions into the blood serving these organs. The consequent increase in blood H^+ concentration is normally neutralised by the HCO_3^- ions of the alkaline tide of the blood from the stomach. In addition, the H^+ ions secreted by the stomach into the lumen are neutralised by the HCO_3^- ions present in the digestive juices (bile, pancreatic juice and intestinal juice) acting in the small intestine (Fig. 2.9). This balance can be upset by gastric resection that restricts acid production. Feedback control mechanisms normally regulate the secretion of H^+ and HCO_3^- ions to keep the pH values in the gut lumen within appropriate limits. Many metabolic functions in the body are extremely sensitive to pH change, and the pH of body fluids such as plasma must therefore be maintained within a very narrow range.

Abnormalities can occur in the acid–base balance of patients who have undergone partial gastrectomy, but the body usually compensates for these disturbances. After removal of the stomach, the alkaline tide obviously does not occur, but H^+ ions are still transported into the blood during a meal from the secreting pancreas, liver and intestines, and the blood tends to become acidic. This metabolic acidosis can be compensated in the short term by the respiratory system that responds with an increase in the rate and depth of breathing. This results in CO_2 being blown off from the blood. The reaction:

$$H^+ + HCO_3^- \rightarrow H_2CO_3 \rightarrow CO_2 + H_2O$$

is consequently driven to the right, and the H^+ ion concentration in the blood falls towards normal. However, full compensation of the acidosis takes longer and depends on processes in the renal tubules that conserve HCO_3^- and secrete acid. In the presence of impaired renal function, the patient's blood tests would show a low pH, low HCO_3^- concentration and a low pCO_2. In a compensated patient, acidotic urine would be excreted following a meal.

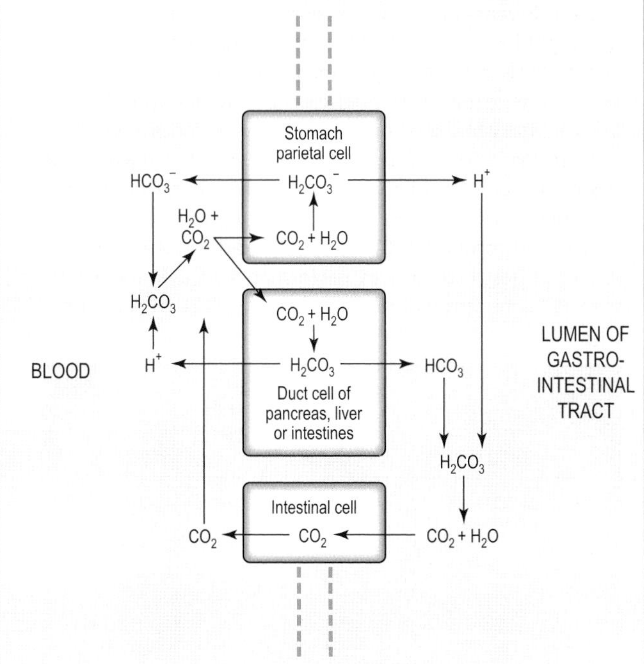

Fig. 2.9 Neutralisation of acid in the blood and in the intestinal lumen.

Intestinal consequences of gastrectomy

Patients post-gastrectomy commonly develop sensations of dizziness, palpitations and sweating after meals, which is attributed to activation of the sympathetic nervous system. If the stomach is removed, a normal-sized meal moves rapidly into the small intestine due to the reduction in storage capacity. This results in the absorption of nutrients at an abnormally rapid rate. However, there may be insufficient time for the meal to be completely digested and absorbed before it is moved on along the intestines.

Case 2.2

Part 4 Gastric cancer—cont'd

Hypoglycaemia

If a meal has a high carbohydrate content, the absorption of glucose can be so fast that the homeostatic mechanisms for attenuating the increase in blood glucose concentration during absorption are disturbed. Normally the blood glucose rises to a maximum level at 30–60 min after the meal has been ingested. An increase in blood glucose stimulates insulin secretion from the pancreas into the blood. This hormone lowers the blood glucose by promoting glucose uptake into muscle and adipose tissue. Normally the blood glucose returns to normal after 1.5–2 hours (Fig. 2.10). The insulin concentration also returns to normal. This is normally a finely tuned feedback control system. However, if the blood glucose concentration rises too rapidly, the blood insulin concentration also rises rapidly to reach an abnormally high level in the plasma (see Fig. 2.10). This results in rapid clearance of the blood glucose, but it can overshoot to an abnormally low level (hypoglycaemia). Hypoglycaemia is associated with sweating and fainting, which are seen after meals in a patient who has undergone gastrectomy. Salivary amylase is normally inactivated by acid in the stomach; therefore, after removal of the stomach, the concentration of active amylase in the small intestine can be abnormally high. This enhances the rate of glucose production in the lumen and uptake into the blood glucose. The hypoglycaemia that ensues could thereby be exacerbated. Sympathetic nerves are stimulated by low blood glucose and so hypoglycaemia causes symptoms associated with activation of the sympathetic nervous system; palpitations, sweating, vasoconstriction and pallor.

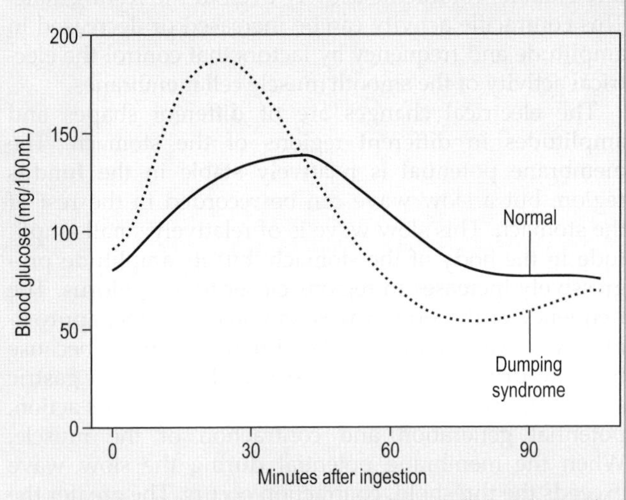

Fig. 2.10 Effect of eating an average-sized, high-carbohydrate meal on the concentration of blood glucose in a normal adult *(solid line)* and in a patient who has undergone gastrectomy *(dashed line)*.

Extracellular fluid volume

Another consequence of the rapid entry of material into the small intestine is a rapid loss of fluid into the GI tract that results in a reduced intravascular volume. This happens because the contents of the intestinal lumen become hyperosmotic due to the breakdown of macromolecules in the food, being dissolved in an abnormally low volume of digestive juices. The presence of a hyperosmotic solution in the intestines results in the transport of water from the blood, down its osmotic gradient into the lumen. The loss of water from the body can result in a dangerous fall in the extracellular fluid volume. A concomitant fall in the intravascular volume results in hypotension that will exacerbate the fainting sensation caused by hypoglycaemia. Furthermore, the passage of hypertonic chyme through the small intestine into the large intestine will impair water absorption in the colon, resulting in diarrhoea.

The symptoms that develop when a meal enters the small intestine too rapidly are collectively known as 'dumping syndrome'. All of these symptoms can be prevented by reducing the size of meals and thereby restricting the transit of food into the small intestine.

as the migrating motor complexes (MMCs). This contractile activity is essential to ensure that the stomach mucosa remains healthy by sweeping inert matter and sloughed epithelial cells out of the stomach. It also prevents stagnation and bacterial accumulation.

Although only a small amount of material is ejected through the sphincter each time the antrum contracts, immediately after the food has entered the duodenum the back-pressure helps to close the sphincter. Thus, the function of the sphincter is to allow the carefully regulated emptying of gastric contents, and also to prevent regurgitation of the duodenal contents that contain bile into the stomach. The latter is important as the gastric mucosa is highly resistant to acid but may be damaged by bile. The duodenal mucosa, on the other hand, is resistant to bile but may be damaged by acid. Too rapid emptying of gastric contents can lead to duodenal ulcers, whereas regurgitation of duodenal contents may possibly contribute to gastric ulcers.

Control of motility in the stomach

In the stomach, pacemaker cells are located in the longitudinal muscle in the greater curvature region of the fundus. The basal electrical rhythm (spontaneously oscillating membrane potential) generates action potentials in the pacemaker cells, and these are transmitted through the sheets of smooth muscle. The muscle therefore exhibits contractile activity even in the resting state. This contractile activity can be increased or decreased in amplitude and frequency by factors that control the electrical activity of the smooth muscle cell membranes.

The electrical changes are of different shapes and amplitudes in different regions of the stomach. The membrane potential is relatively stable in the fundus region, but a slow wave can be recorded in the rest of the stomach. This slow wave is of relatively small amplitude in the body of the stomach, but its amplitude progressively increases in regions closer to the pylorus. The frequency of the slow waves remains the same, approximately 3 waves/min, in the different regions because they are driven by the same pacemaker cells. In gastric smooth muscle, there is a threshold potential for action, potential generation and contraction of the muscle. When the membrane potential during the slow wave exceeds the threshold, contraction occurs. The greater the depolarization and the longer the membrane potential remains above the threshold, the more action potentials are generated and the greater the tension developed.

The action potentials in the antrum exhibit an initial rapid depolarisation phase followed by a long plateau phase. The rapid depolarisation phase is caused by Ca^{2+} entry into the cells through voltage-gated channels and the plateau phase is due to entry of both Ca^{2+} and Na^{+} through slower voltage-gated channels. The influx of Ca^{2+} leads to muscle contraction. In the terminal antrum, action potential spikes occur on the plateaus of the slow waves. Trains of action potentials that occur during the plateau phase elicit vigorous contractions in the antrum and these can lead to gastric emptying. Factors that regulate gastric motility include:

- Stretching or distension of the stomach walls increases tension (the myogenic reflex) and gastric motility.
- Increased levels of circulating gastrin stimulates motility.
- Stimulation of the vagus nerve leads to a greater force of contraction.
- Stimulation of the adrenergic sympathetic nerves to the stomach decreases motility. Sympathetic nerves are activated during exercise and therefore the motility of the GI tract decreases.
- Increased levels of CCK in the blood results in hyperpolarisation of the membrane, fewer action potentials, and relaxation of the muscle.

Control of the pyloric sphincter

The mucosal and muscle layers of the stomach and duodenum are discontinuous due to the presence of a ring of connective tissue on the duodenal side of the pyloric sphincter. The basal electrical rhythm of the duodenum is faster (approximately 10/min) than that of the stomach. The duodenal bulb contracts rather irregularly because it is influenced by the basal electrical rhythm of both the stomach and the duodenum. However, the activity in the antrum and duodenum is coordinated, and when the antrum contracts, the duodenal bulb is relaxed. The pylorus is densely innervated by parasympathetic (vagal) and sympathetic nerve fibres. The sympathetic nerves release noradrenaline, which acts on adrenergic receptors to increase the constriction of the sphincter. Relaxation of the sphincter is due to impulses in peptidergic fibres in the vagus that release VIP. It is discussed later that a major trigger for release of CCKs is the presence of fat in the duodenum; hence, this acts as a feedback mechanism to limit the volume of chyme released from the stomach.

Control of gastric function by food

Motility in the stomach is controlled partly by blood glucose levels. When the blood glucose concentration falls during fasting, gastric smooth muscle is stimulated. Peristaltic contractile activity increases, but not gastric emptying. These contractions can be strong enough to cause 'hunger pains'. They are due to impulses in the vagus nerve that is sensitive to low blood glucose.

Acid is secreted at a low rate even when the stomach is empty. The basal rate is approximately 10% of the maximum rate. However, the basal rate is not constant as it shows a diurnal variation: it is lowest in the morning and highest in the evening.

When a meal is eaten, the mechanisms which control the secretion of gastric juice and the motility and emptying of the stomach interact in a complex manner to coordinate the functions of this organ. The control of gastric function during a meal can be conveniently divided into three main phases depending on the location of the food:

1. The cephalic phase occurs before the food reaches the stomach. It is a response to the approach of food (i.e., smell or sight of food) or the presence of food in the mouth.
2. The gastric phase occurs in response to food when it reaches the stomach.
3. The intestinal phase occurs in response to food material in the intestines, mainly the duodenum and upper jejunum.

In practice, for much of the time during a meal, ingested material is present at different locations at the same time.

The cephalic phase

During the cephalic phase, gastric acid and pepsinogen secretion is activated by the thought, sight or smell of food, and by the presence of food in the mouth. The mechanisms of control of gastric secretion during the cephalic phase are summarised in Fig. 2.11. Emotions also influence gastric secretion. The response to the sight and smell of food is a conditioned reflex, or a learned response, based on previous experiences of eating food. Therefore, this enhanced secretion would only occur if one liked or wanted a particular food. Depression and loss of appetite can suppress this cephalic reflex.

The taste and feel of food in the mouth also elicit secretion of gastric juice before the food reaches the stomach. This is a non-conditioned reflex. The gastric juice secreted during the cephalic phase is rich in pepsinogen, but also contains some acid. The secretion of both pepsinogen and acid is due to impulses in the vagus nerve. Stimulation of the nerves releases acid both directly from parietal cells and indirectly via the release of gastrin (see Fig. 2.11). Less than half the acid produced in response to a meal is secreted during the cephalic phase. The importance of the vagus nerve and the cephalic phase is exemplified in those rare patients who undergo a vagotomy, which results in diminished gastric acid. Furthermore, during the cephalic phase, motility is also reduced, including gastric emptying. Pain, depression, fear and sadness also inhibit gastric motility.

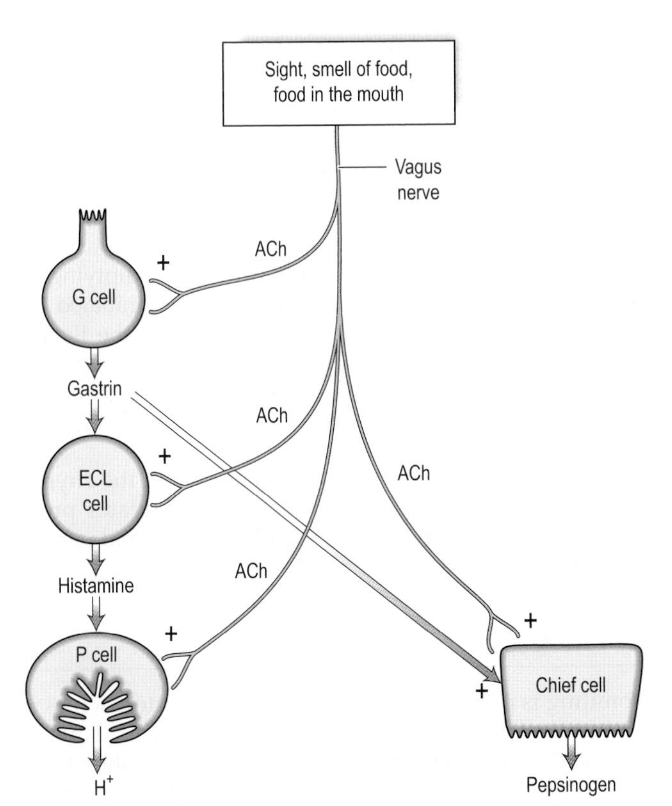

Fig. 2.11 Cephalic phase of control of gastric secretion. *ACh, acetylcholine; ECL, enterochromaffin-like; P, parietal.*

The gastric phase

The gastric phase, which can last between 3 and 4 hours, accounts for more than 50% of the acid secreted during a meal. The control of secretion during the gastric phase is summarised in Fig. 2.12. The amount of secretion depends on the chemical content and volume of food. Secretion of gastric juice is in response to chemicals in the food and to distension of the walls of the stomach by food. The products of protein digestion, especially peptides and amino acids (in particular tryptophan and phenylalanine), and caffeine and alcohol stimulate gastric secretion. These secretogogues are sensed by endocrine cells which behave as chemoreceptors or 'taste' cells. The G cells sense peptides and amino acids. Distension, another stimulus that increases acid secretion, is detected by pressure receptors or nerve endings in the mucosa. Distension is not as powerful a stimulant as the chemical constituents of food. The low pH in the stomach inhibits acid secretion, although pepsinogen secretion is stimulated. The D cells sense H^+ ions. The regulation of gastric secretion in this phase is via coordinated neural, hormonal and paracrine mechanisms. The neural signals are conducted in extrinsic nerves of the vagus nerve and in intrinsic nerves of the enteric nerve plexi.

During the gastric phase, the stomach empties at a rate that is proportional to the volume of material within it. This is due partly to the effect of distension; the chyme stimulates pressure receptors in the wall of the stomach, which trigger impulses in nerves in the internal nerve plexi. It is probably also due to the direct effect of stretching the smooth muscle. There is also a vagal mechanism

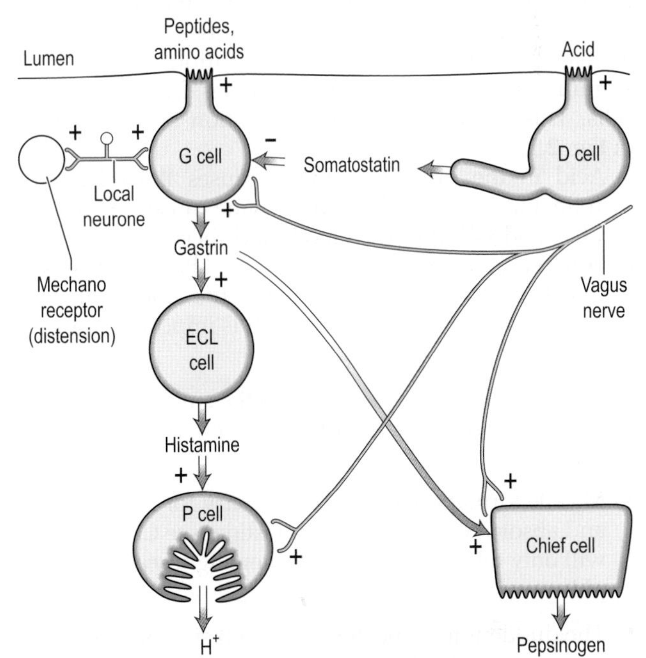

Fig. 2.12 Gastric phase of control of gastric secretion. *ECL, enterochromaffin-like; P, parietal.*

involved in the response to distension, but in the gastric phase (unlike the cephalic phase), impulses in the vagus nerve increase peristalsis and gastric emptying. In this case, it is the cholinergic nerve fibres in the vagus that are activated. However, excessive distension inhibits contractility, thereby allowing a longer time for the digestive processes to operate. Release of gastrin into the blood in response to peptides and amino acids also causes potentiation of peristalsis.

Gastric emptying is brought about by strong periodic contractions of the antrum, potentiated by gastrin in the stomach and acetylcholine in the vagus nerve. The pyloric sphincter relaxes when the antrum contracts and allows a portion of the gastric chyme into the duodenum. The relaxation of the sphincter is probably due to impulses in peptidergic nerve fibres which release VIP in the vagus nerve.

The intestinal phase

The intestinal phase of gastric function is largely inhibitory. Gastric secretion and motility are both inhibited. In the duodenal phase, the food is mixed with the digestive secretions of the pancreas and liver. The inhibition of gastric emptying by food in the duodenum enables the duodenal contents to be processed before more material enters it from the stomach.

Although food in the duodenum is largely inhibitory as far as gastric secretion is concerned, there is an early stimulatory phase in response to slight distension of the duodenum, probably due to the release of gastrin from endocrine cells in the walls of the duodenum. However, appropriate stimulation of the duodenum inhibits gastric secretion. Inhibitory stimuli include distension of the duodenum, fats and peptides in the chyme, increased acidity and hypertonic solutions. All of these stimuli cause the release of hormones from endocrine cells. This phase of control of secretion is summarised in Fig. 2.13.

Acid in the duodenal chyme causes the release of secretin and fat in the duodenal chyme causes the release of CCK and GIP into the blood, and these hormones all inhibit secretion of gastric juice (see above). This is a feedback mechanism that prevents the duodenal contents becoming excessively acidic. It is important for several reasons:

- Digestive enzymes, which act in the small intestine, require neutral or acidic pH values for optimum activity.
- Micelle formation, which is necessary for fat digestion and absorption in the small intestine (see Chapter 6), will only take place at a neutral or slightly alkaline pH.
- The duodenum is the most common site for ulcer formation in the digestive tract and acid is the primary cause of ulceration in this region. The reduction of acid secretion begins when the pH of the duodenal contents falls to 5.0, and it is complete at a pH value of approximately 2.5.

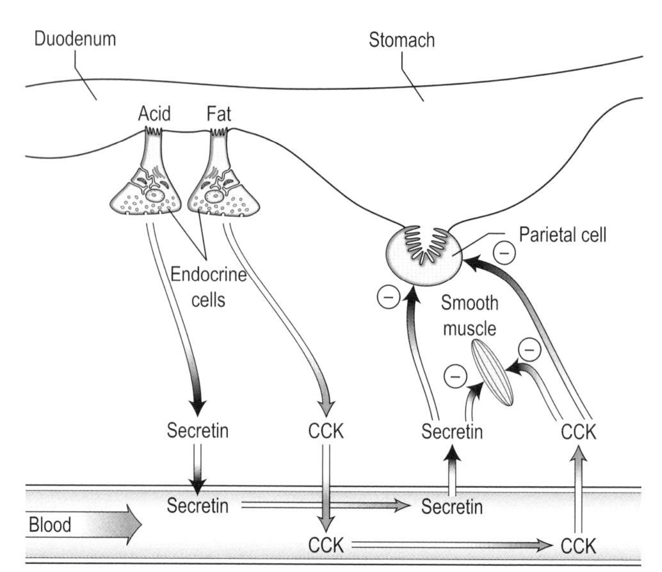

Fig. 2.13 Intestinal phase of gastric control. *CCK, cholecystokinin.*

pH control in the GI tract helps to maintain the blood pH within normal limits. The effects of hypersecretion of acid on acid–base balance are described in Case 2.2.

Motility in the stomach can be influenced by food in the duodenum, ileum and colon. Distension of the duodenum inhibits gastric motility via two mechanisms:

1. An enterogastric reflex which employs nerve fibres in the vagus nerve, and
2. A slower humoral mechanism involving the release of hormones from the walls of the duodenum into the blood. These hormones are collectively known as enterogastrones. They include CCK and secretin (see Fig. 2.13).

When food material reaches the ileum, the emptying of the stomach is delayed. This is a neural reflex initiated by activation of mechanoreceptors in the walls of the ileum, which trigger action potentials in nerve fibres in the internal nerve plexi. Interestingly, when food enters the stomach, the motility of the ileum is increased. Thus, the ileogastric reflex operates in both directions.

There is also a neural reflex response when the chyme enters the colon; distension of the colon activates pressure receptors which triggers impulses in internal nerves to delay gastric emptying.

Vomiting

Vomiting is part of the protective role of the stomach as it protects the body from ingested toxic substances. Thus, it augments the other protective mechanisms of the stomach including acid and pepsin secretion that inactivate ingested aerobic bacteria, and mucin secretion that protects the columnar epithelium.

Vomiting or emesis is the forceful ejection of gastric contents, and sometimes duodenal contents, through the mouth. It is a reflex that is usually preceded by a feeling of nausea. This can be accompanied by salivation, sweating, pallor, a fall in blood pressure, pupillodilation, increased heart rate and irregular breathing. It is usually also preceded by retching in which the gastric contents are forced into the oesophagus without entering the pharynx. A series of retches of increasing strength often precedes vomiting.

The vomiting reflex is controlled by the vomiting centre in the reticular formation in the medulla oblongata and the chemoreceptor trigger zone (CTZ) in the area postrema that resides in the floor of the fourth ventricle near to the vagal nuclei that innervate the GI tract. The reflex response involves stimulation of the respiratory and abdominal skeletal muscles as well as the smooth muscle of the GI tract. A large number of different areas of the body have receptors that provide afferent inputs to the vomiting centre to trigger vomiting. Major stimuli that can trigger vomiting include:

- Stimulation of sensory nerve endings in the stomach and duodenum (e.g. by solutions of copper sulphate and hypertonic sodium chloride).
- Drugs, such as cytotoxic drugs (e.g. cisplatin used in the treatment of cancer), and L -dopa used to treat Parkinson's disease.
- Endogenous substances produced as a result of radiation damage, infections or disease.
- Touch receptors at the back of the throat.
- Disturbances of the vestibular apparatus (known as motion sickness).
- Stimulation of the sensory nerves of the heart and viscera (uterus, renal pelvis, bladder, testicles).
- A rise in intracranial pressure.
- Nauseating smells, sights and emotional factors acting through higher central nervous system centres.
- Endocrine factors (e.g. increase in oestrogen concentration in morning sickness).
- Migraine.
- Circulatory syncope.

Case 2.3 Part 1 Excessive vomiting

A 55-year-old woman with a 15-year history of type 1 diabetes mellitus presented with a 4-month history of progressive nausea, vomiting, early satiety and weight loss. Her vomiting can often be severe and contains food ingested several hours before. She was on a basal bolus regimen of subcutaneous insulin; however, her diabetes was not well-controlled. She also suffered from retinopathy and peripheral neuropathy as a consequence of her diabetes. She did not take any antimotility drugs. On examination, she had mild epigastric distension and tenderness. She was admitted to hospital as she had developed dehydration and electrolyte imbalances due to her vomiting.

Acid–base status

The measurements made on the patient's blood included pH, HCO_3^- concentration, pCO_2 and K^+ concentration. If the vomiting were not suppressed, the patient's blood gas analysis would indicate metabolic alkalosis (i.e., high pH, high $[HCO_3^-]$, normal or mildly elevated pCO_2).

Case 2.3 Part 2 Excessive vomiting

She underwent an upper GI endoscopy which revealed a large volume of food and fluid in her stomach despite a 6-hour fast. There was no evidence of gastric outlet or duodenal obstruction. She underwent a barium meal and follow-through (Fig. 2.14) and a scintigraphic gastric emptying study which confirmed significantly delayed gastric emptying. A diagnosis of gastroparesis was made, and she was treated with a short course of metoclopramide as it acts an antiemetic and a prokinetic. Her diabetes control was optimised, and this improved her symptoms significantly.

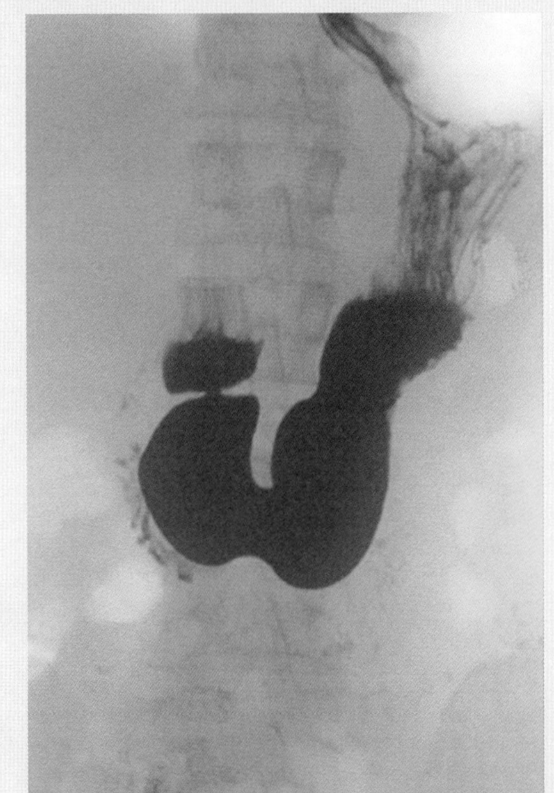

Fig. 2.14 Barium meal shows a distended stomach with minimal passage of contrast into the small bowel. This suggests gastroparesis in a patient with a normal upper gastrointestinal endoscopy.

The disturbance in acid–base balance is brought about because the HCO_3^- transported into the blood, from the secreting parietal cells in the stomach would not be neutralised sufficiently by the H^+ ions transported into the blood as a result of the secretion of alkaline pancreatic juice, bile and intestinal juice, which is not affected by persistent vomiting. Compensation for this alkalosis by the lungs and kidneys would become inadequate due to the persistent loss of H^+ ions.

Electrolytes

Hypokalaemia (a low blood K^+ concentration) may also be present in this patient because K^+ would be exchanged for H^+ in the kidneys (to partially correct the blood pH) and lost in the urine. Hypokalaemia affects nerve function (importantly, including that in the heart) and can lead to kidney damage. Alkaline K^+ salts like K^+ acetate, K^+ citrate or K^+ bicarbonate could be administered to correct the disturbance in plasma K^+ concentration.

Gastroparesis

Gastroparesis is a syndrome of delayed gastric emptying of solids and liquids in the absence of mechanical obstruction. Patients can present with symptoms of nausea, vomiting, early satiety, bloating and epigastric pain. There are multiple causes associated with gastroparesis, including diabetes mellitus, medications (such as opiates and tricyclic antidepressants) and gastric surgery. However, no obvious cause is identified in over half of patients with gastroparesis. An upper GI endoscopy is performed to rule out a mechanical cause for delayed emptying and can often reveal moderate amounts of food or fluid despite fasting. In patients with suspected gastroparesis, an assessment of gastric motility is necessary to establish this diagnosis. This can be achieved by a nuclear medicine scan called a scintigraphic gastric emptying study, where a radioisotope-labelled meal is consumed with imaging of the stomach immediately after the meal and again at 2 and 4 hours after ingestion. Delayed gastric emptying is defined as gastric retention of greater than 10% at 4 hours and/or greater than 60% at 2 hours. Management of gastroparesis consists of diet modification with avoidance of fatty and spicy foods and optimisation of diabetic control. In patients with continued symptoms, therapy with prokinetics and antiemetics may be considered. If these symptoms remain refractory, other options may include tube feeding beyond the stomach (percutaneous jejunostomy), surgical jejunostomy parenteral nutrition and gastric electrical stimulation.

EXOCRINE FUNCTIONS OF THE PANCREAS

3

Chapter objectives and clinical presentations

After reading this chapter, review your learning by considering the following:

1. Can you describe the macroscopic and microscopic anatomy of the pancreas and relate these to function?
2. Can you detail the components of pancreatic juice and how they aid in the digestion process?
3. Do you understand how pancreatic enzymes are secreted in a way such that autodigestion does not occur?
4. Are you able to describe the processes that regulate secretion from the exocrine pancreas?

Also, you should be familiar with the following clinical presentations:

- Cystic fibrosis
- Acute pancreatitis
- Chronic pancreatitis
- Pancreatic cancer

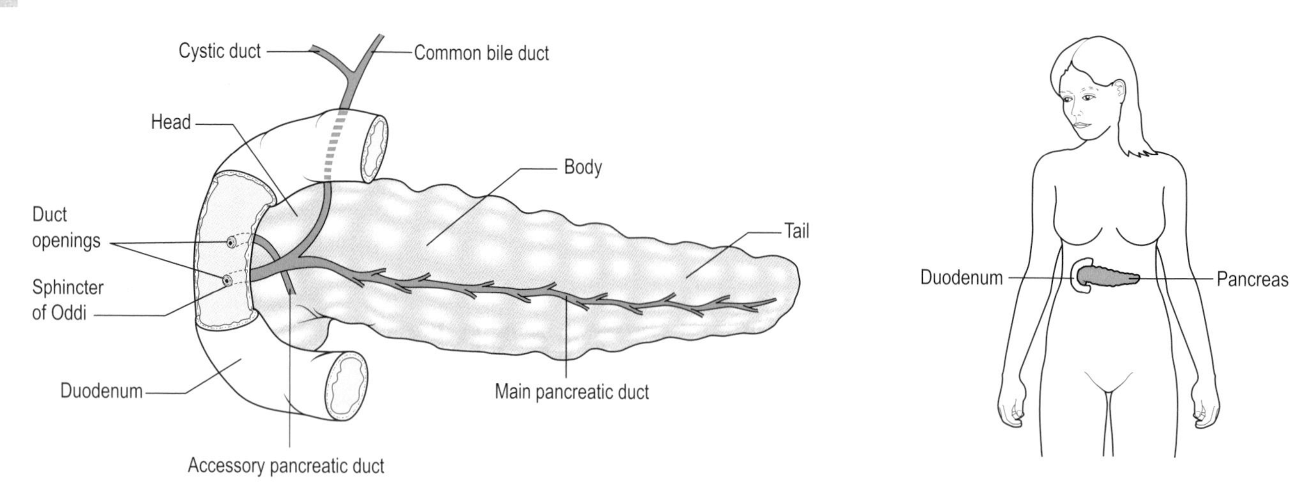

Fig. 3.1 The pancreas and its innervation and blood supply.

Clinical outlook

Patients with disorders of their pancreas often present with abdominal pain, weight loss and malabsorptive symptoms such as diarrhoea. Diseases of the pancreas may present acutely with acute pancreatitis due to gallstones or alcohol intake or over a longer period with chronic pancreatitis due to alcohol or cystic fibrosis. Patients may also present with epigastric pain and weight loss as symptoms of pancreatic cancer.

Introduction

The pancreas contains exocrine tissue that secretes pancreatic juice, a major digestive secretion and endocrine tissue that secretes hormones such as insulin and glucagon. These hormones are important in the control of metabolism and their roles in the absorptive and postabsorptive metabolic states will be discussed in Chapter 9. This chapter will be mainly concerned with the exocrine secretions of the pancreas, their functions and the mechanisms whereby the secretory processes are controlled.

Pancreatic juice finds its way into the duodenum via the pancreatic duct that opens into the duodenum at the same location as the common bile duct (Fig. 3.1). Entry of both pancreatic juice and bile (originating from the gallbladder) into the duodenum is controlled by the sphincter of Oddi. The smooth muscle of the sphincter contracts between meals so that the junction is sealed. When a meal is being processed in the gastrointestinal (GI) tract, the sphincter muscle relaxes and allows the pancreatic juice and bile into the small intestine. Pancreatic exocrine dysfunction may be due to disorders of the pancreas itself, or due to blockage of the ducts which prevents the exocrine secretions reaching the duodenum. Duct blockage may also result in impaired bile flow from the liver, which can result in jaundice.

In the small intestine, pancreatic juice, bile and the juices (secreted by the walls of the intestines) mix with the fluid (chyme) arriving from the stomach (see Fig. 7.1). Pancreatic juice provides most of the important digestive enzymes. In addition, by virtue of its bicarbonate content, it helps to provide an appropriate pH in the intestinal lumen for the enzymes to act on their nutrient substrates. The functional importance of the pancreas to the digestive processes can be illustrated by the problems arising in chronic pancreatitis and cystic fibrosis in which pancreatic tissue is destroyed.

Anatomy and morphology

The pancreas is an elongated gland, 14–21 cm in length, that lies in the abdominal cavity. It weighs around 100 g and can be divided into three regions: the head, the body and the tail (see Fig. 3.1). The head is an expanded portion that lies adjacent to the C-shaped region of the duodenum to which it is intimately attached by connective tissue, and to which it is connected by a common blood supply. The body and tail extend across the midline of the body toward the hilum of the spleen. The pancreatic duct extends through the long axis of the gland to the duodenum. Pancreatic juice empties from this duct into the duodenum via the ampulla of Vater. Bile via the common bile duct from the liver also enters the duodenum at the ampulla of Vater by passing through the head of the pancreas. This is why inflammation (pancreatitis) and tumours (pancreatic cancer) involving the head of the pancreas are commonly associated with jaundice, as a consequence of blockage of the common bile duct, which can lead to impaired liver function.

Exocrine tissue

The exocrine units of the pancreas are tubuloacinar glands that are organised like bunches of grapes (Fig. 3.2), in a similar manner to the units in the salivary glands. The exocrine units surround the islets of Langerhans, the endocrine units of the pancreas. For this

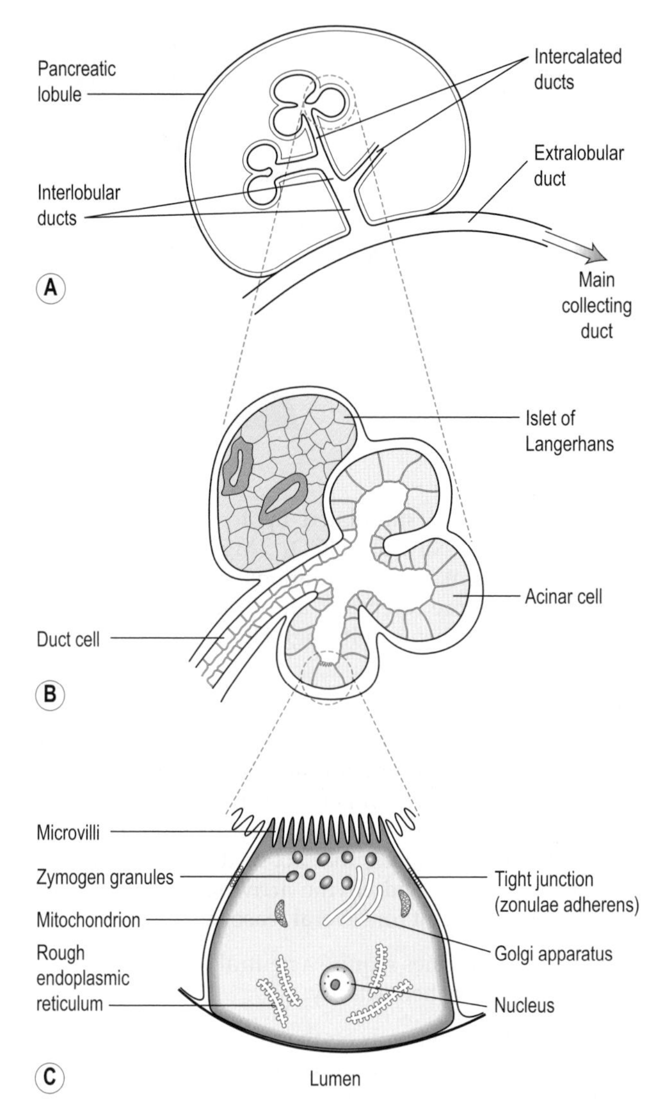

Fig. 3.2 (A) A lobule of the pancreas indicating the duct system. (B) The relationship of an exocrine unit and an islet of Langerhans. (C) An acinar cell.

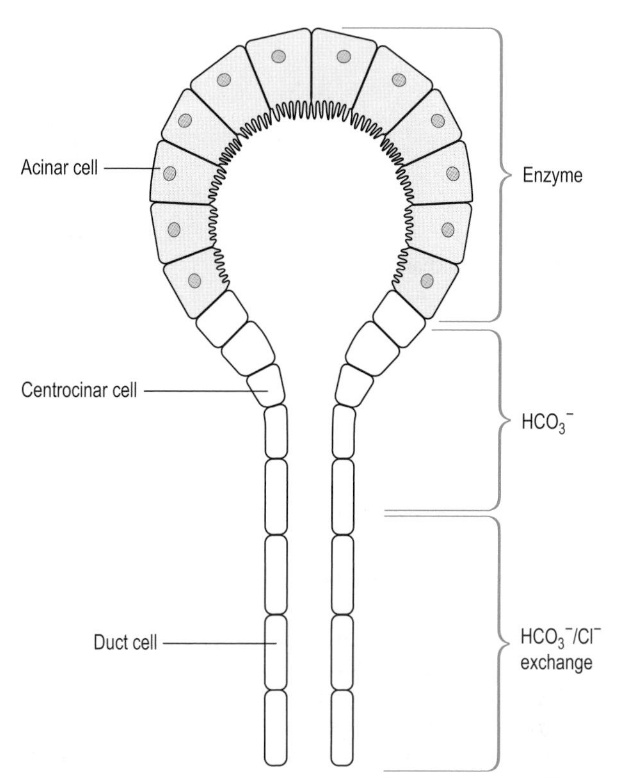

Fig. 3.3 Secretory unit showing the cellular locations of the different secretions.

reason, destructive diseases such as chronic pancreatitis involve impairment of both exocrine and endocrine function. A thin layer of loose connective tissue surrounds the gland. Septa extend from this layer into the gland, dividing it into lobules and giving it an irregular surface. Larger areas of connective tissue surround the main ducts and the blood vessels and nerve fibres that penetrate the gland. Small mucous glands situated within the tissue surrounding the pancreatic duct secrete mucus into the duct.

Histology of the exocrine tissue

Fig. 3.2 shows the structure of a pancreatic lobule. The exocrine units of the pancreas or pancreatins, each consist of a terminal acinar portion and a duct (Fig. 3.3). The duct that drains the acinus is known as an intercalated duct. These empty into larger intralobular ducts. The intralobular ducts in each lobule drain into a larger extralobular duct that empties the secretions of that lobule into still larger ducts, and the latter converge into the main collecting duct, or the pancreatic duct.

Most pancreatic tissue is devoted to its exocrine function, in which digestive enzymes are produced. The cells responsible for enzyme synthesis are acinar cells, which make up around 85% of the pancreas. The word 'acinar' is derived from the Latin word 'acinus', meaning 'grape', as they are cellular aggregates that form bundles like clusters of grapes. The acinus is a rounded structure consisting of acinar cells (see Fig. 3.3). These cells secrete the digestive enzymes of the pancreatic juice. They display all the features characteristic of a cell specialised for protein production (in this case, digestive enzymes), including an abundance of rough endoplasmic reticulum, Golgi apparatuses and numerous zymogen granules that contain the pancreatic enzymes (or, specifically, their precursors, as detailed later). The zymogen is released into the lumen and travels through the various ducts ending up in the lumen of the small intestine as described above. The acinar cells are tightly linked through various cell-cell junctions. Tight junctions separate the fluid in the lumen of the acinus from the fluid in the intercellular spaces that bathes the basolateral surfaces of the cells. Importantly, the tight junctions are impermeable to macromolecules in the luminal fluid, such as digestive enzymes, but permit the exchange of water and

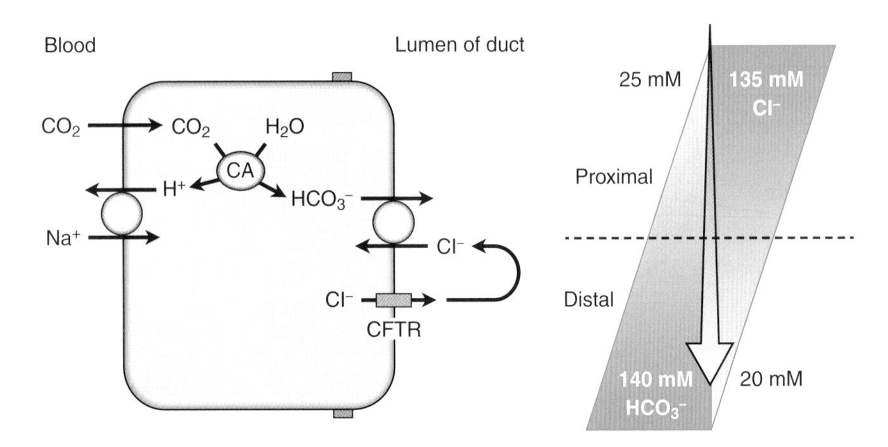

Fig. 3.4 Cellular mechanisms involved in the production of HCO_3^- and H^+ in a duct cell. CA, carbonic anhydrase; CFTR, cystic fibrosis transmembrane conductance regulator. Pancreatic duct with the variation in the composition of pancreatic juice with respect to Cl^- and HCO_3^-.

ions between the interstitial spaces and the lumen of the acinus.

The intercalated duct begins within the acinus. This is a unique feature of secretory glands. The upper duct cells within the acinus are known as centroacinar cells (see Fig. 3.3). These cells are continuous with those of the short, intercalated duct that lies outside the acinus and drains it. The intercalated ducts are lined by flattened squamous epithelial cells (referred to here as duct cells). Similarly, these duct cells possess tight junctions, separating the duct lumen from the intercellular spaces and function to exclude large molecules from the spaces. The acinar cell secretions, which are ultimately modified by the duct cells, flow from the intercalated ducts to the intralobular ducts and then into the main pancreatic duct.

Pancreatic juice

Between meals, pancreatic secretions occur at a low rate (0.2–0.3 mL/min) which markedly increases during ingestion (4.0 mL/min). The total daily secretion is approximately 2.5 litres. The pancreatic juice entering the duodenum is a mixture of two types of secretion: an enzyme-rich secretion from the acinar cells and an aqueous alkaline secretion from the ducts. Thus, if the ducts are ligated near the acini, which results in acinar cell degeneration, the secretion of the alkaline component of the juice is largely unaltered, but the secretion of enzymes is markedly reduced. The alkaline secretion originates largely from the centroacinar cells and the duct cells of the intralobular and small interlobular ducts. These relationships are illustrated in Fig. 3.3.

Alkaline secretion

Composition

The cells of the upper ducts secrete an isotonic juice which is rich in bicarbonate but contains only traces of enzymes. There is a continuous resting secretion of this juice, but it can be stimulated up to 14-fold during a meal. It contains Na^+, K^+, HCO_3^-, Mg^{2+}, Ca^{2+}, Cl^-, and other ions present in concentrations similar to those of plasma. It therefore resembles an ultrafiltrate of plasma, but is alkaline by virtue of its high HCO_3^- content.

Functions

The pancreatic juice arriving in the duodenum is mixed with the chyme by contractions of the smooth muscle of the small intestine. The function of the alkaline pancreatic secretion, together with the other alkaline secretions (bile and intestinal juices) that act in the small intestine, is to neutralise the acid chyme arriving from the stomach. This is important for several reasons:

- Pancreatic enzymes require a neutral or slightly alkaline pH for their activity;
- Fat absorption depends on the formation of micelles in the intestinal lumen, a process which only takes place at neutral or slightly alkaline pH values; and
- The pancreatic juice protects the intestinal mucosa from excess acid which can lead to the formation of ulcers. This (peptic) ulceration most commonly occurs in the first part of the duodenum before the acidic chyme has mixed with the alkaline pancreatic juice.

Cellular mechanisms of secretion

The mechanisms involved in the production of intracellular HCO_3^- in the centroacinar and upper duct cells are illustrated in Fig. 3.4. The initial intracellular step involves the reaction of CO_2 with water. Secreted H^+ ions react with HCO_3^- ions in the blood perfusing the gland and this generates CO_2, some of which diffuses into the duct cell. In the cell, CO_2 combines with intracellular water to generate carbonic acid in a reaction catalysed by carbonic anhydrase, an enzymes present in the centroacinar and upper duct cells. The carbonic acid dissociates into HCO_3^- and H^+. Whilst bicarbonate is being secreted the partial pressure of CO_2 (pCO_2) in the cells is lower than that in the blood as it is being used up in the production of HCO_3^- ions, and the higher the rate of secretion, the greater the downhill gradient for diffusion of CO_2 into the cell. The HCO_3^- ions are secreted across the luminal membrane by Cl^-/HCO_3^- exchange, and the H^+ ions are secreted into the blood. Thus, for every HCO_3^- ion that is secreted into the duct lumen, one H^+ ion is secreted into the blood. Therefore, the blood flowing through the pancreas becomes transiently acidic when it the pancreas is secreting HCO_3^-. The H^+ ions in the blood help to neutralise the 'alkaline tide' produced during a meal by the secreting stomach (see Ch. 2), by combining with plasma HCO_3^- to produce CO_2. In conditions involving a pancreatic fistula, loss of HCO_3^- must be carefully monitored.

The exchange mechanism in the centroacinar and upper duct cells, whereby HCO_3^- is secreted in exchange for Cl^-, obviously depends on the presence of Cl^- in the fluid in the lumen. This is achieved by flux of Cl^- ions out of the cell into the lumen via a chloride conductance channel known as the cystic fibrosis transmembrane conductance regulator (CFTR). HCO_3^- secretion thus critically depends on the activity of CFTR, a cAMP-dependent anion channel localised in the apical membrane. In the proximal part of pancreatic ducts close to acinar cells, HCO_3^- secretion across is largely mediated by a Cl^-/HCO_3^- solute exchanger (Pendrin L1). In more distal ducts, most of the HCO_3^- secretion is mediated by HCO_3^- conductance of CFTR. It is a defect in the CFTR that results in impairment of the secretory process and disruption of pancreatic function in cystic fibrosis (Case 3.1: 1). As water transport would normally follow the ion transport (down the osmotic gradient), the defective ion secretion in these conditions results in a viscous fluid in the ducts with a high concentration of protein in the pancreatic ducts which can block the lumen. This results in secondary pancreatic damage. The main features of the ion transport relationships in the pancreatic duct cell are shown in Fig. 3.4.

Variation in composition with flow rate

The concentration of bicarbonate in the pancreatic juice that enters the duodenum is around 140 mM (note the concentration in a patient with cystic fibrosis is commonly around 25 mM). The electrolyte composition of the juice varies with the flow rate. Fig. 3.4 shows the changes in concentrations of HCO_3^- and Cl^- ions with increasing rates of flow. There is a reciprocal relationship between the concentrations of the two ions. The concentration of HCO_3^- increases with increasing flow rate and the concentration of Cl^- decreases. The sum of the concentrations of the two ions is kept constant by the action of the ion exchange pumps. As the HCO_3^- concentration increases, the juice becomes more alkaline.

The changes in the ionic composition of the juice with rate of flow are due to the presence of transport systems in the membranes of the duct cells. The primary alkaline juice secreted at the tops of the ducts is modified as it is passed down the ducts by transport systems in the cells lower down in the extralobular ducts and in the main ducts. At high flow rates, the time the juice spends in contact with the cells is not sufficient for appreciable modification via HCO_3^-/Cl^- exchange and other processes to take place. Therefore, the composition of the juice produced at high flow rates resembles that of the primary secretion more closely than juice secreted at low flow rates.

Case 3.1 Cystic fibrosis part 1

A 12-year-old boy who was suffering from cystic fibrosis was taken to the outpatient clinic for his regular check-up. Cystic fibrosis is an inherited autosomal recessive disorder. The primary defect is a mutation in the gene that encodes CFTR. CFTR is responsible for cAMP-regulated Cl^- conductance in the membranes of secretory cells of epithelia. The defect causes impaired Cl^- transport that is predominantly a problem in the wet surfaces of the respiratory tract, but also causes severe problems in the pancreas. It also manifests in the reproductive tract and sweat glands. The boy's condition had been diagnosed soon after birth and he had both respiratory tract and pancreatic involvement. He had been asked to bring a sample of his stool. This was pale-coloured, poorly formed and oily in appearance. It was sent to the laboratory for analysis to assess his pancreatic function. His exocrine pancreatic insufficiency was being treated with a pancreatic enzyme preparation and the anti-ulcer drug omeprazole.

Defect and diagnosis

In the pancreas, the CFTR defect is associated with defective secretion of chloride into the ducts, and therefore reduced water transport so that the fluid in the ducts becomes viscous. This leads to the formation of protein-rich plugs which can obstruct the proximal intralobular ducts, resulting in secondary pancreatic damage (a process similar to that which occurs in chronic pancreatitis). Thus, the digestive enzymes do not reach the duodenum. The tests performed on the stool sample would show a high fat content. Chymotrypsin or trypsin content would also be high. Over 80% of patients have steatorrhoea due to pancreatic dysfunction and meconium ileus (obstruction of the small intestine by impacted material) is common in newborns (Fig. 3.5).

The same process of mucous plugging results in blockage of the bronchioles. This leads to recurrent respiratory infection and eventually to respiratory failure. These bron-

Continued

Case 3.1 Cystic fibrosis part 1—cont'd

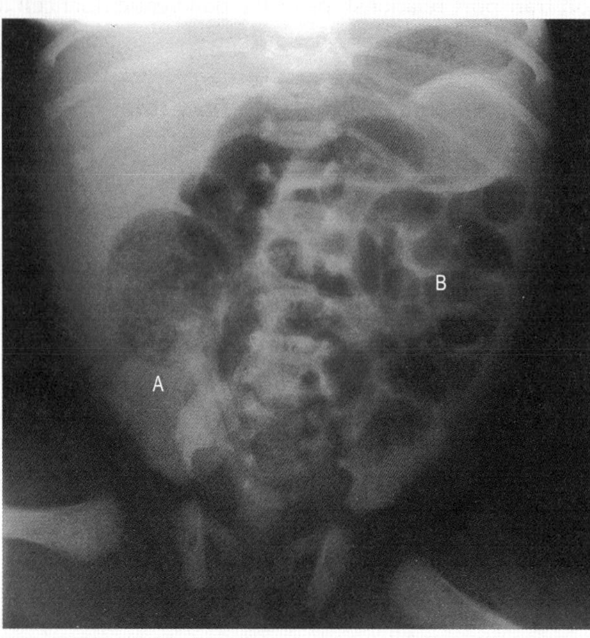

Fig. 3.5 Plain abdominal X-ray taken from an infant with cystic fibrosis. The meconium stool has obstructed the bowel and can be seen in the caecum (A). The proximal small bowel loops have dilated (B) and are filled with gas.

chopulmonary and GI manifestations usually alert the clinician to the possibility that the child has cystic fibrosis. The condition can be diagnosed by DNA analysis or the presence of a high Na^+ concentration (over 60 mmol/L) in sweat. The latter is due to the impaired Cl^- transport in the secretory cells of the sweat glands as water transport into the sweat depends on an osmotic gradient.

Pancreatic enzymes

The pancreas produces pancreatic juice that consists of a mixture of more than two dozen digestive enzymes in the pre-activated form, called zymogens. It should be noted that enzymes are not the sole proteinaceous secretion from the pancreas, and it has recently been identified that up to 285 proteins could be identified in normal pancreatic secretion (or that commonly associated with digestive function). Interestingly, studies have found that pancreatic juice from pancreatic cancer patients differs markedly in composition. Such changes, if readily characterised, could be useful for improving diagnosis.

As detailed above, the protein-rich secretion (which contains zymogens) produced by acinar cells, meets the bicarbonate rich fluid produced by more distal pancreatic duct cells. Trypsinogen is the most important zymogen. Once activated, it becomes trypsin, the key enzyme that then activates all other zymogens. This includes proteolytic enzymes (trypsin, chymotrypsin, carboxypeptidase and elastase) and phospholipase A. Lipase, α-amylase, ribonuclease and deoxyribonuclease are secreted as active enzymes. The release of enzymes as inactive precursors ensures that the activated enzymes do not autodigest the pancreatic tissue. Enzymes released in an active would not cause pancreatic cellular damage because there is no starch, glycogen or triglyceride substrate in pancreatic tissue.

Once released from the pancreas into the duodenum and subsequently into the ileum, the activity of these enzymes diminishes as they themselves become degraded; the stability towards degradation is considerable amongst these enzymes. In healthy people, 74% of the amylase activity, 22% of the trypsin activity and 1% of the lipase activity survives intestinal transit. The importance of the pancreatic enzymes for nutrition can be illustrated by consideration of the impairment of function and the treatments employed in chronic pancreatitis and cystic fibrosis.

Secretion of enzymes and precursors

The mechanism of secretion in the acinar cell is illustrated in Fig. 3.6. The enzymes or precursors are synthesised on the rough endoplasmic reticulum of the cell. The molecules are then released into the cisternae of the endoplasmic reticulum. Buds containing enzymes or enzyme precursors break off the cisternal membranes and coalesce in the region of the Golgi complex to form 'condensing vacuoles'. The Golgi complex also sorts and targets newly synthesised proteins into various cell compartments; digestive enzymes are transported to the zymogen

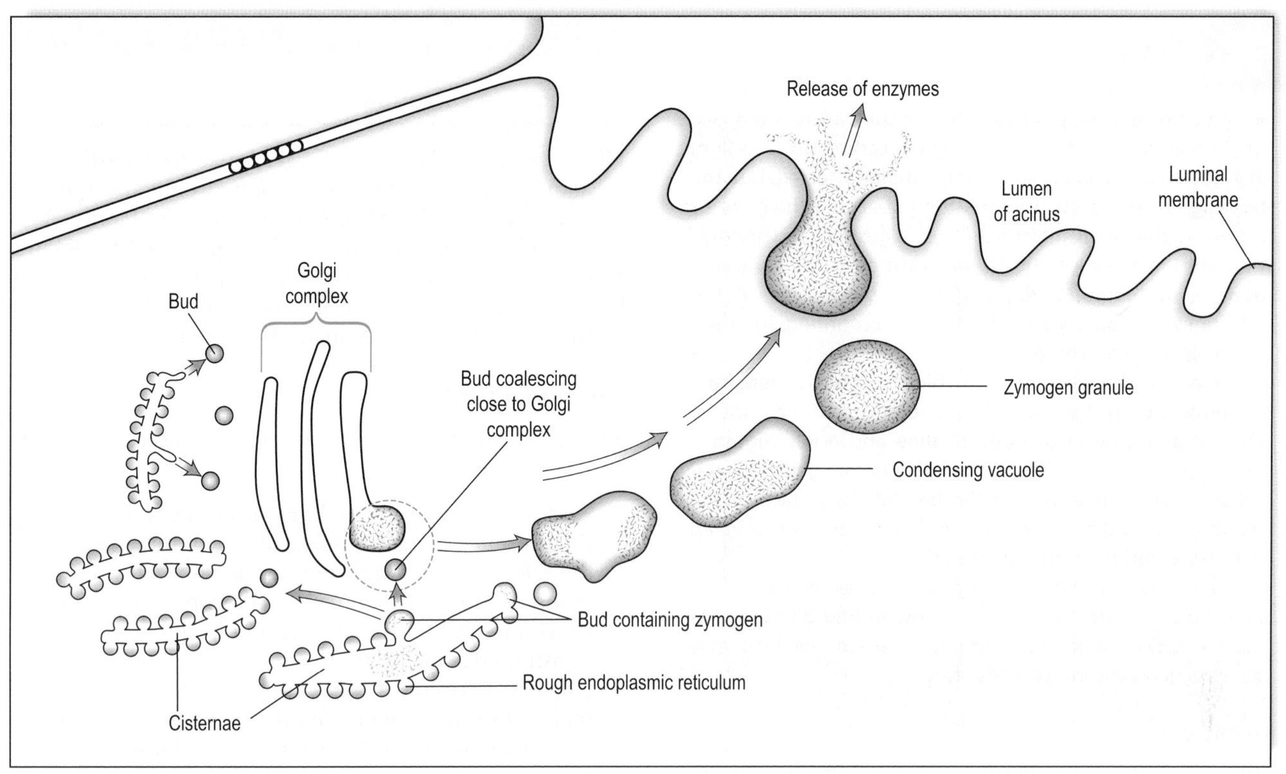

Fig. 3.6 Mechanism of enzyme secretion in the acinar cell.

granules. The vacuoles migrate towards the luminal membrane. If cells are stained for zymogen, the vacuoles appear more and more densely stained as they approach the surface. At the luminal membrane, the membranes that surround the zymogen granules fuse with the cell membrane and the vesicles break open to release their contents, a process known as exocytosis. The different enzymes are packaged together in each zymogen granule, and they are probably released together in constant proportions. The zymogen granule membrane is rapidly recycled from the surface membrane.

It is exocytosis, rather than the synthesis or sequestration of the enzyme proteins, that is under physiological control by hormones and neurotransmitters. Exocytosis is triggered by an increase in intracellular Ca^{2+}. The rise in intracellular Ca^{2+} when the cell is stimulated is via influx from the extracellular spaces or release from intracellular stores.

Activation of enzyme precursors

The enzyme precursors secreted by the acinar cells are activated in the lumen of the duodenum and jejunum. Trypsinogen is converted to trypsin plus a short peptide in a reaction catalysed by enterokinase, an enzyme in the brush border of the epithelial cells of the small intestine. Once a small amount of activated trypsin has been formed, it can catalyse the conversion of more trypsinogen to trypsin. Trypsin is a powerful proteolytic enzyme that can convert chymotrypsinogen, procarboxypeptidase, proelastase and prophospholipase A to their activated forms. Thus, once a small amount of trypsin is formed, a catalytic chain reaction occurs (Table 3.1).

Table 3.1 Activation of enzyme precursors in the small intestine

Precursor	***Active enzyme***
Trypsinogen	trypsin 1 peptide
Chymotrypsinogen	chymotrypsin 1 peptide
Proelastase	elastase 1 peptide
Procarboxypeptidase	carboxypeptidase 1 peptide
Prophospholipase A	phospholipase A 1 peptide

In acute pancreatitis, a condition which can be life-threatening, activated enzymes are present in the pancreatic ducts leading to destruction of the pancreatic tissue. Several mechanisms to prevent this from occurring are employed, including:

- Enterokinase, which initiates the cascade of zymogen activation, is not found in the pancreas but rather is localised on the brush border of the small intestine.
- The secretory granules containing zymogen are impermeable to proteins. Thus, the zymogens and active digestive enzymes are sequestered from

Case 3.1 Cystic fibrosis part 2

In cystic fibrosis, the primary defect in the pancreas is a lack of Cl^- secretion leading to defective bicarbonate secretion. The secretion of enzymes is not initially affected but the blockage of the ducts prevents them reaching their site of action in the small intestine. Thus, digestion and absorption are impaired leading to malnutrition if the condition remains untreated. Undigested fat is passed out of the intestines and appears in the stools, accounting for their pale colour (steatorrhoea).

Although the secretion of bicarbonate is impaired, abnormalities in the patient's acid–base status may not be present as secretion of both alkaline and acidic digestive juices are affected (plasma Cl^- ions are exchanged for intracellular bicarbonate ions on the basolateral surface of the parietal cell, and the intracellular Cl^- ions are then coupled with H^+ secretion on the apical surface.

In advanced disease, the pancreas may become damaged and there may be a deficiency in insulin and glucagon. As insulin is the dominant hormone, diabetes mellitus may develop (as in chronic pancreatitis).

Treatment

There is currently no cure for this condition. The pulmonary problems dominate the condition in most cases; however, the management of the pancreatic insufficiency is necessary to maintain overall nutrition and growth. The treatment is the ingestion of a pancreatic enzyme preparation by mouth. The enzymes are usually administered in enteric-coated form that renders them resistant to degradation by acid in the stomach. The coating is susceptible to degradation in the alkaline environment of the small intestine, where the enzymes are consequently released at their usual site of action. Degradation of the enzymes by gastric acid can still be a significant problem but this can be minimised by concomitant treatment with an acid suppressant.

proteins in the cytoplasm and other intracellular compartments.

- Enzyme inhibitors such as the pancreatic trypsin inhibitor SPINK1 are co-packaged in the secretory granule. SPINK1 can inhibit any activated trypsin which may find its way into the ducts by complexing with it. This trypsin inhibitor is a 56-amino acid peptide that inactivates trypsin by forming a relatively stable complex with the enzyme near its catalytic site
- The condensation of zymogens, the low pH, and the ionic conditions within the secretory pathway further limit enzyme activity.
- The alkaline pH (8.0–9.5) and low Ca^{2+} concentration in pancreatic secretions promote the degradation rather than the activation of trypsinogen.

Control of secretion

Bicarbonate secretion

HCO_3^- secretion increases in response to ingestion of a meal and is regulated by multiple neuronal and humoral mechanisms. Ductal HCO_3^- secretion is not only regulated by hormones and cholinergic nerves detailed below, but constituents and the environment within the lumen of the duodenum also have an influence. These include intraductal pressure and Ca^{2+} concentration.

Hormonal control

Several hormones are responsible for pancreatic bicarbonate secretion:

1. Secretin: A low duodenal pH (around pH 4.5, due to the presence of gastric acid within chyme) stimulates the release of secretin from duodenal S cells into the blood. In turn, this stimulates the pancreatic duct cells to secrete HCO_3^-. It is now recognised that secretin additionally potentiates enzymatic secretion.
2. Cholecystokinin (CCK): As detailed later, CCK is the major stimulator of enzymatic secretion from acinar cells. The direct effect of CCKs on ductal secretion is low.
3. Purines: Duct cells express many purinergic receptors at both their apical and basolateral membranes. These receptors are stimulated by purinergic ligands released from nerve terminals and zymogen granules (in the luminal space). The role of purinergic receptor activation in HCO_3 secretion is still under investigation.

Neuronal control

Pancreatic secretion is also regulated by the enteric nervous system. Acetylcholine is the major neurotransmitter acting on pancreatic ducts at both M1 and M3 muscarinic receptors. This leads to increased secretion from duct cells. Additionally, this cholinergic stimulation enhances ductal secretion stimulated by secretin.

Zymogen secretion

As with HCO_3^- secretion, several factors influence the secretion of zymogens from acinar cells.

Hormonal control

1. CCK: CCK is the major hormone that stimulates the secretion of the enzyme component. CCK is produced by I cells localised in the small intestine. CCK and gastrin compete for the same receptor on the acinar cell; gastrin also increases acinar secretion (Fig. 3.7). Although the main function of secretin is acting on the duct cell to produce HCO_3^-, it can also act on the acinar cell to increase intracellular levels of cAMP (see Fig. 3.7). Vasoactive intestinal peptide (VIP) can also

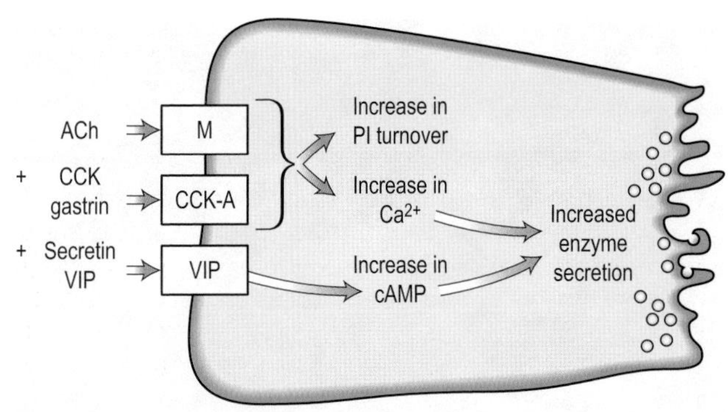

Fig. 3.7 Cellular mechanisms of control in the acinar cell. M, muscarinic receptor; PI, phosphatidylinositol.

mediate this effect too, and because of the increase in cAMP, the effect of CCK and gastrin is potentiated. Consequently, the enzyme secretion is greater when the two types of secretagogue are acting together.

2. Somatostatin: Somatostatin, which is present in δ-cells in the islets of Langerhans of the pancreas, is a powerful inhibitor of pancreatic secretion. It acts in a paracrine manner to inhibit the release of the exocrine alkaline and enzyme-rich secretions, as well as the pancreatic hormones insulin and glucagon. In addition, it inhibits the release of several GI hormones, including CCK, secretin and gastrin. Somatostatin-28 is the dominant isoform in the GI tract, whereas somatostatin-14 is stored within the pancreatic δ-cells. Analogues of somatostatin such as octreotide are used clinically to treat specific hormone-secreting neuroendocrine tumours.

Nervous control

Parasympathetic innervation plays a major role in the regulation of pancreatic functions, and patients who have undergone a vagotomy results in an almost complete abolishment their pancreatic exocrine secretion. Stimulation of cholinergic fibres in the vagus nerve enhances the rate of secretion of enzyme fluid secretion. The effects of sympathetic nerve stimulation on pancreatic exocrine secretions are not as clear. Stimulation of the sympathetic nerves is likely to inhibit secretion, mainly by reducing the blood flow to the gland (via vasoconstriction of the arterioles) that decreases the volume of juice secreted. However, stimulation of the sympathetic nerves to the pancreas depresses the enzyme content of the secretion as well as the volume of juice secreted.

Control of secretion during a meal

The control of the secretion of pancreatic juice during a meal depends on the volume and composition of the food. Ingested material at different locations within the GI tract affects the control of the secretions in different ways. The control during a meal can be divided into three phases, according to the location of the food or chyme:

1. The cephalic phase, due to the approach of food or the presence of food in the mouth.
2. The gastric phase, when food is in the stomach.
3. The intestinal phase, when food material is in the duodenum.

Cephalic phase

The sight and smell of food, or other sensory stimuli associated with the impending arrival of food, elicit increased pancreatic secretion via a 'conditioned' reflex. Around 20%–25% of the total pancreatic exocrine secretion occurs during the cephalic phase. The presence of food in the mouth stimulates secretion via a 'non-conditioned' reflex. The control during this phase is therefore nervous. It is mediated by impulses in cholinergic fibres in the vagus nerve. The juice secreted is mainly the enzyme-rich secretion, containing very little HCO_3^-.

In response to vagal stimulation, the acinar cells also secrete kallikreins, which catalyse the production of bradykinin, a vasodilator. This results in increased blood flow to the pancreas, and increased volume of secretion.

Gastric phase

Entry of food into the stomach initiates the gastric phase and is associated with approximately 10% of pancreatic secretion. Secretions induced during this phase consist mainly of enzymes suggesting a greater role for acinar cells in this phase. Activation of chemoreceptors in the walls of the stomach by peptides and the activation of mechanoreceptors causes the release of gastrin from G cells into the local circulation. Stimulation of cholinergic nerves is also involved in this phase of control.

Intestinal phase

The cephalic and gastric phases 'prime' the pancreas for the intestinal phase. In this phase, enhanced blood flow to the pancreas is established and exocrine secretion is initiated. Most of the pancreatic secretory response (50%–80%) occurs during the intestinal phase and is regulated by hormonal and neural mechanisms. Consequently, the intestinal phase of control is the most important phase of the response to food. Acid stimulates the release of secretin from S cells in the walls of the intestine and this hormone stimulates the duct cells to secrete the alkaline fluid. This is a feedback control mechanism that helps to control the pH of the duodenal contents. CCK is released from I-cell activation by proteins and fats and their partial digestion products: peptides and fatty acids. CCK stimulates the acinar cells to secrete enzymes in addition to causing gallbladder contraction and relaxation of the sphincter of Oddi. Of note, trypsin in the duodenum inhibits the release of enzymes via inhibition of CCK release. This is another feedback control mechanism, which limits the quantity of enzymes present in the intestines and may have some protective function.

Acute pancreatitis

Acute pancreatitis is a condition in which the pancreatic tissue is destroyed by digestive enzymes. Patients present with severe pain in the upper abdomen (epigastrium) which may radiate to the back. Most attacks of this acute disease (approximately 75%) are mild but in some more severe cases the condition can result in haemodynamic instability and multi-organ failure. The physiological mechanisms underlying acute pancreatitis are not completely understood. It is characterised by the presence of activated enzymes in the pancreatic ducts. The consequence of this is autodigestion of the pancreatic tissue.

In acute pancreatitis, activated trypsin in the ducts of the pancreas proteolytically activates more trypsinogen and other proteolytic enzyme precursors (chymotrypsinogen, proelastase and procarboxypeptidase) and prophospholipase A.

The active enzymes digest the pancreatic tissue. When the walls of the acini on the surface of the pancreas are digested, the enzymes leak into the abdominal cavity and a generalised peritonitis results. In 5% of cases, the condition is extremely serious, and the blood vessels are digested by pancreatic elastase resulting in internal bleeding and eventually ischaemia (due to hypotension) and anaemia. The condition is then known as haemorrhagic necrotising pancreatitis, which has an 80% mortality rate.

The exocrine pancreas produces and secretes digestive enzymes that are only activated on reaching the duodenum. However, although small amounts of trypsinogen are spontaneously activated, several mechanisms are in place to remove activated trypsin. These include binding with pancreatic secretory trypsin inhibitor (PSTI, or SPINK1) and autolysis of prematurely activated trypsin. In acute pancreatitis there is intra-acinar activation of these proteolytic enzyme which leads to pancreatic inflammation. Several mechanisms have been proposed with instability of vacuoles within the acinar cell that release large amounts of activated trypsin overwhelming normal defence mechanisms. This results in pancreatic autodigestion which in turn sets up a cycle of further activated enzymes being released from damaged cells.

Acute pancreatitis is often caused by excessive alcohol intake and gallstones that are often lodged in the biliary ducts at the ampulla of Vater and prevent the closure of the sphincter of Oddi. This process may allow duodenal juice containing activated enzymes to reflux into the pancreatic duct. Infections, pancreatic tumours, treatment with certain drugs and specific genetic defects may also have a causative role in acute pancreatitis. In relation to excess alcohol consumption, recent evidence suggest that acinar cells are able catabolise ethanol and produce acetaldehyde and fatty-acid ethyl esters, both of which are cytotoxic.

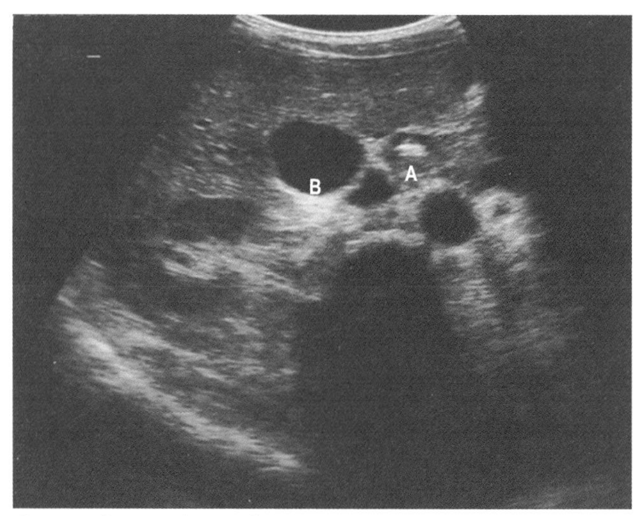

Fig. 3.8 Ultrasound scan of the biliary tree, showing a calcified stone in the common bile duct (A) which is dilated around the stone. The adjacent gallbladder is also seen (B).

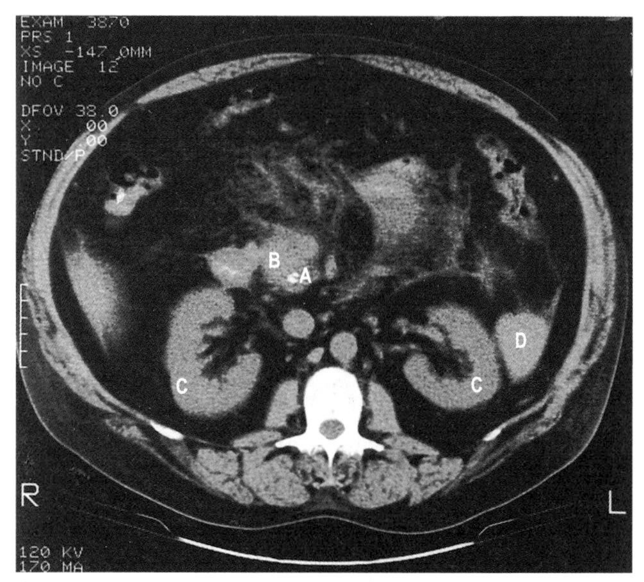

Fig. 3.9 Computed tomographic scan of the same patient as Fig. 3.8, showing the calcified stone at the lower end of the common bile duct (A) lying within the swollen head of the pancreas (B). The kidneys (C) and spleen (D) are also visible.

The diagnosis of acute pancreatitis depends on the presence of high concentrations of α-amylase in the blood. This enzyme, together with others, leaks from the lysed pancreatic cells into the blood. α-Amylase may also be present in the urine because it is not adequately reabsorbed in the kidney tubules. An ultrasound scan (Fig. 3.8) of the abdomen may reveal the presence of biliary gall stones. Computed tomography (CT) scanning (Fig. 3.9) enables the extent of necrosis to be assessed. Hypocalcaemia may also be present. This is partly due to loss of albumin, with bound Ca^{2+}, in the protein-rich exudates from the pancreas. This exudation also causes a rise in the haematocrit due to loss of plasma volume.

Case 3.2

Chronic pancreatitis

A 40-year-old man who had been a heavy drinker for many years went to see his general practitioner. He had made two previous visits over the past year complaining of recurrent episodes of abdominal pain. Although the pain had been intermittent at first, it was now continuous. The doctor ascertained that the pain originated in the epigastrium and radiated through to the back. The patient had lost a considerable amount of weight since his last visit. The doctor noticed that he was mildly jaundiced. Arrangements were made for the patient to be admitted to hospital for tests.

An X-ray examination and serum and urine analyses were performed. The patient's stools were collected over three days. These were pale-coloured and bulky, indicating a high fat content (steatorrhoea). He was told to abstain from food the next morning so that a glucose tolerance test could be performed.

The blood tests showed increased bilirubin and alkaline phosphatase. The glucose tolerance test showed an abnormally high and prolonged rise in serum glucose, and urine analysis confirmed the presence of glucose (glycosuria), indicating that the patient was diabetic. The presumptive diagnosis was chronic pancreatitis. The patient was prescribed pethidine to control the pain. He was advised to abstain completely from alcohol and to eat regular meals. Fig. 3.10 shows a CT scan of the abdomen of an individual with chronic pancreatitis.

Defect and causes

The primary malfunction in chronic pancreatitis is defective ductal secretion of bicarbonate and water, which results in a high protein concentration in the pancreatic juice in the ducts. The protein precipitates and forms plugs, with consequent dilatation of the proximal ducts. A high pressure is generated behind the blockages causing pain. Secondary back pressure may lead to disruption of the ductal epithelium and result in destruction of the pancreatic tissue. This can lead to an inflammatory and fibrotic process in and around the pancreatic tissue. This in time leads to pancreatic insufficiency due to destruction of islet cells and acinar glands. The pancreas lies close to the coeliac plexus and inflammation around these autonomic nerves results in chronic back pain.

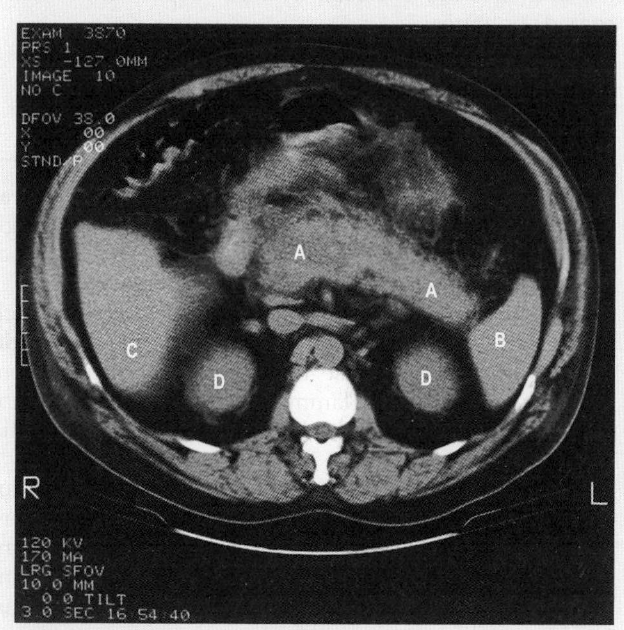

Fig. 3.10 Computed tomography: cross-section of the abdomen showing a swollen pancreas caused by pancreatitis (A) lying posteriorly on the abdominal wall. The spleen (B) and lower border of liver (C) and kidneys (D) are also seen.

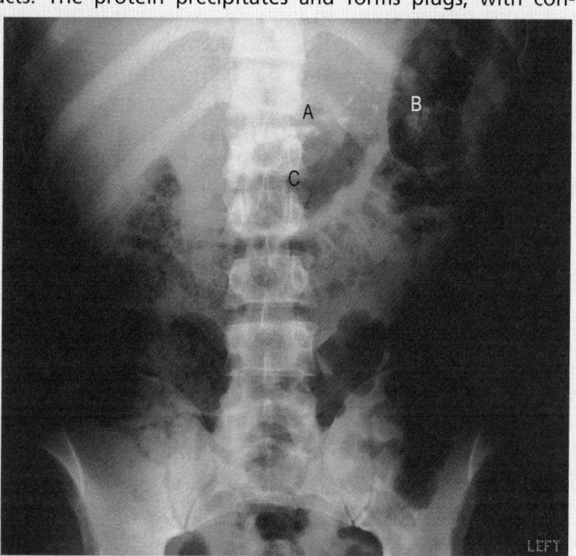

Fig. 3.11 Plain abdominal X-ray showing calcified stones in the pancreatic duct (A) from a patient with chronic pancreatitis secondary to alcoholism. Gas in the left colon (B) and overlying stomach (C) are also seen.

Chronic pancreatitis is characterised by progressive damage to the pancreas with permanent destruction of pancreatic tissue. Exocrine and endocrine pancreatic insufficiency usually follow. However, owing to the tremendous reserve of pancreatic tissue, the insufficiency may be subclinical, and tests of pancreatic function may be necessary to reveal it. The histopathology indicates irregularly distributed fibrosis, reduced number and size of islets of Langerhans, and variable obstruction of pancreatic ducts of all sizes. Protein precipitation initially occurs in the lobular and interlobular ducts, leading to the formation of plugs that calcify by surface accretion. Concentric lamellar protein precipitates appear in the major pancreatic ducts, and these also calcify to form stones. A specific protein, called stone protein, a normal constituent of pancreatic juice, which has a high affinity for Ca^{2+}, is the major protein present in the stones. The calculi contain calcium bicarbonate or hydroxyapatite (calcium phosphate and calcium bicarbonate). The stones can be seen in X-rays (Fig. 3.11). The chronic inflammation may extend to adjacent organs, including the duodenum, common bile duct, stomach antrum and transverse colon.

Acute pancreatitis can occasionally lead to complications such acute fluid collections, pseudocyst formation, and necrosis. Treatment of acute pancreatitis is primarily supportive and removal of the initiating cause such as alcohol or an obstructing gallstone. Patients require strict fluid replacement in view of excessive fluid losses, enteral or parenteral feeding and occasionally antibiotics. In some cases, patients may develop multi-organ failure requiring organ support in an intensive care unit during the period of recovery.

There is a history of excessive alcohol intake in up to 80% of patients with chronic pancreatitis but there are rare autosomal dominant inherited forms and autoimmune pathologies for the disease. The incidence of the disease is low, being approximately 56/100,000 per year in the UK. Onset is usually in middle aged. The disease is approximately 3 times more common in males than females. Most patients with alcohol dependency already have sustained permanent structural and functional damage to the pancreas by the time of their first attack of abdominal pain. Moreover, morphological changes are evident at post-mortem examination in many alcoholics who had no symptoms of pancreatic disease during life. Removal of the causative factor leading to development of pancreatitis (such as alcohol) is one of the mainstays in preventing further damage to the pancreas. Treatment of chronic pancreatitis is in the form of pain control, treatment of pancreatic insufficiency by replacement of exocrine pancreatic enzymes and any resultant vitamin deficiencies that may ensue.

Impairment of functions

Both exocrine and endocrine secretions of the pancreas are impaired in chronic pancreatitis. The blockage of the secretory ducts and loss of acinar tissue lead to a decrease in both alkaline juice and enzymes. The reduced alkaline secretion leads to: (1) reduced activity of enzymes in the small intestine which results in malabsorption and weight loss, (2) impaired micelle formation (essential for adequate lipid absorption) which leads to steatorrhoea, and (3) possibly duodenal ulceration because of the high acidity.

Destruction of islet tissue can lead to decreased secretion of insulin and glucagon, which are both involved in the control of glucose metabolism. Insulin lowers the blood glucose by increasing the uptake of glucose into tissues whilst glucagon increases blood glucose by stimulating glucose release from the liver. Thus, the two hormones have opposite effects on blood glucose concentration, although the effect of insulin is dominant.

Insulin is normally released from the pancreas in response to an increase in blood glucose concentration during a meal. The glucose tolerance test measures the insulin response to ingestion of a glucose solution. The insulin response is impaired early in chronic pancreatitis, that is, the time taken for the increased blood glucose to return to normal is prolonged. Overt diabetes eventually develops in many patients.

Physiological consequences, treatment and management

The main consequences of malabsorption and diabetes mellitus are malnutrition and weight loss. Lack of alkaline secretion can lead to alkalosis because the 'alkaline tide' in the blood which results from gastric acid secretion during a meal (see Chapter 2) is normally partially neutralised by the 'acid' tide resulting from the secretion of alkaline juice by the pancreas. However, in chronic pancreatitis, the alkalosis is normally compensated by respiratory and renal mechanisms.

Treatment is usually non-surgical in uncomplicated chronic pancreatitis. The need for complete abstention from alcohol is emphasised. Pain relief is initially via treatment with a non-steroidal anti-inflammatory drug (NSAID) such as aspirin, and then, if necessary, via opiates. Nutritional support in the form of simple nutrients (amino acids, glucose, fatty acids) may be advised. Oral pancreatic extract can be prescribed to replace the pancreatic enzymes. Usually, the extract is enriched with lipase as the secretion of this enzyme tends to decrease more rapidly than that of proteolytic enzymes. The enzyme preparation can be administered together with an acid suppressant since acid will inactivate the enzymes. Alternatively, the enzymes can be administered in the form of granules within which the enzymes are enclosed in a pH-dependent (enteric coated) polymer.

Pancreatic and digestive diseases associated with diabetes mellitus

High blood sugars may be a presenting or prominent feature of some digestive and pancreatic diseases. Although these are primarily GI disorders, they can lead to destruction of the islet cells which produce and secrete insulin.

These include some classical pancreatic problems such as after pancreatic surgery. Clinicians may need to begin insulin treatment almost immediately post-operation. Similarly, pancreatic inflammation (pancreatitis) or neoplasia (tumours) may result in severe hyperglycaemia needing insulin.

A common genetic condition is haemochromatosis which affects both the liver and pancreas. There are autoimmune causes of diabetes (called late-onset autoimmune diabetes in adults, or LADA) which are more common in patients with autoimmune conditions of the gut (such as coeliac disease, pernicious anaemia, or autoimmune hepatitis).

Therefore, the digestive disease symptoms together with a high sugar should lead to a suspicion of insulin deficiency caused by one of these underlying conditions.

Pancreatic cancer

Pancreatic cancer is the 10th most common cancer in the UK, accounting for 3% of all new cancer cases with approximately 10,000 new cases diagnosed annually. Similar to other cancers, it is predominantly a disease of the aged with approximately half of all cases diagnosed in people aged 75 and over. Alarmingly, the incidence of pancreatic cancer has increased by approximately 10% in the UK over the last decade. There is some evidence to suggest that a subset of pancreatic cancers are associated with deprivation and more common in White and Black people than in Asian people. While it is the 10th most common cancer, it is the 6th most common cause of cancer death in the UK, accounting for 6% of all cancer deaths. Pancreatic cancer has an approximate 7% 5-year survival which exemplifies the aggressive nature of the disease and the fact that it tends to present very late in the disease progression when curative treatment is not feasible in the majority.

Risk factors

The estimated lifetime risk of being diagnosed with pancreatic cancer is approximately 2% and is associated with tobacco smoking (2.2-fold increased risk compared to never-smokers) and being overweight or obese (12% of all pancreatic cancers are caused by being overweight or obese). Other lifestyle factors which have been linked to the development of pancreatic cancer are alcohol and red or processed meat. Thus, unsurprisingly, approximately one-third of all pancreatic cancers are thought to be preventable. The disease is also associated with a family history and a variety of genetic factors. It is predicted that risk of pancreatic cancer is approximately 70% higher in people with a first-degree relative with the disease and 45% higher in individuals with a first-degree relative with prostate cancer. Other diseases which are linked to pancreatic cancer include Peutz-Jeghers syndrome (100-fold higher risk), familial atypical multiple mole melanoma syndrome (10%–40% higher risk), and hereditary non-polyposis colorectal cancer (nine-fold higher risk). Other genetic aberrations which are associated with pancreatic cancer include BRCA1 and BRCA2 mutations.

Surgical resection

Resection of the pancreas is a technically challenging procedure carried out both for inflammatory diseases of the pancreas (pancreatitis) and for pancreatic cancer.

Case 3.3 Pancreatic cancer

A 58-year-old man presented to his general practitioner with a 4-month history of chronic upper abdominal pain. He reports losing two stone in weight unintentionally over this period. More recently, he also noticed yellowing of his sclera. He is otherwise well and denies any significant past medical history. He smokes 20 cigarettes a day and has done so over the last 10 years. On examination, his abdomen was soft and non-tender with no palpable masses. His blood tests revealed elevated bilirubin and deranged liver enzymes. A CT scan was requested, and this revealed a tumour rising from the head of his pancreas with some associated lymphadenopathy suggestive of pancreatic cancer. The tumour had caused a degree of obstruction to his common bile duct resulting in his jaundice. He was referred to the hospital where after further evaluation he underwent a Whipple procedure (pancreaticoduodenectomy); an operation to remove the head of the pancreas, duodenum, gallbladder and bile duct. He remained on surveillance follow-up to identify early recurrence of cancer.

Most pancreatic tumours arise in the head of the pancreas. When they are diagnosed at an early stage they can be treated successfully by removal of the head and neck of the pancreas. Because the pancreas receives a joint blood supply with the duodenum, it is safer to remove the duodenum together with the head of the organ. This requires the common bile duct, tail of the pancreas and stomach to be re-joined with a loop of jejunum. Safely joining the bowel to the pancreas is a hazardous procedure. This is partly because the tissue of the pancreas is soft and friable but also because activated digestive enzymes released from the pancreas interfere with the healing process at the anastomosis. Following this major procedure, patients will have impaired fat and protein metabolism. This is not usually due to insufficient pancreatic secretion, but rather to premature stomach emptying without coordinated secretion from the pancreas and liver. It can be partially overcome by preservation of the pyloric sphincter (pylorus-preserving Whipple's procedure).

Total pancreatectomy is in one respect a safer operation because anastomosis to the remaining pancreas is not required. It does, however, involve the loss of all endocrine and exocrine secretions from the pancreas. For satisfactory digestion of food, it is necessary to add pancreatic enzyme supplements to the diet. In addition, these patients are diabetic, and because there is loss of both insulin and glucagon, control of their diabetes is especially difficult, sometimes referred to as brittle diabetes.

LIVER AND BILIARY SYSTEM

4

Chapter objectives and clinical presentations

After reading this chapter, review your learning by considering the following:

1. Can you describe the role of the liver in the digestive process and the excretion of waste metabolites and toxic substances?
2. What is the relationship between the structure of the hepatobiliary tract and its function in the secretion and storage of bile?
3. Can you detail the mechanisms of secretion of the important components of bile and their recycling via the enterohepatic circulation?
4. Do you understand the mechanisms of control of bile secretion and its release into the duodenum?

Also, you should be familiar with the following clinical presentations:

- Alcoholic liver disease
- Drug overdose (Paracetamol)
- Jaundice
- Gallstone disease

Clinical outlook

Common presentations with liver and biliary disease include jaundice, abnormal liver enzyme tests, abdominal pain and swelling of the abdomen. Patients with liver disease may present with acute liver failure from viral hepatitis, paracetamol overdose, chronic liver disease secondary to chronic alcohol use or autoimmune liver disease. Patients with biliary disease may present with gallstones with obstruction of their biliary tree or gallbladder, or biliary cancer (cholangiocarcinoma).

Introduction

The numerous functions of the liver can be divided into two categories:

1. The processing of absorbed substances and synthetic reactions, and
2. Processes of secretion and excretion.

This chapter is concerned with the secretory and excretory roles of the liver. The most important exocrine functions of the liver are:

- The provision of bile acids and alkaline fluid for the digestion and absorption of fats, and for the neutralisation of gastric acid in the intestines;
- The degradation and conjugation of waste products of metabolism;
- The detoxification of poisonous substances; and
- The excretion of waste metabolites and detoxified substances in bile.
- Detoxified substances and waste metabolites are eliminated from the body either in the bile, via the gastrointestinal (GI) tract, or via secretion from the liver into the blood for subsequent excretion by the kidneys.

The liver has an enormous functional reserve capacity and therefore the clinical manifestation of liver disease implies considerable damage to the organ.

Within this chapter the functions of the liver are outlined through 3 clinical cases: alcoholic liver disease, paracetamol overdose and gallstone disease.

Overview of the functioning of the hepatobiliary system

The anatomical arrangement of the liver, gallbladder and biliary tract is shown in Fig. 4.1. The liver is continually secreting substances both into the blood and into the bile. Bile is both a secretory fluid and an excretory medium.

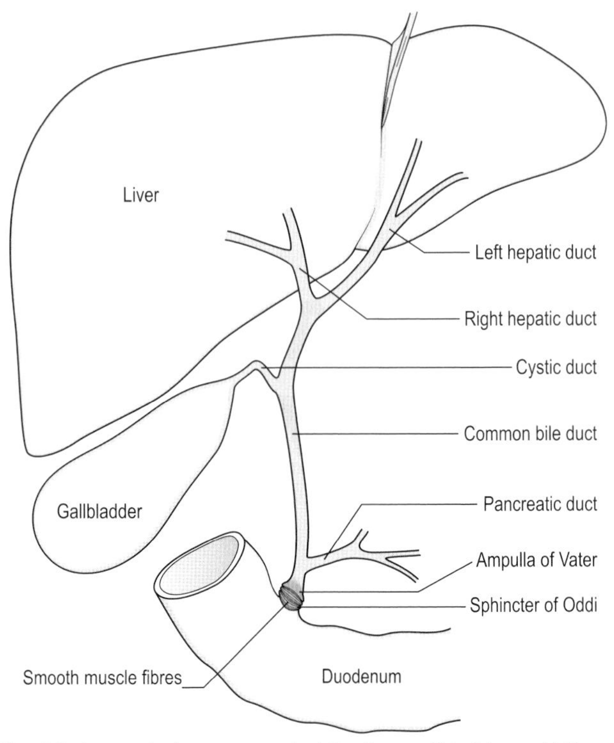

Fig. 4.1 Anatomical arrangement of the liver, gallbladder and biliary tract.

In humans, it is stored between meals in the gallbladder, where it is concentrated. The most common location for gallstones and thus gallstone-related disease is the gallbladder. During a meal, bile is released from the gallbladder into the cystic duct which drains into the common bile duct. The bile enters the small intestine at the level of the duodenum. Its entry into the small intestine is controlled by a smooth muscle sphincter called the sphincter of Oddi.

The gallbladder is surrounded by smooth muscle. Between meals, when the gallbladder smooth muscle is relaxed, the sphincter of Oddi is closed, preventing the bile from entering the small intestine. Consequently, the bile passes into the gallbladder where it is stored and concentrated. Contraction of the gallbladder forces the bile into the common bile duct. At the same time, the smooth muscle in the sphincter of Oddi relaxes, and the sphincter opens to allow the bile to enter the duodenum. Food in the duodenum is the main stimulus for gallbladder contraction. Food, predominantly fat in the lumen of the duodenum, stimulates cholecystokinin (CCK) release from I cells which in turn triggers gallbladder contraction.

Anatomy and morphology of the liver

The liver is the largest single organ in the body. It accounts for approximately 2%–3% of average body weight in adults. It consists of right and left lobes (Fig. 4.2A), the right lobe being 6 times the size of the left in the adult.

The liver is composed of lobules (Fig. 4.2B). In the centre of each lobule is the central canal, in which lies a hepatic vein, which is a tributary of the inferior vena cava. Columns of liver cells (hepatocytes) and sinusoids radiate out from the central canal. Several portal tracts lie at the periphery of each lobule. Each tract (or 'portal triad') contains a bile duct, a branch of the portal vein and a branch of the hepatic artery.

The liver has a double blood supply: the hepatic artery supplies the liver with oxygenated blood from the lungs and the portal vein supplies it with nutrient-rich blood from the intestines. The arterial blood and portal venous blood comprise approximately 20% and 80%, respectively, of the total blood supply of the liver. The arterial blood and the portal venous blood mix together in the liver sinusoids. The sinusoidal blood drains away via the hepatic veins to the vena cava. This direction of flow is determined by the relatively higher pressure of the blood in the portal vein compared to the central vein.

In liver cirrhosis, scar tissue replaces normal healthy tissue. This scar tissue distorts the normal structure and regrowth of liver cells and blocks the flow of blood through the organ.

The liver is covered by a fibroconnective tissue capsule known as the capsule of Glisson, from which thin connective tissue septa enter the organ to divide it into lobes and lobules. The capsule is covered by peritoneum, except in an area known as the 'bare area' which is in direct contact with the diaphragm.

The secretory system of the liver begins with minute tubules, called the canaliculi. These are formed by oppositely aligned grooves in the contact surfaces of adjacent hepatocytes (Figs. 4.2C and 4.3). The membrane of each liver cell contributes to several bile canaliculi. Bile secreted into the canaliculi flows in the opposite direction to the flow of blood in the sinusoids. The canaliculi drain into terminal bile ductules. The ductules converge to form intralobular ducts, and these converge to form interlobular ducts, which in turn converge to form the right and left hepatic bile ducts. These converge outside the liver to form the common hepatic bile duct.

Histology

The major type of cell in the liver is the hepatocyte that is an epithelial parenchymal cell. The hepatocytes are arranged in plates which branch and anastomose to form a three-dimensional lattice (Fig. 4.2). Between the plates are the blood-filled sinusoids. In this respect, the liver resembles an endocrine gland. There is usually only one layer of hepatocytes between the sinusoids.

The sinusoidal spaces differ from blood capillaries in that they are of greater diameter and their lining cells are not typically endothelial. The basal lamina around the sinusoids is incomplete and this enables direct access of the plasma to the surface of the hepatocyte. This allows

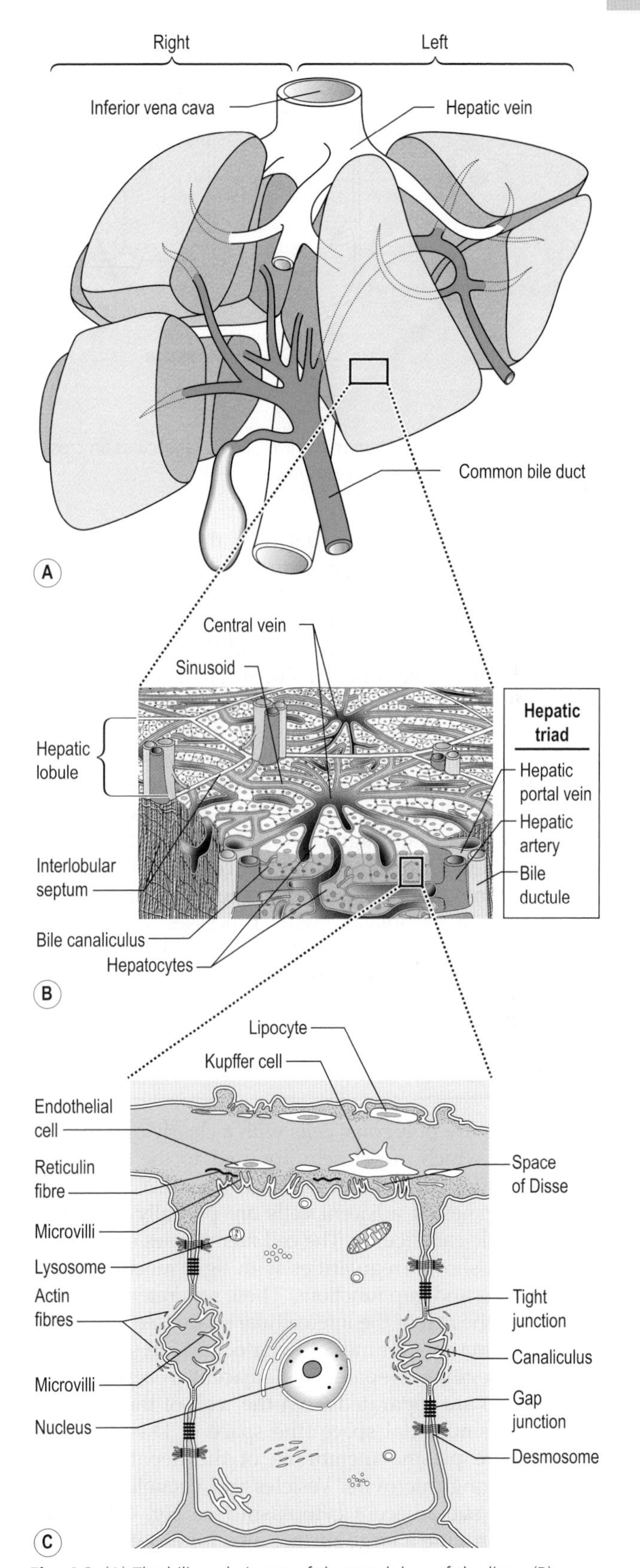

Fig. 4.2 (A) The biliary drainage of the two lobes of the liver. (B) Lobular structure of the liver, illustrating the biliary secretory system and the dual blood supply. (C) Features of the hepatocyte, and its relationship to adjacent cells and the sinusoid.

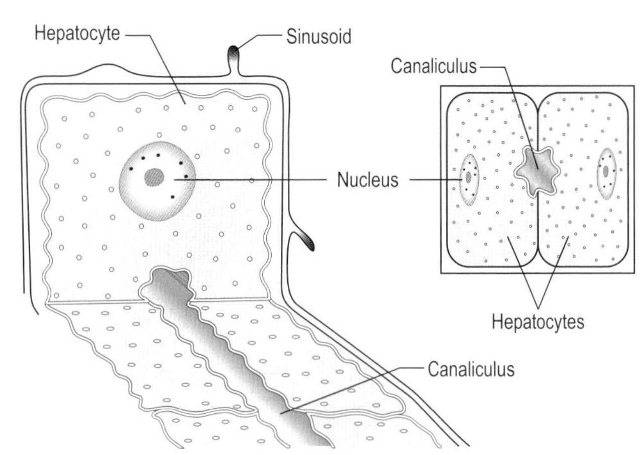

Fig. 4.3 Early secretory system of the liver. Inset: canaliculus (in cross-section) formed by adjacent hepatocytes.

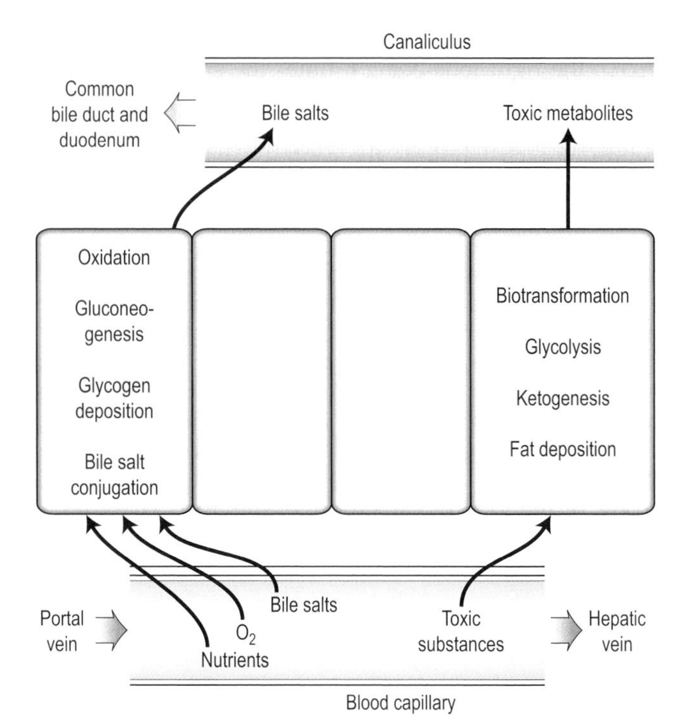

Fig. 4.4 Major functions of periportal and perivenous hepatocytes.

active metabolic exchange between the blood and the cells (see Fig. 4.2C). The perisinusoidal space is an interstitial space that contains reticular and collagenous fibres. The two main cell types are present in the sinusoidal lining are endothelial cells and Kupffer cells. They lie in a mesh of fine reticular fibres. The endothelial cell has small, elongated nuclei and greatly attenuated cytoplasm. The cytoplasm may interdigitate with cytoplasmic processes from adjacent cells of the same type or another type. They contain few organelles but numerous pinocytotic vesicles. They also contain large fenestrae that are not closed by a diaphragm. Kupffer cells are phagocytic and often contain degenerating red cells, pigment granules and iron-containing granules. They have large nuclei and extensive cytoplasm, with processes that extend into, and sometimes across, the sinusoidal space. They increase in number when required for phagocytosis, possibly by differentiation of the endothelial type of cell.

Hepatocytes

Hepatocytes are polygonal cells with a clearly defined cell membrane, which are closely apposed to the cell membranes of adjacent hepatocytes (see Figs. 4.2C and 4.3). The membranes of adjacent cells are partially separated to form a bile canaliculus. The cell membranes of adjacent hepatocytes show irregularities with tight junctions, spot desmosomes and gap junctions. These separate the canaliculus from the rest of the intercellular space (see Fig. 4.2C).

The plasma membranes of hepatocytes are specialised in certain regions. Hepatocytes adjacent to a sinusoidal blood space are separated from the wall of the sinusoid by the perisinusoidal space (the space of Disse); at this location, the plasma membrane of the hepatocyte has numerous long microvilli. Vesicles and vacuoles are present in the sub-adjacent cytoplasm (see Fig. 4.2C). The microvilli provide a large surface area for absorption and secretion.

The nuclei in different hepatocytes vary considerably in shape and size and the cells are binucleate in some cases. Clumps of basophilic material are present in all cells. There are numerous small mitochondria throughout the cytoplasm of the hepatocyte. The structure of all hepatocytes is broadly similar, but the cytoplasm of the cells shows a gradual variation with the distance of the cell from the periphery. The differences are related to the differences in functional activity of the peripherally and centrally positioned cells. The hepatocytes closest to the afferent blood supply, the 'periportal' cells, are exposed to the highest concentrations of nutrients and oxygen, whereas those in the central region, the 'perivenous' cells near to the efferent outflow, are exposed to the lowest concentrations. The periportal cells are the most active in the uptake from the blood of bile salts and in the secretion of many bile constituents into the canaliculi as well as in oxidative metabolism and gluconeogenesis (Fig. 4.4).

After feeding, glycogen is deposited first in the periportal cells. It is only after a carbohydrate-rich meal that the more centrally located perivenous cells store glycogen. Moreover, when the blood sugar concentration falls, glycogen is removed first from the perivenous cells. The perivenous cells, which are exposed to depleted plasma, are the more active in biotransformation reactions and the secretion of potentially toxic xenobiotic and endobiotic substances. They are also more active in glycolytic and ketogenic reactions. Under certain conditions, fat is deposited in the hepatocytes, and it appears first in the more centrally disposed cells. Thus the cytosol of a given hepatocyte exhibits differences in composition at different times in relation to feeding and whether fat or glycogen has been deposited.

The canaliculus

The lumen of the canaliculus is approximately 0.75 µm in diameter. Microvilli project from the canalicular membrane into the lumen, providing a large surface area for secretion. Membranes of adjacent hepatocytes are joined by tight junctions near the canaliculus (see Fig. 4.2C). These junctions are leaky and permit paracellular exchange between the plasma and the canaliculus.

The canaliculus is involved in transport of substances into the lumen, but it is also a contractile structure. Actin filaments are present in the microvilli, and both actin and myosin fibres are present in the cytoplasm surrounding the canaliculus. Contractions of the canaliculi can be stimulated by extracellular ATP. The contractions involve actin–myosin interaction as in smooth muscle cells. They probably pump bile towards the ducts. Atony (lack of contractile function) of the canaliculus causes cholestasis (reduced bile flow).

The junctions of the bile canaliculus with the bile ducts at the periphery of a lobule consist of an intermediate structure called the ductules or canals of Hering. Here, the hepatocytes that form the canaliculus are gradually replaced by smaller cells with dark nuclei and poorly developed organelles. These are the ductule cells which are in direct contact with the basal lamina. The lumen of the ductule eventually joins that of a bile duct in the portal area.

Extrahepatic ducts

The extrahepatic ducts are lined by tall columnar epithelium that secretes mucus. There is a layer of connective tissue beneath the epithelium, with numerous elastic fibres, mucous glands, blood vessels and nerves. In the common bile duct there is also a layer of smooth muscle cells. These cells are sparse in the upper region of the duct but form a thicker layer of oblique and transverse fibres in the regions of the sphincter of Oddi (also known as the hepatopancreatic sphincter) near the duodenum (see below).

Liver cirrhosis

In cirrhosis of the liver, scar tissue replaces normal healthy tissue and blocks the flow of blood from the portal vein through the organ. This leads to reduced synthesis of proteins and other molecules by the liver and reduced oxidative capacity. Metabolism of bile constituents, drug detoxification and secretion and excretion of bile constituents become inadequate to maintain health.

Causes of liver cirrhosis

- Chronic alcoholism. This is the primary cause of liver cirrhosis in the Western world.
- Chronic hepatitis C, B or D. Hepatitis C virus causes low-grade damage, which over the course of many years can lead to cirrhosis. This is a major cause of liver cirrhosis. It was commonly transmitted by blood transfusion before routine testing for hepatitis C virus was available. Hepatitis B virus is the most common cause of liver cirrhosis in developing countries but is less common in more developed countries.
- Autoimmune disease. The immune system attacks the liver, causing inflammation and tissue damage which can eventually lead to cirrhosis. These conditions include autoimmune hepatitis and primary sclerosing cholangitis.
- Inherited diseases including α1-antitrypsin deficiency, haemochromatosis, Wilson's disease, galactosaemia and glycogen storage diseases.
- Drugs, toxins and infections. Severe reactions to prescription drugs, prolonged exposure to environmental toxins and parasitic infection (with schistosomes) can also cause liver cirrhosis.

Clinical management

The signs and symptoms of liver cirrhosis include fatigue, weight loss, nausea, abdominal pain, spider-like blood vessels on the skin, oedema of the legs and abdomen (ascites), jaundice, gallstones, itching (due to bilirubin being deposited in the skin) and a tendency to bleed easily (due to reduced clotting factor synthesis in the liver).

The treatment of liver cirrhosis depends on the cause of the condition and the complications experienced. The damage cannot be reversed but the progression of the disease can be arrested or delayed by cessation of alcohol abuse or medication to treat infections and other causes. When liver damage is so pronounced that the liver stops functioning, a transplant is necessary. The survival rate after liver transplantation is over 90% now that effective immunosuppressive drugs are available.

Bile

Composition and functions

Bile is secreted at a rate of 250–1000 mL/day in the adult. It is isosmotic with blood plasma. It is a composite of two different secretions: one originating in the hepatocytes, and the other in the cells that line the bile ducts (Fig. 4.5). The two secretions mix in the ducts.

Secretion of the duct cells

The secretion from the duct cells is a watery alkaline fluid that is rich in bicarbonate. It comprises approximately

Case 4.1 Alcoholic liver disease

A 54-year-old man presented to the acute medical unit with a 3-week history of progressive jaundice and abdominal swelling. He reported consuming over 80 units of alcohol a week for the last 3–4 years after losing his employment. He was unkempt, appeared tremulous on examination and was visibly jaundiced with evidence of fluid in his abdomen (ascites). His blood tests revealed elevated bilirubin and prothrombin time, and low albumin. He underwent an ultrasound scan of his abdomen, and this revealed a shrunken liver, a large spleen and a large amount of free fluid in his abdomen. His serological liver screen ruled out viral, autoimmune and other metabolic causes of liver disease. A diagnosis of alcoholic liver disease was made. On admission, he was commenced on intravenous vitamin B compounds, an alcohol detoxification regimen, diuretics and appropriate nutrition. Fluid from his abdomen was sent for further analysis. He underwent an upper GI endoscopy, and this revealed that he had multiple dilated veins in his oesophagus – known as oesophageal varices. He was started on a beta-blocker to prevent these from bleeding. He was strongly advised not to drink alcohol and was discharged home once stable with plans for outpatient following.

Excessive alcohol intake can be associated with several manifestations in the liver including cirrhosis and alcoholic hepatitis. Patients with an intake of 30 or more grams per day of alcohol are at increased risk of cirrhosis. However, unfortunately, most patients at presentation would have already developed fairly advanced liver disease with these presentations often being a result of a complication of their liver disease, such as variceal bleeding. Patients may present with various symptoms including fatigue, weight loss, nausea, abdominal pain, spider-like blood vessels on the skin, ascites, gallstones and jaundice. Laboratory tests that should be obtained in patients with suspected alcoholic liver disease include liver enzymes, bilirubin, albumin, coagulation studies and a full blood count. If ascites is present, patients should undergo an ascitic tap (diagnostic paracentesis) to confirm that the ascites is due to portal hypertension (serum-to-ascites albumin gradient ≥11 g/L) and rule out evidence of spontaneous bacterial peritonitis. Further tests should be done to rule out other causes of liver disease as described earlier.

Pharmacologic options for alcoholic liver disease are limited. Therefore, avoidance of alcohol remains the primary form of treatment and its ongoing use is an important risk factor for progression of liver disease. Treatment goals including ensuring abstinence from alcohol is established and maintained, liver function is stabilised and complications such as varices and hepatocellular carcinoma are appropriately investigated and managed. Liver transplantation is an option in appropriately selected patients with advanced liver disease and alcoholic liver disease remains one for the leading indications for transplantation in the Western world.

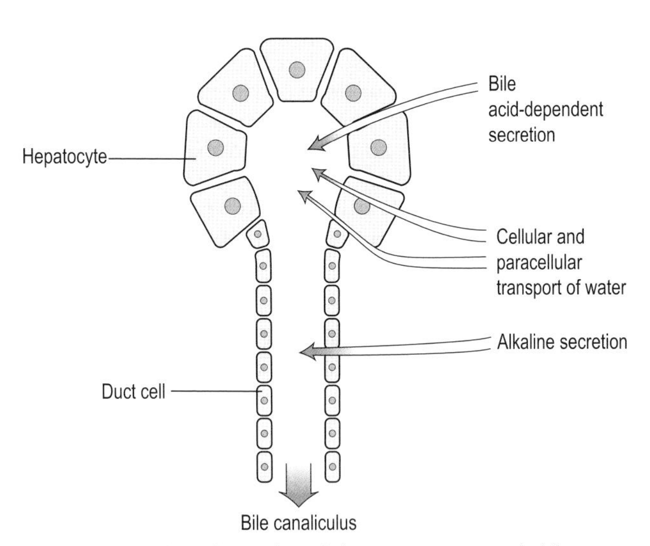

Fig. 4.5 Sites of secretion of the two components in bile.

25% of the total bile volume. Its function is, first, to provide an appropriate pH for the process of micelle formation (see below), which requires a neutral or slightly alkaline environment. Second, it contributes (together with pancreatic juice and intestinal secretions) to the neutralisation of stomach acid in the intestinal chyme. This is important both for micelle formation and digestive enzyme action in the small intestine. In combination with the alkaline pancreatic secretions, bile assists the neutralisation of acid in the duodenum and protects the mucosa from ulceration. The secretion contains Na^+, K^+, Cl^- and HCO_3^- ions. Its composition is similar to that of alkaline pancreatic juice. At basal rates of secretion, the ionic composition resembles that of plasma. However, as the flow increases upon stimulation (by a meal), the Cl^- concentration decreases and the HCO_3^- concentration increases. This is due to the presence of a Cl^-/HCO_3^- exchange mechanism in the duct cells. At high flow rates, the bile is not in contact with the duct cells for sufficient time, and consequently, less bicarbonate is reabsorbed from the bile, resulting in a more alkaline solution. Thus, the secretion becomes more alkaline at flow rates higher than the basal level.

The volume of the alkaline secretion, unlike the secretion produced by the hepatocytes, is not directly determined by the concentration of bile salts in the blood. It has been termed the 'bile acid-independent' component of bile. The control of this secretion during a meal, like that of alkaline pancreatic juice and the alkaline fluid secreted from Brunner's glands in the duodenum, is via the release into the blood of the hormone secretin from the walls of the duodenum. This occurs mainly in response to the presence of acid in the duodenum. The hormone circulates to stimulate all these alkaline secretions. As it is released in response to acid chyme in the duodenum, this mechanism provides feedback control of the pH of the intestinal contents.

Secretion from the hepatocytes

The hepatocytes secrete a primary juice into the canaliculi. It contains several inorganic monovalent and divalent ions, and various organic substances. The latter include lipids, bile acids, lecithin and cholesterol, all of which are sequestered together in micelles. Bile secretion is a major route whereby cholesterol is lost from the body. The bile acids are essential for the effective digestion and absorption of dietary fats. There are also some proteins in bile, including albumin, polymeric immunoglobulin A (pIgA) that protects the biliary tract and the upper intestines from infection and some plasma-derived enzymes. Bile also contains bile pigments, chiefly bilirubin, that have been conjugated with glucuronic acid. The pigments are breakdown products of haemoglobin. Bile also contains numerous other compounds that are extracted from the blood, metabolised by the liver and excreted. Many of these substances are potentially toxic endogenous or exogenous substances such as steroid hormones, drugs and environmental toxins that have been detoxified and conjugated in the liver. Conjugation serves to increase the polarity of a substance and therefore its solubility in water (see below). Bile remains isosmotic with plasma at different rates of flow. This implies that an increase in secretion of bile acids and metabolites by the liver is accompanied by an increase in water secretion resulting in an increase in bile volume. This is known as the choleretic effect.

Biliary lipids

The structures of the major lipids present in bile are shown in Fig. 4.6.

Bile acids are derivatives of cholesterol. One, two or three alcohol groups are attached to a nucleus with a short hydrocarbon chain ending in a carboxyl group (see Fig. 4.6). Primary bile acids (cholic acid and chenodeoxycholic acid) are synthesised by the hepatocytes. Secondary bile acids (deoxycholic acid and lithocholic acid) are formed by dehydroxylation of primary bile acids in the intestines by bacteria (see Fig. 4.6). Bile acids are usually conjugated in hepatocytes with amino acids, largely glycine or taurine. The conjugated primary and secondary bile acids are reabsorbed actively in the ileum. However, bile acids may be deconjugated by bacteria in the small intestine and colon. Some of the unconjugated bile acids are absorbed by passive diffusion. Bile acids synthesised de novo in the liver and absorbed unconjugated bile acids are reconjugated in the liver. In physiological fluids, bile acids form salts with Na^+ and K^+ ions.

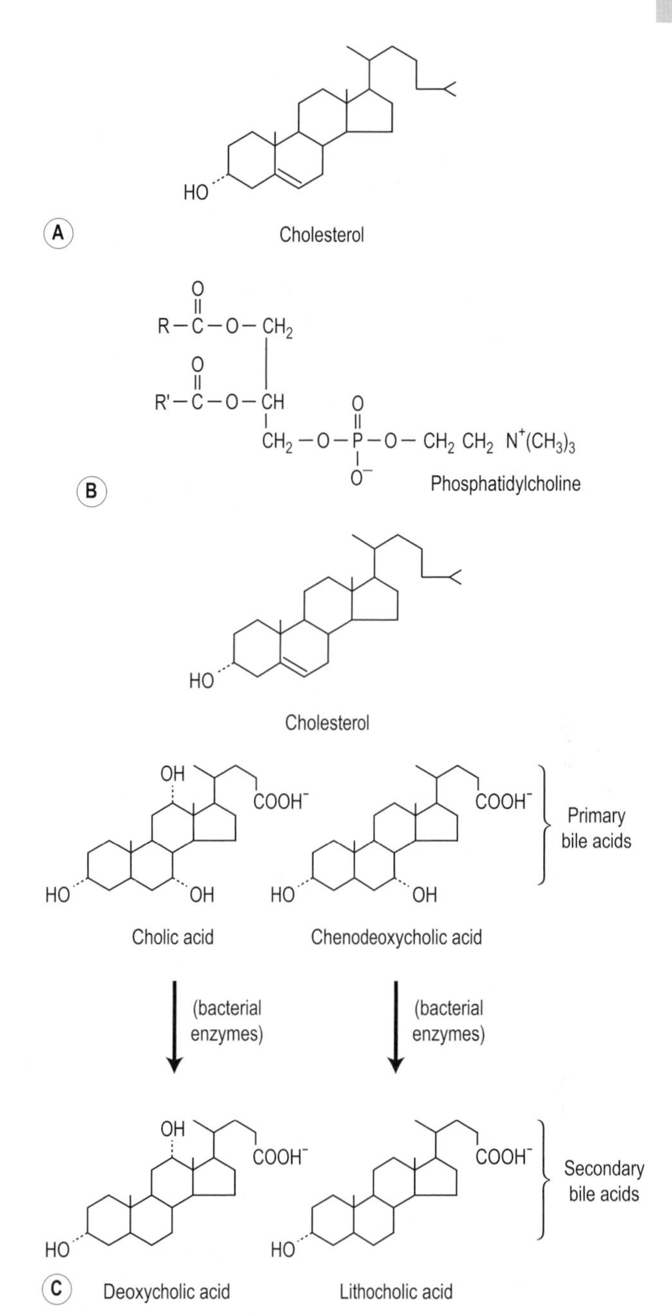

Fig. 4.6 (A) Structure of primary and secondary bile acids and their modification by intestinal bacteria. (B) Structure of phosphatidylcholine (R, palmitic acid; R9, oleic or linoleic acid). (C) Structure of cholesterol.

Uptake of bile salts from the blood into the hepatocyte is an active process that occurs against a concentration gradient (Fig. 4.7). This process derives its energy from a Na^+/K^+-ATPase that pumps Na^+ out of the cell and involves a Na^+/bile salt cotransporter system located in the sinusoidal membrane. The process is driven by the electrochemical gradient for Na^+ set up by the pumping out of Na^+ ions. This sodium-dependent uptake of bile salts utilises the Na^+-taurocholate co-transporting polypeptide, localised in hepatocytes. A mechanism independent of sodium involves polypeptides that transport organic anions. The different bile salts compete,

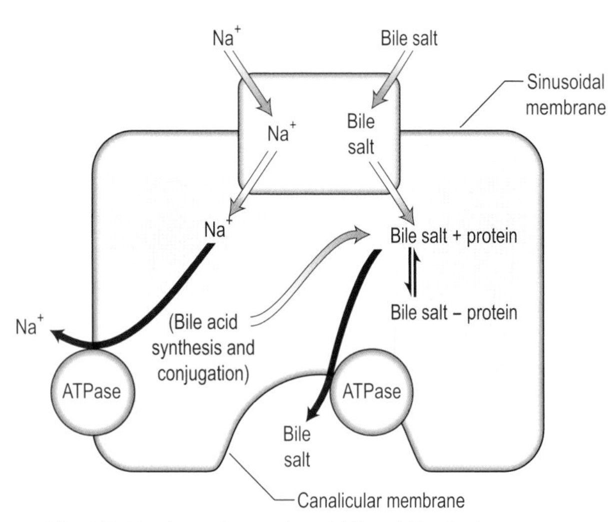

Fig. 4.7 Uptake and secretion of bile acid in the hepatocyte.

indicating that they share the same transporter. Inside hepatocytes, the bile salts bind to protein, thereby keeping the intracellular concentration of free bile salts low. These proteins may be involved in transport of the bile acids through the cell.

Bile salts are secreted into the canaliculus against a considerable electrochemical gradient. The transport across the canalicular membrane is Na^+-independent. The energy may be partly derived from the membrane potential which is approximately 40 mV (negative inside the cell), but an ATPase-dependent pump that is specific for bile acids is present in the canalicular membrane and this is the major mechanism for bile salt transport across this membrane (see Fig. 4.7). It is distinct from the Na^+ gradient-driven bile acid uptake transporter in the sinusoidal membrane.

Bile acids are held in micelles in bile. They can be concentrated several-fold in hepatocyte bile when they are still held in micellar form. Bile acids are powerful detergents, and their sequestration in micelles may reduce their detergent and cytotoxic actions.

The major phospholipid in bile is a phosphatidylcholine (lecithin). The rate of secretion of phospholipids and cholesterols appears to be linearly related to the rate of bile salt secretion. Bile salts are secreted into the canaliculus. The ratio of cholesterols to phospholipids is fairly constant (approximately 0.3 in humans). Some biliary phospholipids and cholesterols are present in bile in vesicles. These vesicles can incorporate bile salts and are gradually converted to micelles.

Micelle formation

Bile salts are essential for the formation of micelles in bile. The bile salt molecule is amphiphilic. The roughly planar ring system is hydrophobic and forms one side of the molecule. The alcohol groups, the carboxyl group and the peptide bond of the bile acid all project from the other side, imparting a net negative charge and therefore a hydrophilic nature to that side of the molecule (Fig. 4.8).

A micelle has a hydrophilic shell region and a hydrophobic core region. Newly formed (primary) micelles are initially composed of bile salt molecules. The bile salts orientate themselves in the micelle with the hydrophobic side in the core and the hydrophilic side in the shell (see Fig. 4.8). Primary micelles can sequester very little cholesterol. However, they take up phospholipids to form mixed micelles. Phosphatidylcholine is also an amphiphilic molecule: the long chain fatty acyl chains form the hydrophobic domain that resides in the core region of the micelle and the phosphorylcholine group forms the hydrophilic domain which projects into the shell region (see Fig. 4.8). Mixed micelles can hold more cholesterol than primary micelles. Larger micelles tend to form in the presence of phosphatidylcholine than in its absence. It is therefore known as a 'swelling' amphiphile. Cholesterol, which is extremely insoluble in water, resides in the core of the micelle. As the net charge on all micelles is negative, they repel each other, thereby preventing coalescence and inducing the formation of a stable suspension. The negatively charged micelle collects an outer shell of cations, mainly Na^+ ions. Micelles are disc-shaped, and their thickness approximates that of a lipid bilayer.

If the concentration of bile acids is too low for micelles to form, cholesterol precipitates out and gallstones form. Properties that influence the behaviour of bile salts towards micelle formation include temperature, concentration and pH. Consequently, the pH of the lumen of the duodenum is important for both enzymatic activity and micelle formation.

Micelle formation determines the volume of bile secreted. An individual micelle may be composed of 20 or so molecules of lipid but constitutes only one osmotic particle. Thus, a simple chemical analysis of the composition of bile does not indicate its osmolarity. Bile is in osmotic equilibrium with blood plasma and any increase in its content of osmotic particles is followed by increased secretion of fluid (the choleretic effect). When biliary lipids are secreted into bile however, micelle formation enables bile to be highly concentrated with respect to its lipid constituents without the enormous increase in volume that would accompany an equivalent secretion of water-soluble molecules.

Conjugation of metabolites and drugs

Several other anions (mostly in conjugated form), in addition to bile acids, appear in bile. Their concentrations may be 10–1000 times that of their precursors in the plasma, indicating that active transport mechanisms exist for the removal of their precursors from the blood or for their secretion into the canaliculus. Some of these anions are of endogenous origin, such as bile pigments or steroid hormones, and others are xenobiotics (a foreign, non-natural chemical) such as drugs, toxins or

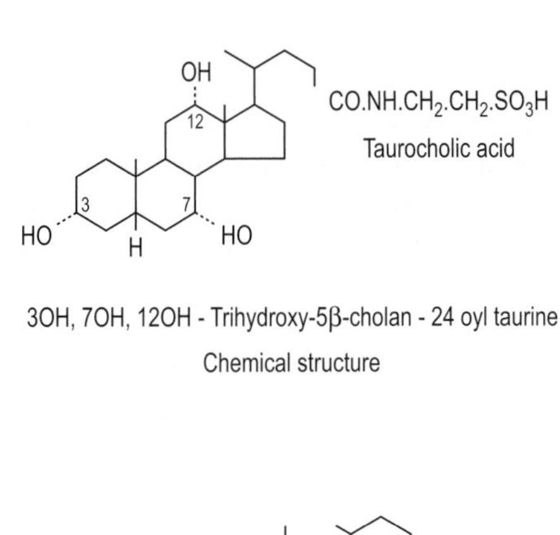

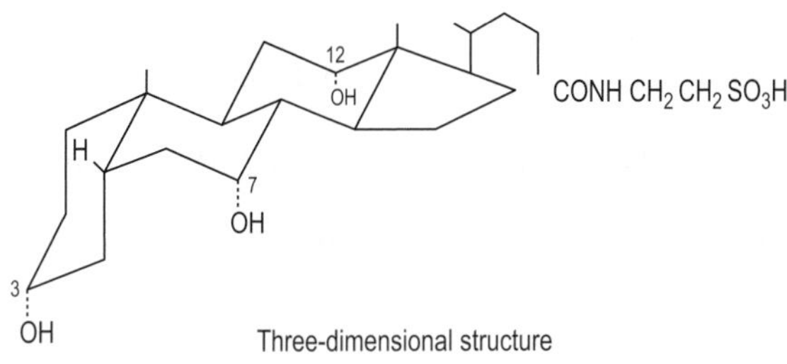

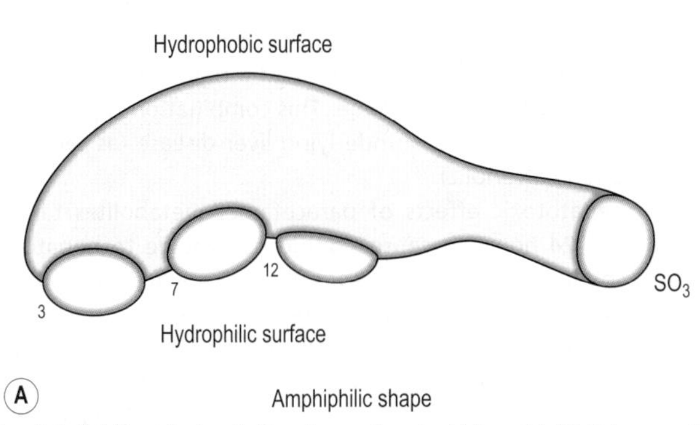

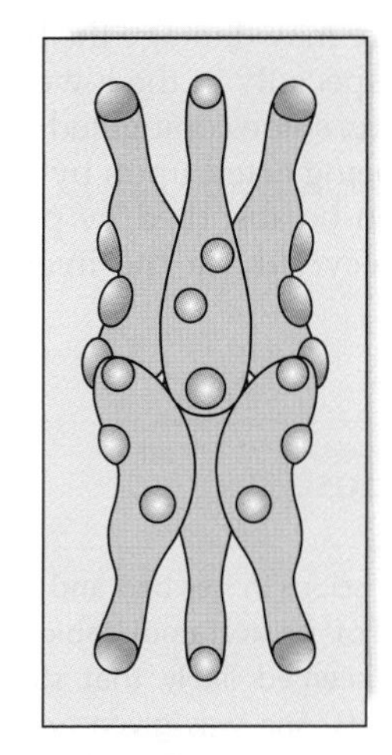

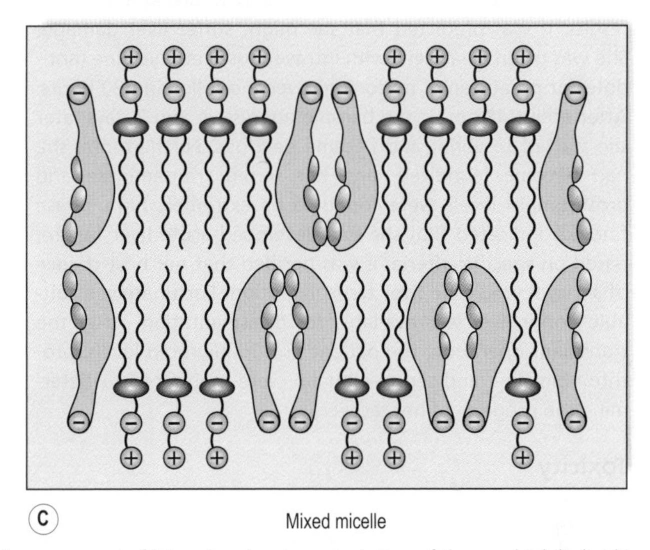

(A) Amphiphilic shape (B) Primary micelle in water (C) Mixed micelle

Fig. 4.8 (A) Electrical polarity of a conjugated bile acid. (B) Primary micelle, composed of bile salts, showing orientation of the amphiphilic lipid in the micelle. (C) Mixed micelle, containing bile acid and phospholipids, illustrating surface net negative charge and outer shell of cations (mainly Na^+ ions).

their metabolites. Many of these organic anions undergo biotransformation in two phases in the liver cells. Fig. 4.9 shows a general scheme for these reactions. Phase 1 metabolism makes the molecule more polar, either through oxidation, reduction or hydrolysis. The most common type of phase 1 reaction is oxidative. These oxidative reactions are catalysed by a complex enzyme system, known as the mixed-function oxygenase system, present in the endoplasmic reticulum. The most important enzyme in this system is cytochrome P-450, a haem protein which is part of the electron transfer chain that catalyses an intermediate hydroxylation step in phase 1 oxidative reactions.

Some drug oxidation reactions involve specific enzymes. Ethanol oxidation, for example, is catalysed by alcohol dehydrogenase and monoamine oxidase inactivates many biologically active amines, including adrenaline and serotonin. Reduction reactions are less common, but one important clinical example is the inactivation of the anticoagulation drug warfarin.

Phase 2 involves conjugation of the anion with a more strongly ionisable group that introduces a negative charge, or increases the negative charge, on the molecule, making it more hydrophilic. The most common phase 2 reaction involves the production of glucuronides. These glucuronidation reactions are all catalysed by UDP-glucuronyl transferase (see Fig. 4.9). Steroid hormones, thyroid hormones, bilirubin and many drugs are converted to glucuronides in the liver. In addition, compounds can be conjugated with amino acids or hexoses, or form sulphates.

These transformations enable the organic anions generated to be handled by anion transporters (see below) in the canalicular membrane. The conjugates are usually more water-soluble and less toxic than their precursors, although some (e.g., 7-O-chlorpromazine glucuronide) may be more toxic, and therefore may damage the biliary system or act as carcinogens (especially in the lower part of the duct system). Furthermore, some conjugated drugs become less hydrophilic after being acted upon by bacteria in the colon. They may then be absorbed by passive absorption in the colon and recycled via the liver (the enterohepatic circulation), in which case they can be difficult to eliminate from the body. Their toxicity is thereby increased. In liver diseases such as cirrhosis, in which the hepatocytes are damaged, there may be an increase in the half-life of a drug because the capacity of the liver to metabolise and secrete it is decreased.

Case 4.2 Paracetamol overdose

A teenager was discovered unconscious in her bed and rushed into hospital. An empty bottle of paracetamol tablets was found in her bedroom, and it seemed likely that she had ingested a whole bottle of tablets. She was given activated charcoal immediately on arrival to casualty. The girl's blood paracetamol levels were monitored for 12 hours, and from the results, it was predicted that she might suffer liver damage. She was given treatment with intravenous acetylcysteine (antidote for paracetamol poisoning) over the following 20 hours. After about 48 hours, she became aggressive and 2 days later she started to vomit and became delirious. Furthermore, she had become jaundiced, and her serum transaminase and prothrombin levels were found to be extremely high. These findings indicated that she had developed acute liver failure; based on specific criteria, it was decided that her best chance of survival would be liver transplantation. Fortunately, a suitable donor liver was available for transplantation. After the transplant operation, the patient's serum bilirubin levels, prothrombin time and serum albumin were monitored to determine the progress of her recovery.

Toxicity

Liver

Paracetamol has potent analgesic and antipyretic actions, but its anti-inflammatory actions are weaker than those of many other non-steroidal anti-inflammatory drugs (NSAIDs). It is given orally. A therapeutic dose of paracetamol is normally metabolised in the liver by conjugation to form soluble glucuronide or sulphate derivatives that can be excreted in the urine. Its half-life in the blood is 2–4 hours. The analgesia and hypothermia are mediated by inhibition of a central nervous system-specific cyclo-oxygenase isoform, COX-3.

High toxic levels of paracetamol cause nausea and vomiting. A dose of approximately 10 g of paracetamol is sufficient to cause toxicity. The damage to the liver is due to the conjugating enzymes becoming saturated, that results in the drug being converted by mixed function P-450 oxidases to N-acetyl-p-benzoquinone imine (NAPBQI). The latter compound causes cell death by:

- Depleting intracellular glutathione, causing oxidative stress (when glutathione is depleted, intermediate metabolites build up and these also contribute to hepatocyte cell death),
- Binding to cell proteins to produce NAPBQI protein adducts,
- Increasing lipid peroxidation and membrane permeability and
- Oxidising SH groups on Ca^{2+}-ATPases resulting in sustained increases in intracellular Ca^{2+} and activation of Ca^{2+}-activated proteases.

Note: Alcohol ingestion should be avoided if paracetamol has been taken for a headache because alcohol is an enzyme inducer and therefore enhances the formation of toxic metabolites of paracetamol. Thus, the combination of a normally safe dose of paracetamol and a high level of blood alcohol can lead to liver damage. This combination is particularly dangerous if there is underlying liver disease (as can be the case in an alcoholic).

The hepatotoxic effects of paracetamol metabolites take more than 24 hours to cause significant damage to hepatocytes. She appeared jaundiced after her relapse because the damaged liver could not excrete bilirubin in the bile. Consequently, it accumulated in the blood. The bilirubin in the blood would be predominantly unconjugated bilirubin because of the widespread damage to the liver cells where it is normally conjugated.

The excessively high concentrations of serum transaminase in the patient's blood and prolonged prothrombin clotting time are other manifestations of liver damage because transaminases are inappropriately released from dying hepatocytes, and liver cell failure results in reduced production of clotting factors such as prothrombin. Determination of these parameters enables the extent of the liver damage to be assessed and its progress monitored.

Other tissues

The patient's aggressive behaviour was due to encephalopathy that can accompany hepatic necrosis. The encephalopathy is due to high concentrations of toxic substances in the blood because of the inability of the liver to detoxify and excrete them. These cross the blood-brain barrier to damage the central nervous system. An electroencephalogram (EEG) can be used to monitor the encephalopathy.

Case 4.2 Paracetamol overdose—cont'd

Paracetamol and other NSAIDs can also cause nephrotoxicity and renal failure. This occurs mainly in patients with diseases where glomerular filtration is compromised, such as heart or liver disease. This effect is due to ischaemia in the kidneys because NSAIDs such as paracetamol inhibit the synthesis of prostaglandins, which are vasodilators.

Treatment

Drugs

Intravenous acetylcysteine was administered to the patient because paracetamol can be conjugated to form sulphates, as well as glucuronides. The sulphation reaction requires glutathione. Acetylcysteine increases glutathione synthesis in the liver, and this increases the conjugation of paracetamol to paracetamol sulphate, which can be excreted. Glutathione itself is not administered because it does not readily penetrate the liver. If the patient is seen soon after ingesting the paracetamol overdose (within 12 hours), liver damage may be prevented by this treatment.

Note: Forced diuresis or renal dialysis would not have been useful in this patient because these procedures do not increase the excretion of paracetamol or its metabolites as the compounds bind tightly to tissues.

Transplantation

A liver transplant was necessary in this patient because, although the ability of the liver to recover function is well-recognised, if over 80% of the hepatocytes have been irreversibly damaged, sufficient function will not be recovered. This degree of damage would have been present in this case.

Determination of blood pH, prothrombin time, kidney function and degree of encephalopathy (altered cognitive state) determines the need for a transplant (based on Kings College Criteria). Similar measures are used to assess the function of the transplanted liver. Following transplantation, the production of clotting factors and albumin is seen within hours. As the new liver becomes functional, the bilirubin levels gradually fall because the liver regains its ability to sequester it from the blood and excrete it into the bile. The process of excreting the bilirubin takes several weeks. Thus, prothrombin time and albumin levels are sensitive tests for monitoring early transplant function.

Determinants of preferential excretion into bile

Some organic anions are excreted preferentially via the bile and some via the urine. The processing of two important drugs to glucuronides is indicated in Fig. 4.9. One of these, the analgesic drug phenacetin, is converted to paracetamol glucuronide, which is secreted by the liver into the blood to be excreted mainly by the kidney. The other, the antipsychotic drug, chlorpromazine, is converted to 7-O-chlorpromazine glucuronide, which is excreted mainly in the bile. In humans, small organic anions of molecular mass less than 500 Da are excreted exclusively by the kidney while bigger anions are preferentially excreted into bile. Conjugation with glucuronic acid or glutathione serves to increase the molecular mass of a substance by 176 Da and 306 Da, respectively and conjugation may therefore increase the likelihood of secretion of the anion into bile. The reason for this discriminatory threshold for excretion in bile is unknown but the anion transporters in the canalicular membrane (see below) may show molecular size specificity. Another possibility is 'molecular sieving' by tight junctions between the hepatocytes; according to this hypothesis, all anions are secreted into the canaliculi, but the small ones leak back into the plasma across the tight junctions.

Transport of organic ions

Transport into the hepatocyte

Organic ions are transported in the blood largely by high-affinity binding to albumin and consequently the concentrations in plasma of the free ions are low.

Uptake of 'cholephilic' anions by the hepatocyte involves membrane carrier proteins with high-affinity binding sites. Competition studies indicate that the carriers are shared by several anions. Thus bilirubin, sulphonamides, salicylates and sulphobromophthalein share the same carrier. This carrier is known as the organic anion transporter (OATP). Transport of anions via this mechanism requires energy and can be against enormous concentration gradients. It involves a chloride antiport system.

Transport into bile

Transport of anions across the canalicular membrane into the bile can be against a 100-fold concentration gradient. The membrane potential difference, which is approximately 40 mV (negative inside the cell), can only account for transport of organic anions against a three-fold concentration gradient. At least three specific

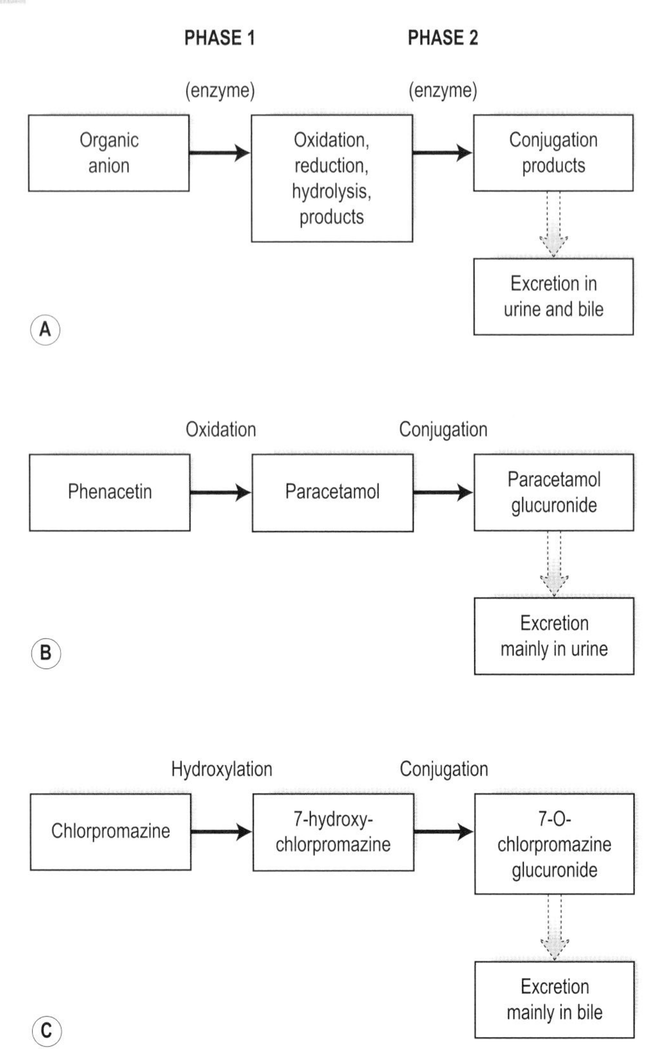

Fig. 4.9 Biotransformation of anions in the hepatocyte. (A) General scheme involving two phases. (B) A drug (phenacetin) which is metabolised in the liver, secreted into the blood and excreted in the kidney. (C) A drug (chlorpromazine) which is metabolised in the liver and excreted in the bile.

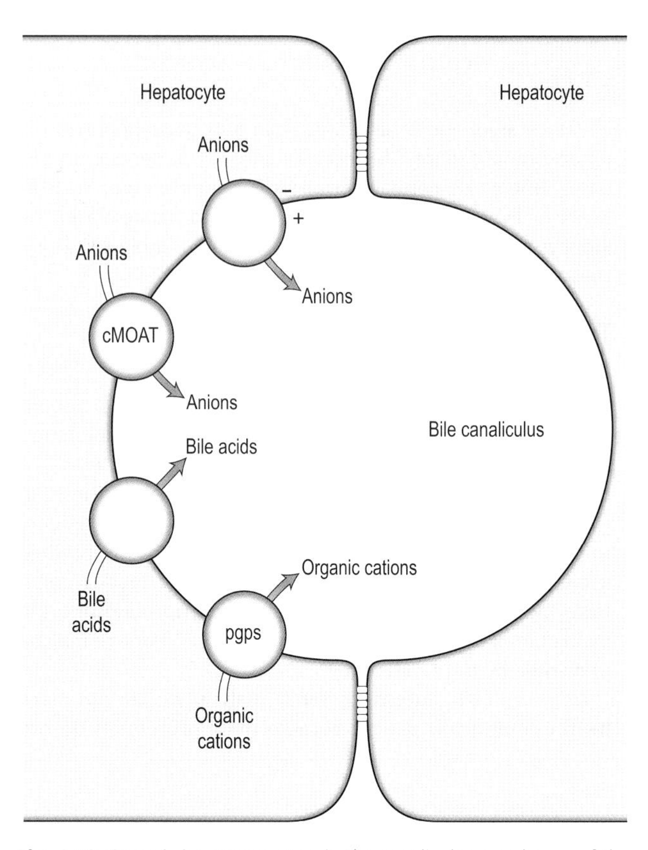

Fig. 4.10 Organic ion transporters in the canalicular membrane of the hepatocyte. *cMOAT, canalicular multiorganic anion transporter; pgps, P-transporters which transport organic cations into bile.*

ATP-dependent active transport mechanisms are present in the canalicular membranes for the transport of organic ions (Fig. 4.10).

The ATP-dependent transporters and the membrane potential-dependent transporter are distinct proteins. The membrane potential-dependent transporter is a glycoprotein. One of the ATP-dependent transporters is responsible for transport of bile acids and has been described above. Another is known as the canalicular multiorganic anion transporter (cMOAT). It transports many organic anions including bilirubin glucuronide and conjugates of various xenobiotics. It does not transport unconjugated bilirubin. The jaundiced mutant (Tr−) rat that exhibits hyperbilirubinaemia is deficient in this transporter. A similar defect is present in Dubin–Johnson syndrome (an autosomal recessive disease resulting in loss of function of multiple drug-resistance protein 2 (MRP2) which is responsible for the section of conjugated bilirubin). The third transporter type is a group of phosphoglycoproteins (Pgps), known as P-transporters, which bind ATP. They transport mainly hydrophobic, neutral compounds, and organic cations into bile. One P-transporter, known as the multidrug transporter 3 (mdr-3), transports many cationic drugs across the canalicular membrane including certain peptides and anti-cancer drugs such as daunomycin. Interestingly, the expression of P-transporters temporarily increases after partial hepatectomy.

Metabolism of bilirubin

Bilirubin, which is reddish orange in colour, is the major bile pigment produced by breakdown of either haemoglobin or myoglobin in the reticuloendothelial system. Fig. 4.11 shows the formation of bilirubin from haem, the porphyrin moiety of haemoglobin. Some of the intermediate product, biliverdin, a green pigment, is also usually present in bile. In bile that has been stored, the bilirubin reoxidises to form biliverdin, and the bile tends to turn green. (These pigments are bound to albumin in the circulation.)

Free bilirubin from the blood enters the liver cells via an anion transporter that exchanges it for Cl^-. Inside the cell, bilirubin is glucuronidated by UDP-glucuronyl transferase to bilirubin diglucuronide which enhances

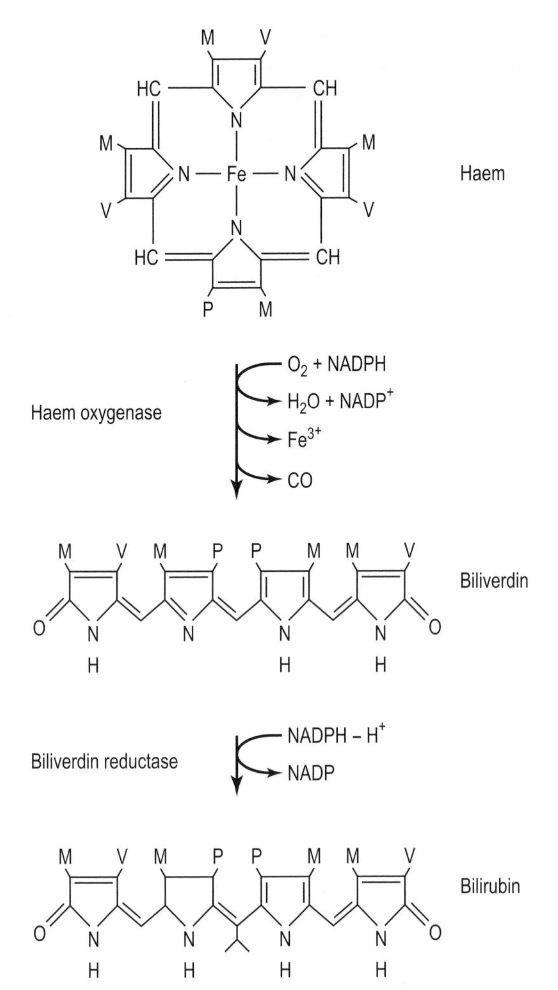

Fig. 4.11 Formation of bilirubin from the enzymatic breakdown of haem. *CO, carbon monoxide; M, methyl; P, propionyl; V, vinyl.*

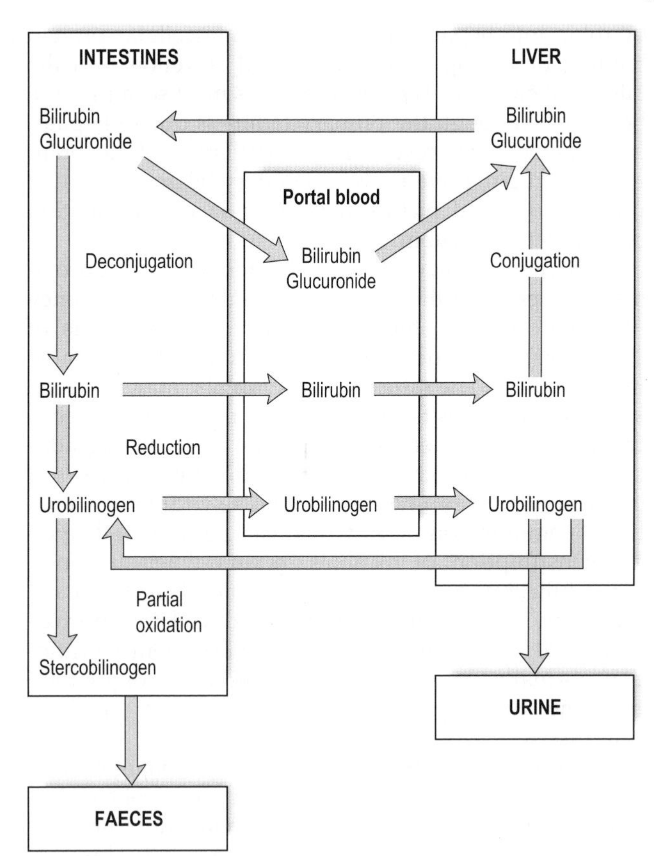

Fig. 4.12 Metabolism and fate of bile pigments in the intestines.

the compounds solubility. This glucuronidated bilirubin is then effluxed via the cMOAT transporter system into bile. If bilirubin subsequently becomes deconjugated in the biliary system, pigment gallstones may form.

Fate of bile pigments in the gastrointestinal tract

After delivery to the intestines, most conjugated bilirubin is eliminated in the faeces. This is because the intestinal mucosa is not very permeable to the conjugated metabolite. However, some conjugated bilirubin may be deconjugated by bacteria in the intestines and the free bilirubin formed can be absorbed to some extent by passive diffusion into the portal blood, because it is more lipid-soluble than conjugated bilirubin. It is then returned to the liver via the enterohepatic circulation (see below). Intestinal bacteria can also convert bilirubin to colourless derivatives known as urobilinogens, which can also be absorbed into the portal blood. These are mostly excreted in the bile, but some are excreted in the urine. Urobilinogen remaining in the gut is partially reoxidised to stercobilinogen, the reddish-brown pigment responsible for the colour of the faeces. Fig. 4.12 outlines the fate of excreted bile pigments.

Failure of the body to excrete bile pigments results in accumulation of the pigments in the blood plasma (hyperbilirubinaemia), causing jaundice. This manifests as yellowing of the skin, sclera and mucous membranes.

Jaundice

Jaundice becomes obvious when the plasma bilirubin concentration exceeds 34 μmol/L. It can be classified into three types, depending on the location of the defect that causes it.

Prehepatic (or haemolytic) jaundice

Excessive haemolysis of red blood cells and haemoglobin breakdown to bilirubin can exceed the capacity of the liver to excrete it. This type of jaundice is most frequently associated with haemolytic anaemia of various types. The bilirubin present in the plasma is largely unconjugated as it has not been taken up and conjugated by the liver.

Intrahepatic (or hepatocellular) jaundice

A variety of defects in the liver itself can also give rise to hyperbilirubinaemia. These include decreased uptake of bilirubin into hepatocytes, defective intracellular protein binding or conjugation or disturbed secretion into the bile canaliculi. This type of jaundice is most seen in acute hepatitis. Although the primary failure is due to hepatocyte damage that results in accumulation of unconjugated bilirubin, there is also secondary biliary stasis that provides a mixed picture with secondary accumulation of conjugated bilirubin.

In Crigler–Najjar disease (incidence of approximately 1 per 1 million) there is an inherited deficiency of glucuronyl transferase and high concentrations of unconjugated bilirubin are present in the plasma, causing jaundice. The affected individuals may develop kernicterus (deposits of pigment in the brain) that can cause nerve degeneration. Exposure to light degrades the pigment, and children born with this disease can be treated by phototherapy. Gilbert's syndrome, a relatively common condition which can be triggered upon the consumption of alcohols, occurs when unconjugated bilirubin accumulates in the blood. In this case, glucuronyl transferase activity is reduced by approximately 70%. This results in mild, intermittent jaundice that normally does not require treatment. Conjugation of some drugs is also usually impaired in these conditions.

At birth, infants have little ability to conjugate bilirubin, but it develops within the first few weeks of life. Thus, some babies are jaundiced soon after birth, as unconjugated bilirubin is not readily excreted. This condition is known as physiological jaundice of the newborn. Exposure to light can be employed in these infants to deplete the excess bilirubin.

Post-hepatic (or obstructive) jaundice

Blockage of the intrahepatic or extrahepatic bile ducts by, for example, gallstones or a tumour, also causes jaundice as the bile is refluxed into the blood. This is commonly referred to as post-hepatic or obstructive jaundice. In this case, the bilirubin is largely conjugated.

A patient with obstructive jaundice commonly presents with dark coloured urine as the conjugated bilirubin is excreted by the kidneys. Furthermore, when the bile ducts are blocked, bile pigments cannot enter the GI tract and consequently the downstream metabolites of bilirubin (e.g., stercobilinogen) are not present in the faeces. Hence, faeces tend to be pale in colour.

Proteins in bile

Most proteins in bile are plasma proteins, although some are derived from cells of the hepatobiliary system. The plasma proteins are mostly synthesised in the liver and secreted into the blood, but some plasma proteins are normally present in bile, including unaltered active enzymes (including alkaline phosphatase) and antibodies.

Some proteins exhibit relatively low bile-to-plasma concentration ratios. Two non-specific pathways exist for protein transport in hepatocytes:

- Paracellular sieving, which is responsible for secretion of smaller proteins, and
- Pinocytosis (membrane vesiculation) followed by transport of the pinocytotic vesicles and exocytosis. This pathway does not discriminate in relation to molecular size.

There are also receptor-linked pathways for the secretion of some proteins. One example is immunoglobulin A (IgA) that is transported by receptor-mediated vesicle transport in the duct cells. This protein provides immunological protection for the biliary and intestinal tracts.

The gallbladder

Anatomy and histology

The gallbladder is a pear-shaped sac. In the human adult, it is approximately 8 cm long and 4 cm wide, but it is capable of considerable distension. It is lined by a mucous membrane that is thrown into numerous folds (rugae) when the gallbladder contracts (Fig. 4.13). As the gallbladder fills with bile, the folds flatten out. The cystic duct conveys the bile to the hepatic duct (see Fig. 4.1).

The wall of the gallbladder is composed of three layers: the mucous membrane, the muscularis and the adventitia (or serosa, see Fig. 4.13). The epithelium of the mucous membrane is composed of high columnar cells with basally located nuclei. The apical (luminal) borders of the cells are provided with microvilli, consistent with their absorptive function. They resemble the absorptive cells of the small intestine. Beneath the epithelial cells is the lamina propria, which is a coat of loose connective tissue. Around the mucous membrane is a thin coat of smooth muscle, the muscularis externa. Most of the smooth muscle fibres run obliquely but some run circularly and some longitudinally. Many elastic fibres are present within the connective tissue between the muscle fibres. Outside this muscle layer is the adventitia (or serosa), which is an outer coat of dense fibroconnective tissue that is covered by peritoneum.

At the neck of the gallbladder, the mucous membrane is thrown into a spiral fold that has a core of smooth muscle (Fig. 4.13). This extends into the cystic duct and is known as the spiral valve. Its function may be to prevent sudden changes in the filling and emptying of the gallbladder.

Functions

The functions of the gallbladder are to store and concentrate bile, and to deliver it into the small intestine during

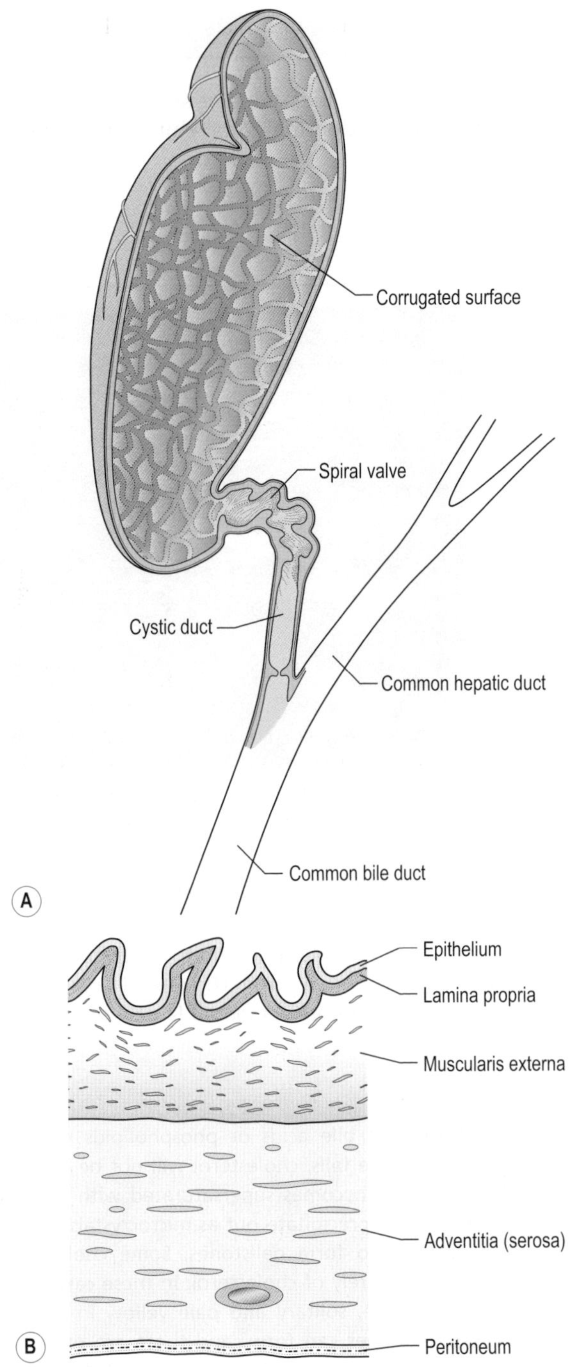

Fig. 4.13 The gallbladder. (A) Structural features. (B) Layers of the gallbladder wall.

a meal. In the human adult, it has a capacity of 30–60 mL. Gallbladder bile is an isotonic solution but some of its components are highly concentrated.

The endothelial cells actively reabsorb Na^+ ions from the bile in exchange for K^+ ions. The Na^+ ions are pumped into the lateral spaces between the epithelial cells. Anions, largely Cl^- and HCO_3^-, follow passively down the electrochemical gradient. The extraction of HCO_3^- ions tends to make the gallbladder bile less

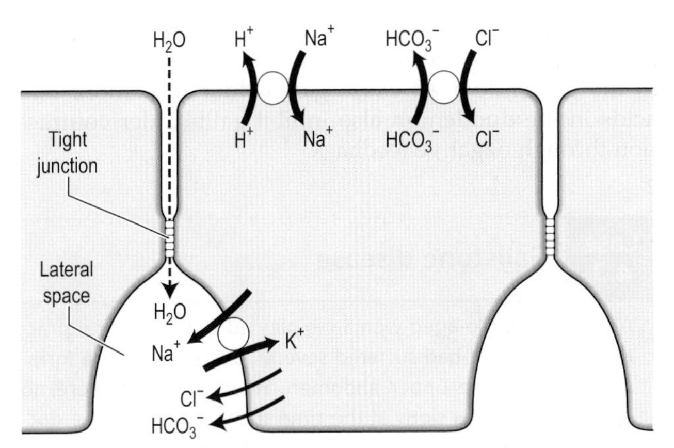

Fig. 4.14 Transport of ions in the gallbladder.

alkaline. Thus, gallbladder bile is less concentrated with respect to Na^+, Cl^- and HCO_3^- than hepatic bile. The pumping of Na^+ out of the endothelial cell at the basal surface keeps its concentration low inside the cell, and this provides the driving force for Na^+ ions to enter the cell via the apical membrane (down their concentration gradient). Transport in the apical membrane occurs partly via exchange for H^+ ions and partly by symport with Cl^- ions. Consequently, water is transported passively down the osmotic gradient and out of the gallbladder. The ions and water then pass through the basement membrane into the blood capillaries (Fig. 4.14).

The organic constituents are highly concentrated in gallbladder bile, but it remains isosmotic with plasma. The bile pigments in hepatic bile impart a golden-brown colour to it, but gallbladder bile is almost black because the pigments are more concentrated. Bilirubin, bile acids, lecithin and cholesterol are 5–10 times more concentrated in gallbladder bile than in hepatic bile.

Gallbladder contraction

The gallbladder exhibits muscle tone and contractions even in the interdigestive period. It also contracts between meals to deliver bile intermittently into the duodenum. The contractions coincide with the migrating motor complex of the small intestine. These fasting contractions may cause mixing of the bile, reducing the likelihood of cholesterol crystals accumulating and forming gallstones.

The major stimulus for gallbladder contraction after a meal is a high blood level of CCK, the hormone that is released in response to fat in the duodenum. It acts on CCK-A receptors on the smooth muscle of the gallbladder. Gastrin, a related peptide, is released by the stomach antrum in response to peptides and stimulates gallbladder contraction. In addition, distension of the stomach antrum stimulates contraction via a nervous reflex. The gastric mechanisms involved in the control of bile release are presumably preliminary to the emptying of chyme from the stomach.

Vasoactive intestinal peptide (VIP), pancreatic polypeptide (PP) and stimulation of the sympathetic nerves to the gallbladder all cause gallbladder relaxation. Bile acids in the duodenum also inhibit gallbladder contraction through negative feedback.

Surgical resection

Removal of the gallbladder (cholecystectomy) is one of the most common abdominal procedures performed in

Case 4.3 Gallstone disease

An obese middle-aged woman explained to her general practitioner that she had suffered several attacks of severe 'gripping' pain in the upper abdomen. However, there were no abnormal physical signs at the time she was seen by the doctor. Upon questioning, she said that the attacks had started after meals. The pain built up gradually to a maximum and lasted for several hours. Her description of the location of the pain indicated that it was epigastric, and in the right upper quadrant of the abdomen. She also said that, during a recent severe attack, her husband had remarked that the 'whites' of her eyes (the sclera) had appeared yellow. In addition, the patient had noticed that her urine became dark in colour, and her stools were pale and greasy-looking and tended to float in the lavatory pan. The doctor suspected that the patient was suffering from gallstones. This was subsequently confirmed by an ultrasound scan, and the patient was referred to a surgeon for a cholecystectomy (surgical removal of the gallbladder).

Detection and cause of pain

Gallstones (biliary calculi) are hard masses that can be present in the gallbladder or the bile ducts (Fig. 4.15). They can be classified broadly into two types:

1. Those composed largely of cholesterol, or
2. Those composed largely of bile pigment.

Cholesterol stones tend to be large (often more than 1 cm in diameter), and several may be present in one individual. The attacks of pain (biliary cholic) experienced following meals are due to transient obstruction of the cystic duct when the gallbladder contracts. The pain in this patient is due to the pressure of the bile behind the stone. However, most individuals with gallstones are asymptomatic and require no treatment.

Gallstones that are sufficiently calcified (20% of all gallstones) can be detected by plain abdominal radiography. These may be cholesterol stones with a calcified shell or pigment stones composed mainly of calcium bilirubinate. Pure cholesterol stones are radiolucent and cannot be detected using this technique.

The simple rapid technique of ultrasonography is usually employed to reveal gallstones (Fig. 4.15). This provides an overall gallstone detection rate of over 90%. It also allows evaluation of the thickness of the gallbladder wall; an abnormally thick wall indicates a diseased gallbladder, usually secondary to chronic inflammation, but occasionally due to a carcinoma.

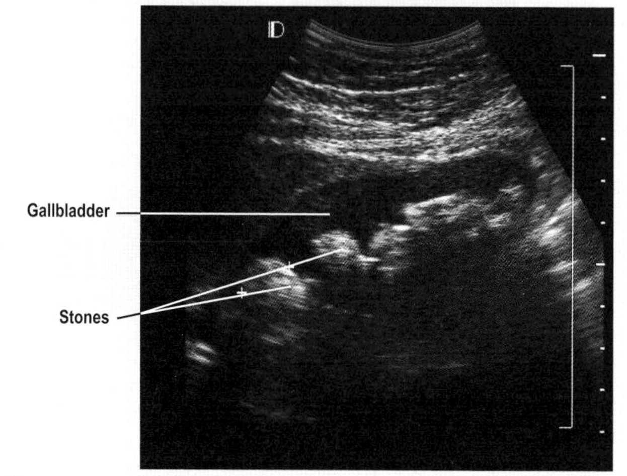

Fig. 4.15 An ultrasound scan showing a distended gallbladder and radio-opaque stones within the lumen.

Gallstones: composition, formation and occurrence

Many compounds can precipitate in bile to form stones, but approximately 80% are formed from cholesterol with a variable Ca^{2+} content. The rest are composed largely of bile pigments and Ca^{2+} salts.

Cholesterol stones

If the concentration of bile acids or phospholipids relative to cholesterol in the bile falls, cholesterol will not be held in micelles. The bile then becomes supersaturated with cholesterol, and this tends to precipitate out as microcrystals. These microcrystals coalesce to form gallstones. Some cholesterol stones are composed purely of cholesterol. In these cases, the stones tend to be large, solitary and pale yellow in colour. Smaller cholesterol stones can form, and these are often of mixed composition but usually contain more than 70% cholesterol. These are also pale yellow and are usually multiple. They vary in size and are laminated, with a dark central nucleus. The cholesterol crystals deposit around this nucleus and then become hardened by the precipitation of organic salts.

Cholesterol gallstones tend to develop when there is a high ratio of cholesterol to bile acids or lecithin in the bile. This can be due to high cholesterol secretion because of a high-fat diet or congenital hypercholesterolaemia. They may also form if there is reduced bile acid secretion because of bile acid malabsorption in the ileum or reduced lecithin secretion. The bile acid

Case 4.3 Gallstone disease—cont'd

pool in an individual is fairly constant (see below) but in people with gallstones it tends to be smaller than average. Gallstone formation may happen at night as bile acid secretion falls (even further) and when blood concentrations are low (see below). The ratio of cholesterol to bile salts and lecithin is raised by a high-fat diet, as fats are converted to cholesterol in the liver. Interestingly, gallstones are common in South American women whose diet includes diosgenin-rich beans, because diosgenin increases cholesterol secretion. Inflammation of the gallbladder may also contribute by increasing reabsorption of bile salts or water in the gallbladder, thereby encouraging the cholesterol to precipitate out in the bile.

Females tend to have a higher cholesterol-to-phospholipid ratio than males, which may account for the fact that 4 times more females than males suffer from gallstones. Genetic and racial factors also appear to be important. Cholesterol gallstones are also found in diseases of the ileum, such as Crohn's disease, which lead to reduced bile salt reabsorption.

Pigment stones

Pigment stones are usually small in diameter (a few millimetres) and dark brown or black in colour. They occur less frequently than cholesterol stones. When they occur, they are usually multiple. They contain 40%–95% pigment and less than 20% cholesterol. They constitute approximately 20% of all gallstones. They can form if there is an overload of unconjugated bilirubin resulting from haemolytic anaemia, burns or crush injury. A high incidence of pigment gallstones is seen in patients with haemolytic states (such as sickle cell anaemia). The bile becomes supersaturated with unconjugated bilirubin, and it precipitates out. The free bilirubin combines with calcium in the bile to form insoluble calcium bilirubinate. This forms the nidus of a stone, and degradation products of bilirubin aggregate on this core to form pigment stones. A deficit in the conjugating ability of the liver can also result in the formation of pigment gallstones. In addition, infecting organisms that contain β-glucuronidase, an enzyme that deconjugates bilirubin glucuronide, can be responsible. Until recently, a form of the disease where highly calcified pigment stones were present occurred in Asian countries (notably Japan). It was caused by infestation of the biliary duct with parasites that contain this enzyme. Its incidence has diminished as hygiene and nutrition have improved. Unfortunately, however, as diets have become 'Westernised', the incidence of cholesterol gallstones has increased. There is also a tendency for pigment stones to form in patients with cirrhosis of the liver due to stasis in the biliary tract.

Fat malabsorption

The pale colour of the patient's stools was due to the absence of stercobilin, and the greasiness was due to the presence of abnormally large quantities of unabsorbed fat. Elimination of excessive amounts of fat is known as steatorrhoea. The fat caused the faeces to float and to smell abnormally offensive because it had been fermented by bacteria in the colon.

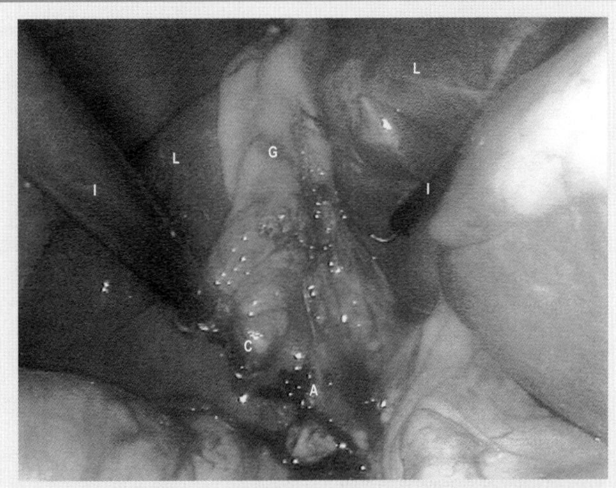

Fig. 4.16 Gallbladder surgery being performed laparoscopically. The gallbladder (G) and divided cystic duct (C) and cystic artery (A) are seen, with the liver (L) lying behind. (I) Instruments for lifting and dividing the gallbladder structures.

Bile acids play an important role in the digestion of lipid and in the absorption of lipid- and fat-soluble vitamins (vitamins A, D, E and K). Consequently, in severe cholestasis such as when the common bile duct is obstructed by gallstones, bile acids are not delivered to the small intestine and therefore lipids are not absorbed. Fat malabsorption causes flatulence and diarrhoea. The duration of the period over which fat malabsorption is present in gallstone disease before it is treated is usually relatively short. For that reason, fat-soluble vitamin deficiency is unusual, except in the case of vitamin K as body stores of vitamin K are very limited. Deficiency of this vitamin leads to deranged blood coagulation.

Restriction of dietary fat reduces steatorrhoea, but then vitamin K supplements are required to prevent clotting abnormalities.

Treatment

Surgery

In gallstone disease, where stones are present in the gallbladder, surgical removal of the gallbladder is often performed using 'keyhole' surgery (Fig. 4.16).

If a gallstone is present in the biliary duct, a procedure called endoscopic retrograde cholangiopancreatography (ERCP) would be performed. This involves passing an endoscope down through the mouth into the duodenum (Fig. 4.17). The sphincter of Oddi is then cut open slightly to allow the stone to be removed.

The digestive processes are not seriously impaired after removal of the gallbladder because hepatic bile simply flows directly into the duodenum. A greater volume of unconcentrated bile enters the intestines, but the extra fluid is

Continued

Case 4.3 Gallstone disease—cont'd

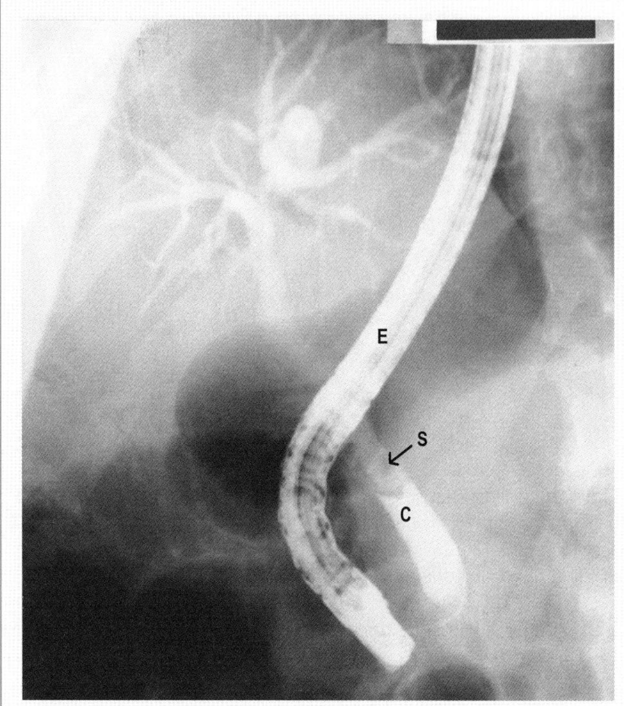

Fig. 4.17 This X-ray shows an endoscope (E) which has been passed into the duodenum. Contrast has been injected (retrograde) into a dilated common bile duct (C), which contains a calculus (S).

absorbed, so dehydration does not occur. One consequence is that bile acids may enter the small intestines more rapidly, and therefore, a higher proportion may be eliminated from the body. However, this reduction in the bile acid pool is normally rectified by increased synthesis in the liver.

Lithotripsy

A non-invasive treatment for gallstones, involving the use of ultrasonic vibrations, known as lithotripsy, can be performed. In this procedure, focused ultrasound waves are used to disrupt the gallstones and the fragments formed are carried in the bile into the small intestines and subsequently eliminated from the body. Lithotripsy is not widely employed because the stone fragments can get lodged in the common bile duct, resulting in obstructive jaundice. (Kidney stones are more commonly treated using this technique.) Newer techniques, such as SpyGlass, allow the stones to be directly treated with either electrohydraulic or laser lithotripsy.

Treatment with bile acids

Gallstones can sometimes be treated by oral administration of oral bile acid supplementation (such as ursodeoxycholic acid), however recent evidence suggests that such agents have very little efficacy. Cholesterol supersaturation in bile in patients with gallstones is usually due to a diminished bile acid pool. The ingested bile acids are absorbed in the ileum and taken up by the liver and then secreted in the bile (Fig. 4.18). Thus, if a bile acid is fed in substantial amounts, the bile acid pool is expanded. This enables more cholesterol to be retained in micelles rather than precipitating in the bile. The bile acids slowly dissolve the gallstones over time, usually several months. These bile acids are effective because they increase cholesterol sequestration in micelles and, unlike cholic acid and deoxycholic acid, they do not suppress bile acid synthesis. Ursodiol also inhibits cholesterol absorption in the intestine and decreases the synthesis of cholesterol in the liver. This causes reduced plasma cholesterol levels, and for this reason, ursodiol has also been considered for the treatment of coronary heart disease.

The main side effect of bile acid treatment is diarrhoea, secondary to incomplete absorption of the ingested bile salts.

Small gallstones disappear relatively quickly with bile acid treatment. However, it is the large stones which are usually responsible for the symptoms of gallstone disease, and so alleviation via bile acid administration means takes a long time. Moreover, most individuals with gallstones present with acute symptoms, which are often associated with a dysfunctional gallbladder. Therefore, the use of bile salt therapy is limited. Furthermore, life-long therapy with bile salts would be required to prevent the stones recurring. Thus, cholecystectomy remains the primary choice for the removal of gallstones.

the Western world. The gallbladder is removed by division of the cystic artery and cystic duct, but the common bile duct is left intact to enable free drainage of bile from the liver into the duodenum. Loss of the storage reservoir for bile salts results in adaptation of bile salt present in the liver. Following surgery, the bile is present in higher volumes from the liver and is released continuously into the duodenum at a slow rate. On ingestion of a fatty meal, liver bile release increases rapidly which compensates for the lack of a gallbladder, and patients can tolerate meals with even a high fat content. An interesting secondary effect from this operation is the increased rate of bile uptake from the ileum into the enterohepatic circulation. This results in a higher proportion of secondary bile acids because of the increased circulation of the bile. There is some evidence to suggest that this may have a potentially carcinogenic effect on the large bowel and there is an association with an increased incidence of colorectal cancer.

Liver cancer

Liver cancer is a relatively rare cancer (18th most common cancer in the UK) accounting for 2% of all new cancers. In the UK, the annual incidence is approximately 6100 with 43% of all new liver cancer cases diagnosed in the elderly (75 and over). Alarmingly over the last decade, liver cancer incidence rates have increased by more than half, and there is a clear association with deprivation. It is a cancer type more common in Asian and Black people than White people. Whilst relatively rare, it is the 8th most common cause of cancer death in the UK, accounting for 3% of all cancer deaths. It has an approximate 5-year survival rate of 13% and, worryingly, liver cancer mortality rates have increased by almost half over the last decade.

Risk factors

Risk factors for liver cancer include smoking (accounting for 20%), alcohol (7%) and being overweight or obese (23%). Thus, unsurprisingly, approximately half of all liver cancer cases in the UK are thought to be preventable. In addition, 10% of hepatocellular carcinoma cases in the UK are caused by hepatitis B or hepatitis C viral infections and, in the vast majority, this is also associated with cirrhosis. Similarly, the risk of cholangiocarcinoma is increased albeit to a lesser extent with hepatitis B virus and/or hepatitis C virus infection.

Surgical resection

Liver resection is being undertaken with increasing frequency, particularly for the treatment of metastases from colorectal cancer. GI tumours most commonly metastasise via the portal venous system to the liver, making this a common site for metastatic disease. The ability of the liver to cope with even major resections is remarkable. It is perfectly feasible to remove 75% of the liver and still retain normal function of the organ. This is in part due to its regenerative properties. These were recognised even by the ancient Greeks. In Greek mythology, the god Prometheus was punished by Zeus, who ordered him to be tied to a rock and have an eagle eat his liver. Prometheus was said to have survived this repeated insult because of the regenerative capacity of the liver.

The sphincter of Oddi

The hepatic bile duct penetrates the wall of the duodenum at the same location as the pancreatic duct. Part of the way through the duodenal wall, the hepatic duct and the pancreatic duct fuse. The lumen of the fused duct is relatively wide, and this region is known as the ampulla of Vater. It opens into the lumen of the duodenum, and at the opening are the duodenal papillae. Circular smooth muscle is associated with the ampulla and with the regions of the hepatic and pancreatic ducts that are associated with it (Fig. 4.1). This constitutes the sphincter of Oddi. The closure of this sphincter prevents bile from entering the intestine. As a result, the bile that is formed while it is closed is diverted into the gallbladder. In addition, there are smooth muscle fibres that run in parallel with the bile and pancreatic ducts. When these fibres contract, the ducts shorten and become wider to increase the flow of the digestive juices through them. The main stimulus for relaxation of the sphincter muscle is CCK. Thus, when the levels of CCK increase in the blood during a meal, the gallbladder contracts and the sphincter of Oddi relaxes, and bile enters the duodenum. These events act in concert to allow bile to enter the small intestine when a meal is being processed in the GI tract.

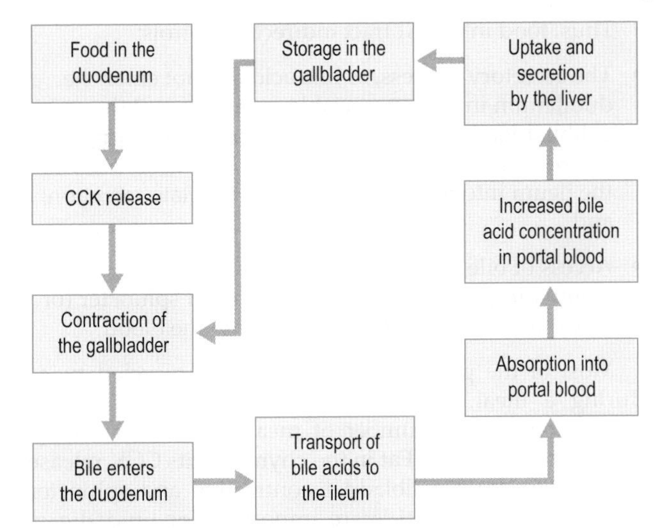

Fig. 4.18 The enterohepatic circulation of bile acids. *CCK, cholecystokinin.*

The enterohepatic circulation of bile acids

Conjugated bile acids are secreted by the liver, released into the duodenum and eventually absorbed in the ileum into the portal blood. They are then taken up by the liver and secreted again. This cycle is continually repeated and is known as the enterohepatic circulation of bile acids. The secretion of the bile acid-dependent fraction of bile from the hepatocytes is not controlled to any great extent by hormones or nerve impulses originating in the GI tract, although CCK may be a weak stimulus. The normal stimulus for increased secretion of bile salts is a high bile salt concentration in the blood (Fig. 4.18).

Bile salts are essentially secreted continuously, but the rate of secretion increases when the blood concentration increases. The concentration in the portal blood normally increases after a meal when the bile acids have been absorbed.

Thus, food in the GI tract indirectly controls:

- The secretory process, as bile acids do not enter the duodenum in any appreciable amounts until the gallbladder contracts and the sphincter (of Oddi) relaxes, when they can subsequently be absorbed in the ileum into the portal blood to stimulate secretion; and
- Access of bile to the chyme in the intestines, by stimulating gallbladder contraction and sphincter (of Oddi) relaxation via CCK release into the blood.

Most of the pool of bile salts may be recycled twice during a meal, and between 3 and 14 times a day depending on the number of meals taken and the fat content of the meals. Fat in the chyme elicits CCK release which stimulates gallbladder contraction and sphincter relaxation. As bile acids are important for lipid digestion and absorption, this control constitutes a positive feedback mechanism. The uptake of bile acids from the intestines enables small gallstones to be successfully treated by oral administration of a bile acid, as this will be secreted by the liver to increase the concentration in the bile and dissolve the stones.

The total bile acid pool (approximately 3.0 g in the adult) is kept constant. The rate of synthesis is normally very low because most of the conjugated bile acids that enter the small intestine are actively reabsorbed and returned to the liver (Fig. 4.18). Normally only a small proportion, approximately 10%, is lost in the faeces. The liver keeps the size of the pool constant by synthesising an amount equivalent to that lost. De novo synthesis is a response to low levels of bile acids in the blood. If, for any reason, bile acids are not reabsorbed in the intestines (e.g., disease of the ileum or surgical removal of part of the distal ileum) then de novo synthesis of bile acids increases. Occasionally, if this increase in the rate of synthesis is not sufficient to compensate for the loss via faeces, then malabsorption of fats and fat-soluble vitamins may arise. A common cause of this is Crohn's disease of the terminal ileum.

Control of the hepatobiliary system during a meal

Several different functions of the hepatobiliary system are under physiological control: secretion of alkaline fluid from the ducts, secretion of bile from the hepatocytes, contraction of the smooth muscle in the wall of the gallbladder to release the stored bile and relaxation of the smooth muscle in the sphincter of Oddi which allows the bile into the duodenum.

The control of alkaline bile secretion (like that of gastric juice and pancreatic juice) during a meal can be divided into three phases according to the location of the ingested material:

1. The cephalic phase, which is the response to the approach of food or the presence of food in the mouth;
2. The gastric phase, which is the response to food in the stomach; and
3. The intestinal phase, which is the response to food in the duodenum.

The bile acid-dependent fraction is essentially secreted continuously, but the gallbladder usually only contracts forcefully during a meal. Thus, although secretion is continuous, bile acids usually only enter the GI tract in appreciable amounts during a meal (i.e., when they are required).

Cephalic phase

The cephalic phase is mediated via impulses in nerve fibres in the vagus nerve. It is due to the sight and smell of food and the activation of taste and touch receptors by food in the mouth. In this phase, there is an increase in the secretion of alkaline bile from the duct cells, which would presumably minimise the effects of increased acid secretion in the stomach during the cephalic phase. Weak contractions of the gallbladder and relaxation of the sphincter of Oddi also occur.

Gastric phase

Peptides in the stomach and distension of the stomach walls cause increased release of gastrin from the pyloric antrum and activation of nerve fibres in the vagus nerve. These influences stimulate alkaline juice secretion from the bile ducts and weak contractions of the gallbladder.

Intestinal phase

The intestinal phase is the most important of the three phases for the control of both the secretion of alkaline bile and the contraction of the gallbladder. It is mediated largely via the peptide hormones secretin and CCK that are released from the walls of the duodenum into the blood. Secretin is released in response mainly to acid in the chyme. It acts on receptors on the duct cells to stimulate the release of alkaline bile. Its action is potentiated by CCK.

CCK is the most potent stimulus for gallbladder contraction. The most potent stimulus for CCK release is fat in the duodenum: when fat is not present in a meal, contraction of the gallbladder is weak. CCK also causes relaxation of the sphincter of Oddi, thereby enabling the bile to flow freely into the duodenum. Bile acids exert a negative feedback control on gallbladder contraction and sphincter relaxation by inhibiting the release of CCK from the duodenum.

THE SMALL INTESTINE

5

Chapter objectives and clinical presentations

After reading this chapter, review your learning by considering the following:

1. Are you able to describe the general anatomy of the small intestine?
2. What cell types exist in the intestinal epithelium? Can you detail their function?
3. Do you know the mechanisms that control secretion within the small intestine?
4. Can you describe how water is absorbed in the small intestine?
5. Can you detail the mechanisms by which sodium and chloride ions are absorbed in the small intestine?
6. Can you describe the different types of motility in the fed and fasted states?

Also, you should be familiar with the following clinical presentations:

- Congenital chloridorrhea
- Diarrhoea
- Cholera

Clinical outlook

Common presenting complaints with disorders of the small bowel include both acute and chronic diarrhoea, bloating, weight loss and abdominal pain. Common diagnoses in Western countries include coeliac disease, gastroenteritis, irritable bowel syndrome and Crohn's disease. Patients may present acutely with dehydration from diarrhoea and vomiting or have a more chronic presentation with abdominal discomfort and weight loss with a change in their bowel habits.

Introduction

In humans, most digestion and absorption occur in the small intestine. Digestion in the stomach is mostly only preparatory. Enzyme- and bicarbonate-rich pancreatic juice originating from the pancreas and bile from the liver enter the duodenum and is mixed with the chyme from the stomach. Intestinal juice is secreted along the entire length of the intestine from glands in the wall. In healthy individuals, digestion is substantially complete when the chyme passes into the colon. In total, around 8.5 L of fluid enters the small intestine over a 24-hour period (2 L of dietary intake in addition to 6.5 L of various secretions including pancreatic secretions, bile, etc.). Approximately 6.5 L of this total fluid is reabsorbed within the small bowel, with the remaining fluid transiting to the colon.

The small intestine is highly evolved to allow efficient digestion and absorption of virtually all nutrients into the blood; consequently, most absorption occurs in the small bowel. The small intestine is also the major site for water absorption, and this is highly dependent on the absorption of ions. The importance of water and electrolyte absorption in the intestines is exemplified in a clinical case of cholera, a condition in which there can be a massive loss of fluid from the body.

Anatomy and structure

The human small intestine is approximately 3.5 times that of the body's length and is a hollow tube 3.5 cm in diameter that is coiled in the abdomen. It leads from the pylorus of the stomach to the colon (Fig. 5.1). The duodenum comprises the first 25 cm of the small intestine, and this region differs from the rest of the small intestine in having no mesentery. The adjacent region is the jejunum with the remaining distal part termed the ileum.

Duodenum

The duodenum has an essential role in mixing digestive juices derived from the liver, pancreas and its own intestinal wall with the chyme from the stomach. It

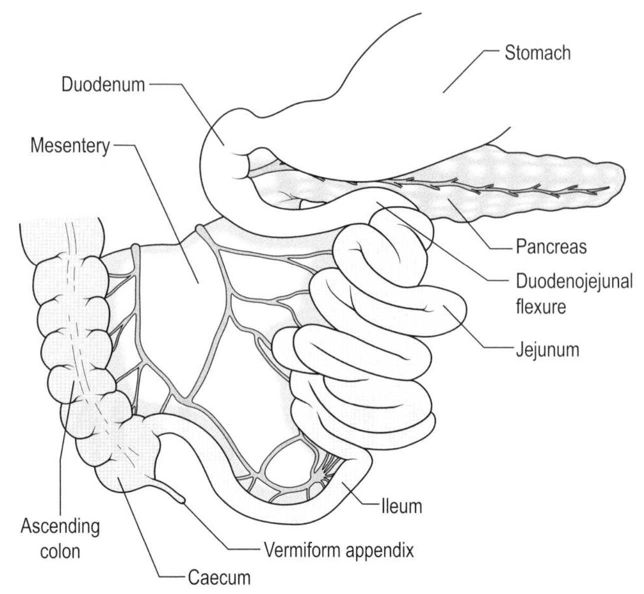

Fig. 5.1 Anatomical arrangement of the small intestine and associated structures.

forms an arc ending in a sharp bend, which is known as the duodenojejunal flexure. The head of the pancreas lies within this arc, with which it shares a blood supply via the pancreaticoduodenal artery (Fig. 5.1). At approximately two-thirds of the way down the descending part of the duodenum are two papillae. The major duodenal papilla is the location of the duct where the bile and pancreatic juice empty into the duodenum via the ampulla of Vater. The opening of the ampulla is controlled by the sphincter of Oddi. An accessory pancreatic duct, present in most individuals, opens at the tip of the lesser papilla.

The surface of the duodenum is folded. The folds are known as plicae circularis (circular folds). Most are crescent-shaped and do not disappear when the intestine is distended. The mucosa of the small intestine is covered with tiny projections, known as villi. These are tongue-shaped in the duodenum.

Two types of glands are present in the duodenal mucosa. At the base of the villi are tubular invaginations that reach almost to the muscularis mucosae, known as intestinal glands or crypts of Lieberkühn (or simply crypts for short). The submucosa of the duodenum contains coiled compound tubular mucous glands known as glands of Brunner that secrete an alkaline fluid rich in mucus. These glands are more numerous in the proximal region of the duodenum. They usually open at the base of the intestinal glands.

Jejunum and ileum

No anatomical feature separates the jejunum from the ileum. The structure of the jejunum and ileum is similar to that of the duodenum. However, there are gradual decreases in diameter, the thickness of the wall and the

Table 5.1 Control of secretion and motility during the intestinal phase

	Effect	*Hormone*
Secretion		
Duodenal (alkaline)	Stimulation	Secretin
Bile (alkaline)	Stimulation	Secretin
Bile (hepatocyte)	None	
Pancreatic juice (alkaline)	Stimulation	Secretin
Pancreatic juice (enzyme-rich)	Stimulation	CCK
Smooth muscle		
Stomach	Relaxation	CCK, secretin
Gallbladder	Contraction	CCK
Sphincter of Oddi	Relaxation	CCK
Intestinal	Contraction	Various

CCK, cholecystokinin.

number of mucosal folds with distance from the duodenum (Fig. 5.2). The folds are absent altogether from the terminal ileum. In addition, the villi gradually become less numerous, smaller and more finger-like with distance from the duodenum. Numerous lymph nodes, called Peyer's patches, are present in the mucosa and submucosa of the ileum. These aggregates of lymphoid tissue monitor intestinal bacteria populations to control the growth of pathogenic bacteria. The junction between the ileum and the large intestine is the ileocaecal junction. It consists of a ring of thickened smooth muscle, known as the ileocaecal sphincter, which reduces reflux from the colon.

The jejunum and ileum are on a mesentery. This contains the arterial blood vessels (branches of the superior mesenteric artery) and the venolymphatic drainage vessels, which are supported in fatty connective tissue and covered by mesothelium.

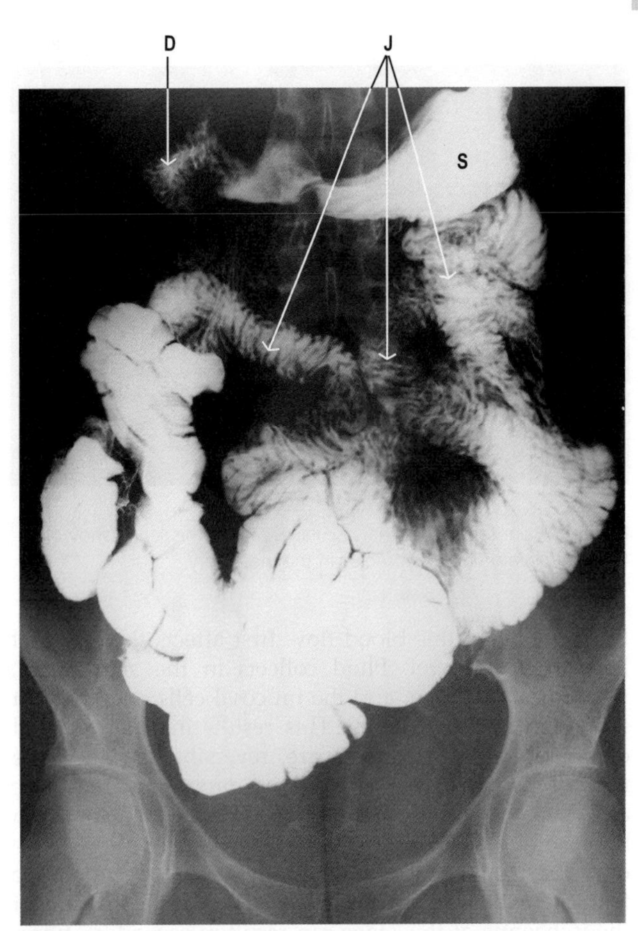

Fig. 5.2 An X-ray of the small bowel taken 2 hours after ingestion of barium. The mucosal outline of the jejunum (J) is clearly seen, showing the dense mucosal folds that maximise the surface area. The stomach (S) and duodenum (D) are also visible.

Blood supply

The major arteries supplying the gastrointestinal (GI) tract are the celiac, superior mesenteric and inferior mesenteric arteries. The celiac supplies duodenum and the superior mesenteric supplies the rest of the small intestine. At rest, approximately 20%–25% of the cardiac output flows to the intestine. Numerous arterial branches form an extensive network in the submucosa that supplies the wall of the intestine (Fig. 5.3).

Nerves, hormones and local paracrine factors control the intestinal circulation. Stimulation of the sympathetic nerves (which follow the arteries) causes vasoconstriction and reduced blood flow, enabling a redistribution of blood away from the intestine. This is particularly important during low cardiac output states such as shock, or during exercise when extra blood is required for skeletal muscle. In the blood vessels of the villi, the vasoconstriction is relatively short-lived. This is due to vasodilator metabolites, such as adenosine, which accumulate during the vasoconstrictor response.

The splanchnic blood flow increases by 50%–300% during a meal (functional hyperaemia). Distension of the walls of the intestine and substances present in the chyme stimulate the blood flow. Other stimuli include products of carbohydrate and lipid digestion in the proximal small intestine and bile acids in the distal ileum. Gastrin, cholecystokinin (CCK), secretin, serotonin and histamine all have the capacity to increase blood flow, and may be involved in this response during a meal. The portal vein carries absorbed constituents away from the small intestine towards the liver.

Ischaemia

Acute ischaemia of the GI tract is a medical emergency. Some 10% of the cardiac output flows to the GI tract.

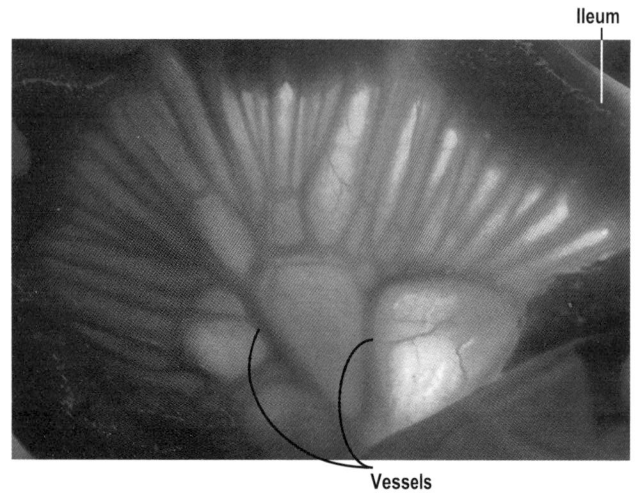

Fig. 5.3 A photograph of the vascular arcade in the ileum, showing the multiple arterial anastomoses in the mesentery.

Interruption of this blood flow first affects the mucosal layer of the bowel. Fluid collects in the submucosa, resulting in oedema, and the mucosal cells quickly start to slough into the lumen. This results in blood-stained diarrhoea. These changes are reversible because the mucosa demonstrates regenerative properties. It can be associated with a fever due to associated bacteraemia because of disruption of the mucosal barrier. Persistence of the ischaemic episode will result in secondary damage to the bowel wall by digestive enzymes. Resolution of the ischaemia at this stage can result in secondary fibrosis and stricturing. Ischaemia that persists beyond a few hours results in loss of integrity of the bowel wall (perforation) and ultimately leakage of intestinal contents into the peritoneal cavity (peritonitis), which can be fatal. Acute ischaemia of the GI tract is a relatively rare event because of the extensive collateral circulation between the mesenteric arteries. Complete occlusion of the superior mesenteric artery, either by thrombosis or an embolic event, may still not lead to infarction because of the collateral blood supply of the coeliac axis and the inferior mesenteric artery.

Ischaemia of the small bowel is more frequently a result of localised venous occlusion. This is seen most often when the bowel is twisted or trapped in a hernia sac. This is made possible because of the mobile nature of the small bowel, the blood supply of which is provided through the mesentery. Here, the arterial pressure is usually sufficient to continue to perfuse the loop of bowel, but the lower-pressure venous drainage is occluded. In this situation, back pressure into the capillary beds results in ischaemia by secondary obstruction to arterial flow.

Circulation in the villi

The blood vessels of the villi (Fig. 5.4) constitute a counter-current exchange system, whereby there is net diffusion of dissolved substances across the interstitium from the venule to the arteriole, or vice versa, depending on which limb has the higher concentration. Thus, oxygen tension is higher in the ascending arterial blood because it is extracted from the blood in the capillaries, and it diffuses from the ascending to the descending limb. This results in a lower oxygen tension at the tips of the villi than at their bases. The relative hypoxia at the tip has been causally implicated in the shedding of the epithelial cells from the tips of the villi.

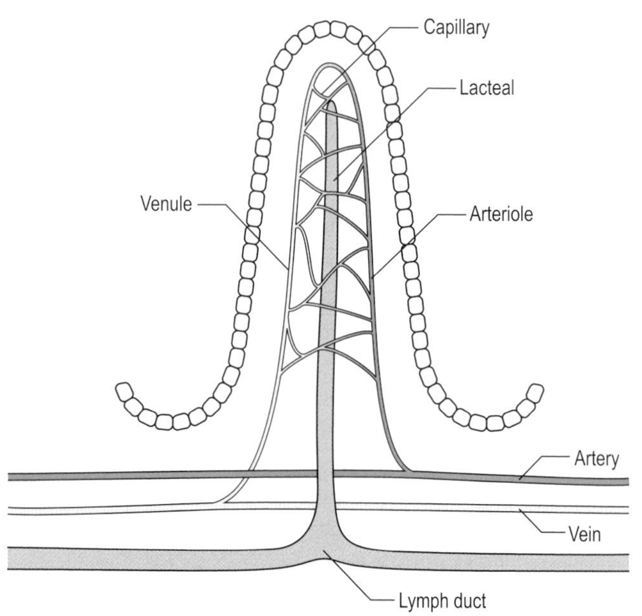

Fig. 5.4 Structural features of the villus.

Surgical resection

The redundant capacity of the small bowel and its ability to adapt, even after major resection, is noteworthy. Even if 60% of the ileum and jejunum are removed, the small intestine retains satisfactory digestive and absorptive capacity. Nutritional support via intravenous feeding (parenteral nutrition) may be required if more than 75% of the ileum and jejunum are removed. This is an unusual situation and is usually only required after a vascular catastrophe when the blood supply from the superior mesenteric artery is lost, and the embryological midgut cannot survive on the collateral circulation from the coeliac and inferior mesenteric arteries. There is insufficient residual digestive and absorptive function to sustain life after such a resection. In addition, the patient will lose considerable quantities of fluid (up to 7 L/day), which also needs to be replaced. It is possible to markedly reduce the secretion using omeprazole, which reduces gastric juice secretion and also reduces secretions in the duodenum as a consequence of the higher pH of the chyme. Segmental resections of the small bowel are frequently and safely performed for conditions such as

Crohn's disease. These segmental resections rarely result in any significant loss of physiological function.

Structure of the intestinal wall

The wall of the small intestine has the same basic structure as other regions of the GI tract. Beneath the serosa is the muscularis externa that consists of two layers of smooth muscle: an outer longitudinal coat and an inner circular coat. Preganglionic parasympathetic nerve fibres of the vagus nerve synapse with the cells of the terminal ganglia in the myenteric plexus. The postganglionic nerves stimulate muscle contraction and gland secretion. Postganglionic sympathetic nerve fibres arising largely from the prevertebral ganglia mostly innervate their target effector cells directly. The submucosal plexus contains a few parasympathetic ganglia of the vagal nerve, but postganglionic sympathetic fibres from the superior mesenteric plexus form the major proportion of the extrinsic nerves present.

Beneath the submucosa is the muscularis mucosae which consists of two thin layers of muscle with some elastic tissue. The inner muscle layer and outer layer consist of circularly and longitudinally disposed fibres, respectively. The muscularis mucosae permits localised movement of the mucous membrane. Small bundles of muscle fibres extend from it to the epithelium. Some of the fibres end on the epithelial basement membrane. Beneath the muscularis mucosa in the lamina propria is a layer of connective tissue that supports the epithelium and contains collagen, reticular fibres and some elastic fibres. It also contains blood capillaries and lymph capillaries that are situated close to the epithelial surface, especially in the villi (Fig. 5.4). It also contains numerous lymphatic nodules. Lymphocytes and plasma cells gain access to this layer across the epithelial membrane. These cells protect the tissue against bacteria that enter across the epithelial membrane.

The brush border/unstirred layer

Despite the mixing processes orchestrated in the small intestine to mix chyme with digestive enzymes and ensure their complete dispersion (see later), the layer of water immediately next to the mucosa is 'unstirred'. Consequently, running along the apical membrane is the 'unstirred layer' or brush border. This acts as an additional barrier to diffusion. This barrier can alter the rate of absorption of water and electrolytes and it can additionally influence the osmotic potential across the membrane.

The villus and crypts

The luminal surface of the small intestine is covered by millions of small projections called villi which extend about 1 mm into the lumen. They consist of a self-renewing population of epithelial cells which absorb nutrients from the lumen and transport them into the blood. The structure of a villus is depicted in Fig. 5.4. Each villus contains a blood capillary network and a blind-ended 'central lacteal' (or lymph vessel). Most of these epithelial cells have numerous cytoplasmic extensions, known as microvilli, at the luminal surface. The microvillous surface of the intestine is known as the brush border. There are approximately 36,000 microvilli per cell, which markedly increases surface area.

Recessed into the mucosa are the crypts. At the centre of these crypts are the progenitor cells from which all cell types found on the epithelium originate. Cells slowly migrate to the top of the villus tips and are eventually shed. The process of migration from the crypts to the tips of the villi occurs over 3–6 days in the human. Thus, most of the intestinal epithelium is renewed every few days. The columnar cells mature as they travel towards the tips of the villi and their functions change.

Cell histology of the villus and the crypt

The following cell types are illustrated in Fig. 5.5.

Columnar absorptive cells/enterocytes

Columnar cells comprise around 80% of all intestinal epithelial cells in the small intestine. Absorptive cells produce digestive enzymes and absorb nutrients. In addition, the cells at the base of the villi produce a glycoprotein cell coat. Some of these glycoproteins are enzymes involved in the digestion of nutrients, such as disaccharides. They act *in situ* but are also active after being shed into the lumen.

Goblet cells

Goblet cells produce mucus which lubricates the surface and protects it from mechanical damage. They additionally produce trefoil peptides which are required for epithelial maintenance.

Paneth cells

Paneth cells are mostly located at the base of the crypts and provide an important antibacterial defence in the small intestine. They are dense with secretory granules of antimicrobial peptides including defensins, as well as lysozyme, phospholipase A and numerous growth factors. Paneth cells uniquely move downwards further into the crypt as they mature (unlike the other epithelial cells). In addition, while most epithelial cells are rapidly turned over, Paneth cells are relatively long-lived and last several weeks.

Endocrine cells

These enteric endocrine cells sense the environment of the lumen. These cells can produce secretin, somatostatin,

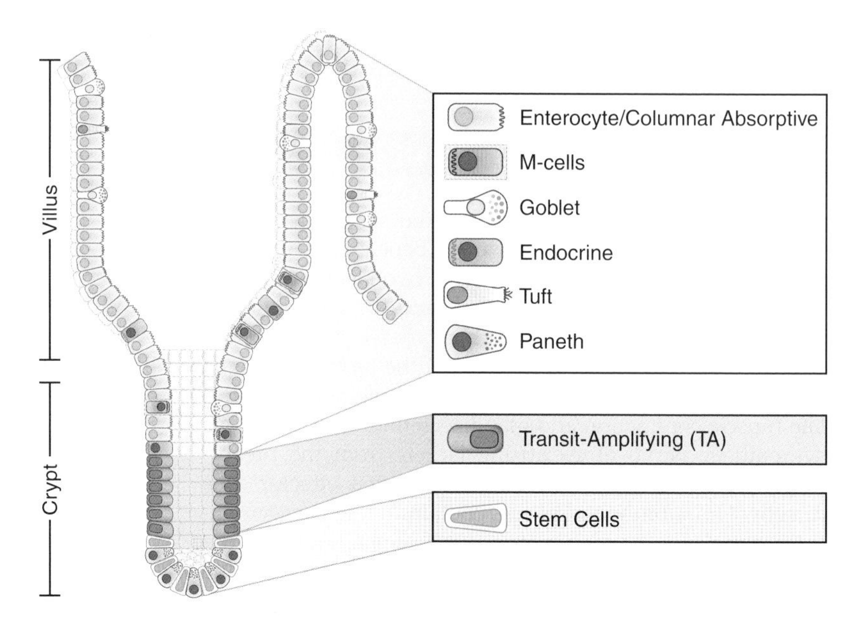

Fig. 5.5 Localisation of the different cell types in the epithelium of the crypts and the villi.

CCK and serotonin. These hormones regulate secretion and motility in the GI tract, liver and pancreas. Endocrine cells comprise about 1% of the cells in the crypts.

Stem cells

Stem cells are found at the very base of the crypts, dividing continuously to replenish all cell types throughout the crypt and villus.

Oligomucous cells

These are precursors to goblet cells. They mature as they distend with mucus whilst migrating up the villus.

Tuft cells

Tuft cells are epithelial cells with a unique tubulovesicular system and apical bundle of microfilaments connected to a tuft of long and thick microvilli protruding into the lumen. They play an important role in the immunological response to intestinal parasites (including helminths and protozoa). Recent studies have found that the number of tuft cells tends to increase in the metaplastic intestine. Their full role and function remain to be fully elucidated.

M cells

M cells cover the surface of the gut-associated lymphoid follicles and function as an interface between the luminal content and the underlying immune cells and thus have a role in mucosal immunity.

Intestinal secretions

An alkaline fluid containing electrolytes, mucus and water is secreted throughout the length of the small intestine. The precise composition of the secretion and the mechanisms that control it vary from one region to another. Normal small intestinal function results in net absorption, although secretion is an important physiologic process. The following two distinct processes establish an osmotic gradient that draws water into the lumen of the intestine: (1) increases in luminal osmolarity due to digested chyme and (2) the secretion of electrolytes from the crypts.

Luminal osmotic pressure due to the influx and digestion of chyme

The chyme that enters the intestine from the stomach is not hyperosmotic. However, as the food components are broken down into smaller constituents, the osmolarity rapidly decreases. Fibrous macromolecules, like starch, contribute little to osmotic pressure in their native intact form. However, as starch is digested, thousands of molecules of maltose are generated, each of which is as osmotically active as the original starch molecule. As these smaller components become absorbed, the osmolarity of the intestinal contents decreases, meaning water can thus again be absorbed.

Electrolyte secretion from crypt cells

Crypt epithelial cells express the cystic fibrosis transmembrane conductance regulator (CFTR). This channel mediates the secretion of water in the lumen of the intestine.

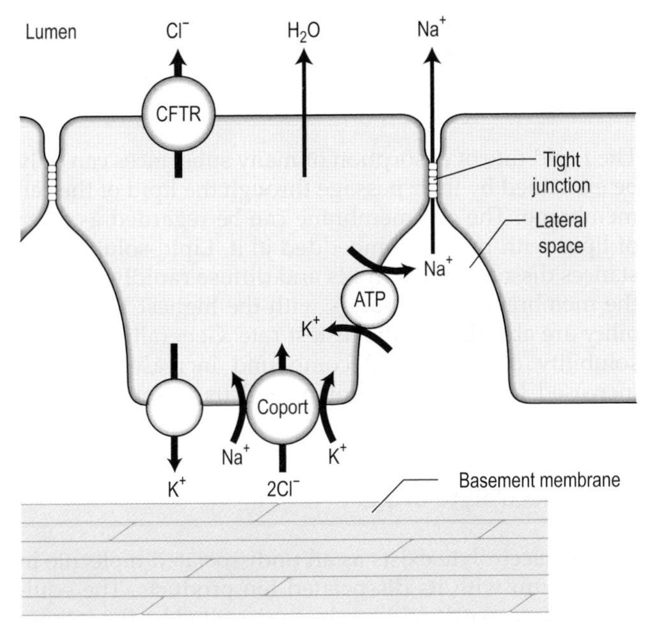

Fig. 5.6 Mechanism of secretion of electrolytes and water by the immature cells of the crypts of Lieberkühn. *ATP, adenosine triphosphate; CFTR, cystic fibrosis transmembrane conductance regulator.*

Firstly, Cl^- is actively transported into the cell via a co-transporter protein that transports one Na^+ ion, one K^+ ion and two Cl^- ions. The transport of Na^+ down its electrical gradient is the driving force for the operation of this transporter. K^+ is transported back out via K^+ channels in the same membrane. This K^+ flux maintains the electrical potential difference (negative inside the cell) across the cell membrane. Activation of adenylyl cyclase by several secretagogues (such as vasoactive intestinal peptide (VIP)) leads to the generation of cAMP which activates the CFTR channel to pump Cl^- ions into the intestinal lumen. Na^+ is then transported via tight junctions into the lumen down an electrical gradient. Secretion of NaCl into the crypt creates an osmotic gradient across the tight junction and water is consequently drawn into the lumen. The mechanisms involved are detailed in Fig. 5.6.

The mechanism of action of cholera toxin is also via increasing intracellular cAMP. In this case, it causes a massive secretion of fluid which results in diarrhoea. Several other bacteria produce toxins that act similarly, which have caused the deaths of billions of people (see later).

Control of secretion in the small intestine

Secretion in the small intestine can be controlled by hormones, paracrine factors and nervous activity.

Hormonal regulation of secretion

A complex array of hormonal mechanisms controls entry and exit of fluid into the GI tract. Serotonin, gastrin, VIP and other hormones stimulate epithelial cells to secrete directly. P-glycoprotein (Substance P) is widely distributed in the small intestine. Substance P alters blood flow, water exchange and intestinal motility to increase secretion.

Neuronal regulation of secretion

Epithelial cells are innervated by secretomotor neurones, mainly from ganglia in the submucosal plexus but also from ganglia in the myenteric plexus. The submucosal neurones release acetylcholine (Ach), VIP, Substance P, serotonin and probably other transmitters to stimulate secretion. Parasympathetic nerves innervate neurones in the enteric nerve plexi. They enhance secretion via ACh release onto neurones in the plexi. Parasympathetic tone contributes to the basal secretion. Reflexes triggered by distension of the lumen of the small intestine and the presence of various substances (glucose, acid, bile salts, ethanol, cholera toxin) in the intestinal chyme stimulate secretion. These reflexes involve intrinsic and extrinsic (parasympathetic nerves) factors.

Noradrenaline inhibits secretion in two ways: it acts directly on epithelial cells (via α-adrenoreceptors) and directly on neurones in the submucosal ganglia to inhibit secretory nerves that stimulate epithelial cells. Somatostatin acts humourally on the crypt cells as an inhibitory neurotransmitter. It is released from the enteric secretomotor nerves and from the nerve fibres that innervate the crypt cells. It inhibits secretion by decreasing the levels of cAMP in the epithelial crypt cells.

Absorption

Most substances are absorbed in the proximal small intestine and most of the contents of the small intestine have normally been absorbed by the time the chyme reaches the middle of the jejunum. However, a few substances such as vitamin B_{12} and bile salts are actively absorbed in the ileum.

Surface area of the small intestine

The rate of transport of materials across the small intestine is proportional to its surface area. The surface area of the small intestine is vast. This organ is therefore well-adapted for absorption. Its area is approximately 600 times greater than that of a simple cylinder of the same length and diameter, by virtue of the presence of mucosal folds, villi and microvilli (Fig. 5.7).

When the surface area is reduced, malabsorption of many substances ensues. In coeliac disease, for example, which is characterised by villous atrophy and therefore reduced surface area, there is malabsorption of many nutrients resulting in malnutrition.

Barriers to absorption

There are several barriers influencing transport from the intestinal lumen to the blood including the unstirred

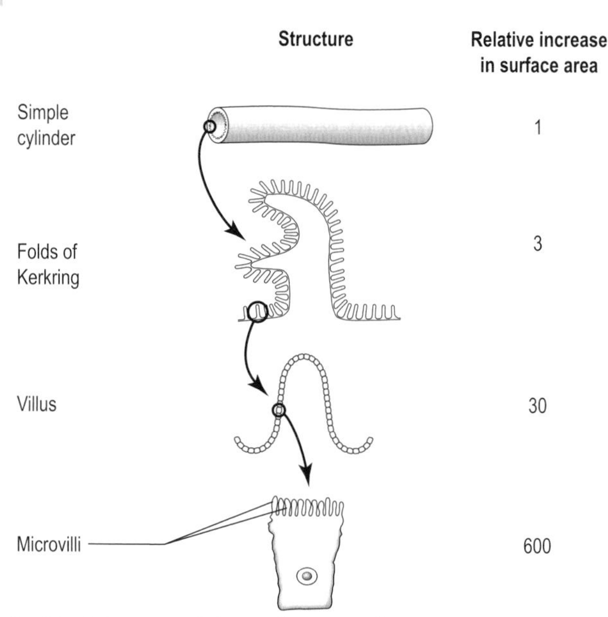

Fig. 5.7 Adaptation of the small intestine for absorption. Comparison of the surface area of a segment of the small intestine with a simple cylinder of the same length and diameter.

layer, the luminal plasma membrane, the cell's interior, the basolateral plasma membrane, the intercellular space, the basement membrane of the capillary and the cell membranes of the endothelial cell of the capillary or lymph vessels.

The luminal border of the enterocyte is the effective barrier for the absorption of many substances, but it is the basolateral border or the endothelial cell membrane for some substances. Transport across some of the plasma membranes involved, like the membranes of the endothelial cells, is via simple passive diffusion. However, for transport across others, special mechanisms such as active transport, facilitated diffusion or pinocytosis (endocytosis) exist.

Potential difference across the small intestine

A potential difference exists across the wall of the small intestine, where the serosal side is positive with respect to the mucosal side. In the case of a charged ion, transport is the net effect of the forces due to the concentration gradient and the potential difference. Thus, net transport of anions from the lumen can occur passively down the electrochemical gradient.

The size of the potential difference varies along the length of the small intestine. The magnitude of the potential difference is determined by the active transport of electrolytes, in particular Na^+, which occurs against the electrical gradient (see below). The magnitude of the potential difference is increased in the presence of glucose that stimulates the active transport of Na^+.

Absorption of drugs

Lipid-soluble drugs

The rapid rate of absorption of many substances can only be explained by their passage through the lipid of the cell membrane. The cell membrane can be regarded as a sea of lipid with proteins embedded in it. Lipid-soluble substances dissolve in the lipids and diffuse rapidly through the membrane. Compounds with the highest lipid solubility are absorbed at the fastest rate. Generally, the lipid solubility of a chemical compound increases with its increased hydrocarbon content and its lesser degree of ionisation.

Weak electrolyte drugs

A weak electrolyte exists as an undissociated molecule in equilibrium with its dissociated ion products. The equilibrium for a weak acid can be represented by the following equation:

$$HA \rightleftharpoons H^+ + A^-$$

HA represents an undissociated weak acid, and A^- its anionic component. The undissociated molecule, since it is not charged, is likely to be more lipid soluble. The barbiturate, phenobarbital, is an example of a weak electrolyte drug. More than 90% of drugs are organic, weak electrolytes, especially those compounded, manufactured or reconstituted as injections in predominantly ionised or salt forms.

The undissociated (HA) molecule is transported rapidly through the lipid membrane. As the undissociated molecule is removed from the lumen, its concentration will drop. As its dissociation constant is under equilibrium, more of the undissociated molecule will form from the dissociated ions. The reassembled HA can then diffuse across the membrane. In this way the substance can be rapidly absorbed. The rate of transport will depend on the proportion of the undissociated compound present in the pH of the small intestinal lumen. In situations where the proportion of non-ionised molecule is increased, the rate of absorption will be high.

Many drugs are weak electrolytes. For a weak acid the rate of absorption can be increased if the pH of the solution is lowered below the pKa value of the acid because the equilibrium will be shifted to the left (as the weak acid will be less likely to be dissociated at these lowered pH environments). The opposite applies to a weak base which has a high pKa. Fig. 5.8 illustrates this for two drugs: 5-nitrosalicylic acid, an aspirin derivative, which is a weak acid, and quinine, which is a weak base. In the upper small intestine, the pH of the chyme tends to be slightly acidic, thereby favouring the absorption of weak acids. Furthermore, some weak acids such as aspirin can be absorbed in the acidic environment of the stomach.

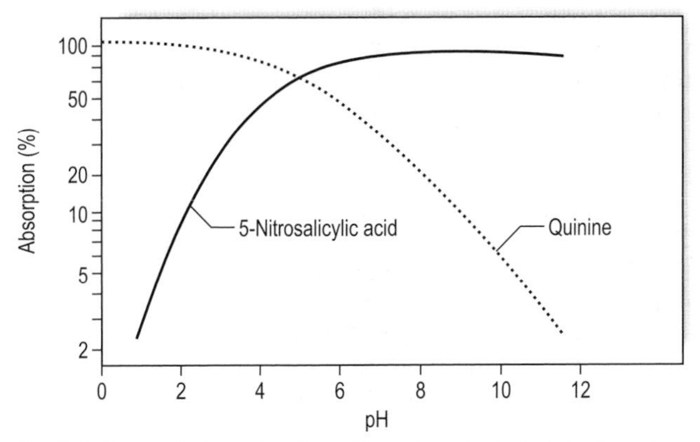

Fig. 5.8 Effect of pH on the absorption of weak electrolyte drugs in the small intestine. Absorption of a weak acid, 5-nitrosalicylic acid (pKa 2.3), and a weak base, quinine (pKa 8.4).

Strong electrolyte drugs

Strong acids (pKa ~ 3.0) and bases (pKa ~ 10) are very poorly absorbed. Clinically important drugs such as the muscle relaxants tubocurarine and hexamethonium that are strong bases must be administered intravenously. However, for others, such as the aminoglycoside antibiotics, their poor absorption is an advantage because they can be used to sterilise the gut before intestinal surgery without producing systemic effects.

Factors that affect gastrointestinal absorption of drugs

Both chemical properties of the drug and GI factors can alter the absorption profile of drugs, including the following:

- Drug concentration: the larger the dose, the quicker it will be absorbed.
- Compound size: the smaller the chemical compound, the quicker it will be absorbed.
- pKa: weak electrolytes are absorbed better than strong electrolytes.
- Lipophilicity: the higher the degree of lipophilicity, the better the absorption.
- Formulation disintegration: slow-release formulations will slow the absorption rate.
- Gastric motility: faster gastric emptying results in faster absorption.
- Intestinal motility: this can increase or decrease the rate of absorption.
- Splanchnic perfusion: Gut perfusion can be a rate-limiting step for rapidly absorbed drugs. If perfusion is impaired, it can impact absorption for all drugs.
- Intestinal content: interaction with other intestinal substances can alter absorption profiles. Chemical properties that can cause a reduced absorption rate include the ability to bind strongly to Ca^{2+} e.g. (for example, tetracycline chelates intestinal calcium forming an insoluble complex).
- Enterohepatic recirculation: hepatic transformation is essential for some pro-drugs (drugs that are activated upon biotransformation by the liver).
- Gut bacteria: metabolism by gut bacteria can alter absorption profiles.

Mechanisms of absorption into the blood or lymph

Some substances are absorbed solely by passive diffusion. Others are absorbed by both passive and specialised mechanisms: at a rapid rate by a specialised mechanism, and at a slow rate by passive diffusion.

A substance that is absorbed into the blood or lymph can be transported across the luminal and basolateral membranes of the enterocyte and, if it is transported into the blood, it crosses the membranes of the endothelial cells of the capillary. In many cases, a given substance is transported across each membrane by a different mechanism. A good example is the transport of Na^+ by carrier-mediated facilitated diffusion across the brush border by active transport across the basolateral border (see below) and via passive diffusion across the endothelial membranes of the capillaries.

Some substances are preferentially absorbed into the blood capillaries of the villi and some into the lacteals (Fig. 5.4). Two properties determine whether a given substance is absorbed into the blood or the lymph: its size and its lipid solubility. Large molecules, particles and lipid-soluble substances are transported into the lymph. Most lipids are sequestered in chylomicrons prior to transport into the lymph, and certain intact proteins can be absorbed in trace amounts in some individuals. Most other small and water-soluble substances are absorbed into the blood.

Transport across the endothelial cells of blood and lymph vessels is always passive and occurs down a concentration or electrochemical gradient. Substances that are absorbed into the lymph eventually gain access to the blood via the thoracic duct. The reasons for a particular substance being preferentially absorbed into the blood or lymph are outlined below.

Absorption into the blood

Both capillaries and lymph vessels are freely permeable to low-molecular-weight water-soluble substances. However, there is an extensive network of capillaries in each villus but only a single lacteal and therefore there is a greater surface area available for transport into the blood than into the lymph and a greater blood volume. Furthermore, blood flow is much greater (approximately

500 times faster) than lymph flow. This ensures the rapid removal of the transported substances, which are carried away via the rapidly flowing blood and helps to maintain a favourable concentration gradient for transport. Thus, most (95%) low-molecular-weight water-soluble substances are absorbed into the blood.

Absorption into the lymph

The endothelial cells of capillaries contain pores (fenestrae) with diameters in the range of 20–50 nM. They also have a basement membrane. The pores are large enough to admit large molecules, but they cannot cross the basement membrane and are therefore excluded from the capillary blood. Lipids are delivered to the lateral spaces as components of large protein-bound particles (chylomicrons), which are excluded from the capillaries for the same reason.

The endothelial cells of the lacteals lack a basement membrane. They do not contain pores, but when they are viewed under the microscope the endothelial cells appear to be displaced relative to each other at their lateral borders (as though movement can occur between adjacent cells). It seems likely therefore that transient gaps form between adjacent cells. Large molecules or particles are probably transported to the lymph between the cells via these gaps. Peristalsis and the pumping action of the villi (see below) aid absorption into the lacteals, probably by promoting the formation of the gaps.

Transport of water and electrolytes in different regions of the small intestine

The cells at the tips of the villi are specialised for water and ion transport while those in the crypts produce net secretion of water and ions. However, the rate of transport varies along the length of the intestine because the villi are larger and the brush border surface is greater per unit area in the proximal region of the small intestine than the distal region (see above). Thus, the fluxes of water and nutrients tend to be greater in the jejunum than the ileum, except where localised special transport mechanisms exist. The surface area in the colon is less than that in the small intestine and therefore less net transport occurs in the colon. Flux of ions and water occurs both transcellularly and paracellularly (involving tight junctions). The tight junctions are leakier in the proximal small intestine than the distal regions. This also results in a greater paracellular flux per unit area in the jejunum than the ileum. The result is that most absorption occurs in the proximal small intestine.

Absorption of water

A healthy individual consumes approximately 2 L of dietary fluid every day. However, in the small intestine this is further mixed with approximately 6.5 L of the various secretions (saliva, stomach juice, small intestinal secretions and bile) which culminates in approximately 8.5 L entering the small intestine every day. Around 80% of this fluid is absorbed before the bolus reaches the colon, outlining the importance of the small intestine in being the primary site for water absorption. The absorption of water across the intestinal border is tightly coupled to the transport of various ions most notably sodium ions.

Initially, active transport of sodium ions occurs into the cell. These ions then pass into the intercellular and lateral spaces, which provides an electrochemical gradient for other ions (notably Cl^- ions) to be absorbed via a passive, paracellular mechanism into these lateral spaces. The net effect is to create a hyperosmotic environment within these spaces which promotes water absorption from the lumen. Thus, water absorption is linked to ion absorption.

In this instance, Na^+ and water will then diffuse into the capillary bed within the villus. The transport of water from the lumen to blood is often against an osmotic gradient, when considered as a whole. This intermediate movement of Na^+ into the enterocyte and out again with water following ensures that the intestine can absorb water into blood even when the osmolarity in the lumen is higher than that of blood.

The transport of water in the small intestine can, however, occur from blood to the lumen. It will be secreted into the lumen if the chyme is hypertonic to plasma and absorbed into the blood if it is hypotonic. The chyme entering the duodenum from the stomach is usually initially hypertonic. Rapid gastric emptying, as may occur after surgery, results in the contents of the small intestine being abnormally hypertonic. This causes an influx of water into the small intestine. If excessive, this can cause severe diarrhoea. The digestion of complex nutrients in the duodenal chyme results in a further increase in osmolarity. The prevailing osmotic forces result in the secretion of water in this region, and the intestinal contents normally become isotonic with plasma in the duodenum.

Absorption of sodium and chloride

The GI tract is responsible for handling fluid containing approximately 800 mmol of sodium and 700 mmol of chloride.

Sodium

There are three main mechanisms of sodium absorption within the GI tract:

1. Nutrient-coupled Na^+ absorption,
2. Electroneutral NaCl absorption through Na^+/H^+ exchange and
3. Electrogenic Na^+ absorption via epithelial Na^+ channels (ENaCs). These are predominantly found within the colon.

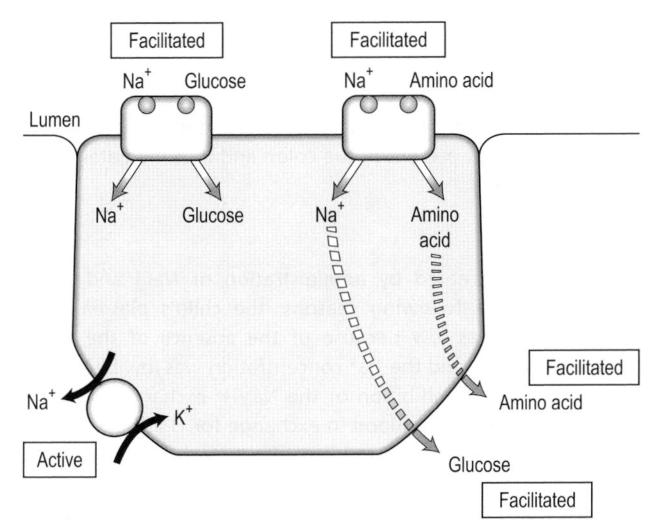

Fig. 5.9 The secondary active transport of Na^+ via the Na^+/glucose and Na^+/amino acid co-transport systems in the absorptive cells of the proximal small intestine.

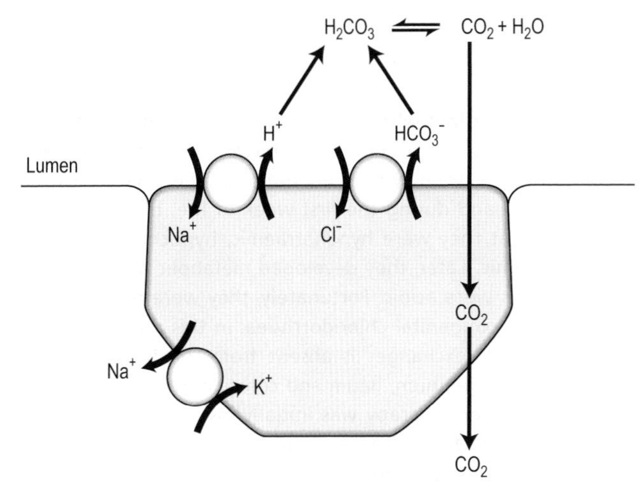

Fig. 5.10 Electroneutral Na^+ absorption. The active transport of Na^+ and Cl^- ions via the Na^+/H^+ exchange and Cl^-/HCO_3^- exchange systems, respectively, in the small intestine.

The transport of sodium across the epithelial cells of the small intestine is by both passive diffusion and active mechanisms. The mucosal surface of the small intestine is electronegative with respect to the serosal surface, favouring the passive transport of Na^+ into the lumen. The electrochemical gradient is largely due to the secretion of Cl^- into the lumen (Fig. 5.6).

Most Na^+ is transported from the lumen of the small intestine into the blood by active mechanisms. This involves the transcellular route. It is usually transported in the absence of a chemical gradient as the chyme in the small intestine is normally isotonic with plasma, but it is obviously transported against the small electrochemical gradient present. The processes involved are illustrated in Fig. 5.9.

The key process is the active transport of Na^+ out of the cell, across the lateral border via a Na^+/K^+ adenosine triphosphatase (ATPase) pump, which simultaneously pumps K^+ into the cell. This maintains the low concentration of Na^+ within the cell. The Na^+ concentration gradient set up by this pump is the driving force for the transport of Na^+ from the lumen of the intestine into the cell. This diffusion across the luminal brush border of the cell is therefore down the concentration gradient. However, transport across this membrane occurs at a faster rate than it would by simple passive diffusion. This is because the Na^+ ions are transported on carrier proteins in the brush border membrane. One of these carriers is the Na^+-dependent/glucose transporter (SGLT1). It only functions if glucose, or galactose (which competes with glucose), is present in the lumen. The transporter has a binding site for glucose and a binding site for Na^+.

In electroneutral NaCl absorption, Na^+ is actively absorbed in exchange for H^+ that is secreted into the lumen via a Na^+/H^+ exchange (NHE) mechanism. This is coupled to a Cl^-/HCO_3^- exchanger where Cl^- is absorbed in exchange for HCO_3^-. Thus, in this mechanism, Na^+ and Cl^- ions are absorbed into the enterocyte in exchange for HCO_3^- and H^+, hence the term 'electroneutral'. The anion exchange mechanism is illustrated in Fig. 5.10. The bicarbonate ion which is central to this mechanism is generated through the actions of carbonic anhydrase using CO_2 and H_2O as additional substrates. This mechanism of Na^+ transport is operational during the fasted state as it is not dependent on the presence of nutrients within the intestinal lumen which drives the nutrient-coupled Na^+ absorption.

The importance of this mechanism is exemplified in congenital sodium diarrhoea, where missense mutations in the gene coding for one of the Na^+/H^+ exchangers have been identified.

The last mechanism, electrogenic Na^+ absorption, which predominantly occurs in the distal colon, involves epithelial sodium channels (ENaCs) which are responsible for sodium absorption. These are regulated in part through mineralocorticoids including angiotensin and aldosterone.

Chloride

There are three main mechanisms of chloride absorption within the GI tract;

1. Via a paracellular pathway,
2. Electroneutral NaCl absorption (as detailed above involving Na^+/H^+ and Cl^-/HCO_3^- exchangers) and
3. HCO_3^--dependent Cl^- absorption.

The paracellular pathway of chloride ion absorption predominantly occurs in the small intestine and is linked to the chloride gradient across the mucosa. The second mechanism of Cl^- ion transport is the electroneutral exchange pathway (detailed above), which culminates in both Na^+ and Cl^- ions. Finally, Cl^- ions can also be exchanged for HCO_3^- ions independent of the sodium proton exchanger in electroneutral NaCl absorption. The importance of this Cl^-/HCO_3^- exchanger is exemplified by the clinical condition congenital chloridorrhoea, where there is a congenital absence of this exchanger.

Case 5.1 Congenital chloridorrhea

A premature infant who was born with a distended abdomen developed diarrhoea soon after birth. The faecal chloride content was extremely high (95 mmol/L). The child appeared dehydrated and during the first week of life, blood analyses showed that they were hyponatraemic, hypochloraemic and hypokalaemic. Later, they developed metabolic alkalosis, and their faeces were acidic. Fortunately, they were quickly diagnosed with congenital chloridorrhoea. In this rare condition, the Cl^-/HCO_3^- exchanger is absent from the luminal membranes of the jejunum, ileum and colon. Intravenous electrolyte replacement therapy was initially instituted, but after a few weeks, electrolyte replacement therapy (a solution of KCl and NaCl) could be given orally.

Defect and consequences

In this condition, the inherited defect is an absence of the Cl^-/HCO_3^- exchanger in the brush border membrane in the small intestine and in the colon. The exchanger transports Cl^- out of the lumen in exchange for HCO_3^- (Fig. 5.10). The Na^+/H^+ exchanger is normal in this condition, but eventually the acidity of the luminal contents inhibits the Na^+/H^+ exchange mechanism as well.

Diarrhoea

If the exchanger protein is absent, Cl^- transported across the gut wall is reduced, and Cl^- is lost in the faeces. The high concentrations of electrolytes present in the lumen cause water to be transported into the lumen by osmosis (osmotic diarrhoea). The absence of the exchanger in the jejunum is less important than its absence in the ileum and colon because water is transported as a consequence of Na^+/glucose and Na^+/amino acid nutrient-coupled mechanisms in the jejunum. These nutrient-coupled systems are not numerous in the ileum and not present in the colon and thus mediates the diarrhoea.

Treatment

The child was treated by administration of NaCl and KCl solution for the following reasons: the child's plasma Cl^- concentration was low because of the absence of the Cl^-/HCO_3^- exchanger, and the Na^+ concentration was low because of the consequent inhibition of the Na^+/H^+ exchanger which transports Na^+ into the blood in exchange for H^+. The K^+ was low because K^+ is transported into the lumen down its concentration gradient. If water accumulates in the lumen, as in diarrhoea, this gradient will favour transport into the lumen, as the contents become more dilute.

Thus, the oral replacement therapy given will correct the hyponatraemia (low blood Na^+ concentration), the hypokalaemia (low blood K^+ concentration) and the hypochloraemia (low blood Cl^- concentration).

Metabolic alkalosis

The exchanger protein that is absent in congenital chloridorrhoea transports Cl^- into the blood in exchange for HCO_3^- that is transported into the lumen. If the exchanger is absent, HCO_3^- accumulates in the blood and causes alkalosis. The Na^+/H^+ exchange system transports Na^+ into the blood in exchange for H^+, which is transported into the lumen. This is normally neutralised by the HCO_3^- transported into the lumen in exchange for Cl^-, but in this case the Cl^-/HCO_3^- exchanger is absent in the membranes and H^+ would be lost in the faeces.

Diarrhoea

Diarrhoea is defined clinically as a loss of excess fluid (>500 mL/day) and solutes from the GI tract, which is typically the passage of three or more abnormally loose or watery stools per 24 hours. The change in consistency of the stool is of greater importance than the number of watery movements. Acute diarrhoea usually resolves within 7 days of onset but can persist up to 28 days. Dysentery is diarrhoea with the visible presence of blood in the stools. The common causes of acute diarrhoea are infectious agents, toxins, drugs, food or anxiety. The mechanisms responsible for loss of fluid can operate in the small intestine or the colon. A common cause of chronic diarrhoea is inflammatory bowel disease (including Crohn's disease and ulcerative colitis).

The different mechanisms of diarrhoea are detailed below. In many cases, there is overlap between the specific mechanisms. Disruption of the osmotic balance between the small intestinal epithelia and the lumen is commonly the reason for water movement into the lumen.

Secretory diarrhoea

In secretory diarrhoea, the secretions of the small intestine are so copious that the capacity of the colon to reabsorb the excessive water is overwhelmed. This diarrhoea is usually caused by infectious agents such as *Vibrio cholerae* or enterotoxigenic *Escherichia coli*. If the bacteria successfully pass through the gastric acid barrier, they can colonise within the small intestine. Here, they produce toxins, specifically enterotoxins. These toxins bind to receptors in the membranes of the secreting crypt cells to increase intracellular cAMP, which stimulates a massive secretion. This is orchestrated as cAMP inhibits or blocks the chloride-linked neutral sodium absorption from the intestinal lumen by the villus cells in addition to directly stimulating chloride secretion by the crypt cells into the lumen. Importantly, the glucose/amino acid-mediated sodium absorption transporters are not affected. Excessive activation of intrinsic neurones in pathological conditions may also cause secretory diarrhoea. Some of these neurones release VIP that increases intracellular cAMP. Others release transmitters such as acetylcholine or substance P that leads to increased intracellular Ca^{2+}, which can also mediate excessive secretion from the crypt cells. The massive secretion of fluid in cholera can cause hypovolaemia.

Case 5.2 Cholera

A father and son both presented to hospital situated in a remote region of Bengal. The father appeared emaciated. He said he had initially been vomiting and suffering from abdominal distention, and now he was suffering from copious diarrhoea. His pulse was barely detectable, but his pulse rate was rapid (100 bpm). His son was also suffering from diarrhoea, but he was less severely affected. The doctor suspected that they were both victims of the latest cholera epidemic. Such epidemics are not uncommon in the region because of contamination of food and drinking water with the bacterium *V. cholerae*. The father was provided with electrolyte fluid via an intravenous drip. His plasma and urine K^+ and HCO_3^- concentrations were monitored. He was also given intravenous tetracycline for 2 days. The son was given some packets containing a mixture of salt (NaCl) and sugar (glucose) and a supply of clean drinking water. He was told to dissolve the salt and sugar in clean water from the hospital supply and to drink large quantities of the solution over the next few days. He was given tetracycline to take by mouth. Both patients recovered within a few days.

Causes, mechanism of action and changes in electrolyte and acid–base balance

Causes

The *V. cholerae* bacterium present in contaminated water and food produces a toxin that elicits a massive secretion of fluid and electrolytes. The effect is produced mainly in the proximal small intestine and the bacteria are harboured in the gallbladder in asymptomatic carriers.

Bacteria are normally destroyed by gastric acid in the stomach, normally providing some protection. Increased susceptibility to the disease is seen in individuals with achlorhydria or those who have had a partial gastrectomy.

Mechanisms of cholera toxin action

Hypersecretion

The increases in cAMP induced by the presence of cholera toxin induces anion secretion whilst also inhibiting sodium chloride absorption. Most pertinently, cAMP inhibits the electroneutral form of Na^+ transport and this in conjunction with the increased anion secretion results in a hyperosmotic luminal environment, which draws fluid into the intestinal lumen. Patients with cholera sometimes produce up to 20 L of watery stool per day.

Hypermotility

Hypermotility of the small intestine can result in water and electrolytes being delivered rapidly into the colon. It can be delivered so fast that the colon may not be able to absorb it before it is lost in the faeces. This mechanism is also involved in conditions such as cholera, as distension of the intestines by the large volumes of secreted fluids stimulates peristaltic activity, which propels the fluid rapidly along the intestines.

Changes in electrolyte and acid–base balance

Secretions of the small intestines contain large amounts of HCO_3^-, Na^+ and Cl^- ions. K^+ is absorbed during a meal, down the concentration gradient set up by the absorption of water. However, when the concentration of K^+ in the lumen is reduced below approximately 25 mM, the concentration gradient favours net secretion into the lumen. This occurs via the paracellular pathway. In diarrhoea, the luminal contents become diluted with respect to K^+ and it is therefore transported into the lumen. Considerable losses of K^+ can occur, leading to hypokalaemia. K^+ is required for cell growth and division, enzyme action, cell excitability, muscle contraction, acid–base balance and volume regulation. Hypokalaemia (reduced serum K^+ concentration) causes hyperpolarisation of cell membranes and reduces the excitability of neurones, cardiac muscle and skeletal muscle. Severe hypokalaemia can cause paralysis, cardiac arrhythmias, decreased ability to concentrate urine and death.

As HCO_3^- is secreted into the lumen, H^+ is transported into the blood, which becomes transiently acidic. Excessive loss of HCO_3^- in secreted intestinal fluid causes a severe acidosis. The transient acidity in the blood is normally neutralised by the alkaline tide that accompanies the secretion of acid in the stomach. However, if there is excessive loss of alkaline fluid from the GI tract, the acidity in the blood is proportionately increased and it cannot be buffered. This metabolic acidosis will be partially compensated in the short term by an increased rate and depth of breathing which results in CO_2 being blown off from the body. Longer-term adjustments are brought about by reabsorption of HCO_3^- in the tubules of the kidney and excretion of H^+.

Rehydration therapy

Individuals suffering from cholera are treated with (1) intravenous fluid and electrolytes or with (2) oral fluid, salt and sugar, depending on the severity of their symptoms.

Continued

Case 5.2 Cholera—cont'd

Intravenous rehydration

The intravenous fluid would consist of water containing electrolytes in concentrations that are isotonic with plasma. The massive fluid loss can lead to dehydration, hypovolaemia, renal failure and death. Particular attention is paid to K^+ and HCO_3^- replacement as excessive losses of these ions can have rapid and dangerous consequences.

Oral rehydration therapy

Whilst cholera toxin supresses electroneutral sodium ion transport, Na^+ can still be absorbed through the nutrient-coupled mechanisms. Consequently, patients with cholera can be successfully rehydrated using a simple oral rehydration therapy based on sodium and glucose. The solution used should be isotonic or hypotonic, as a hypertonic load will create an osmotic gradient for the transport of more water into the lumen. Inflammation and damage to the mucosa are not normally present and the digestion and absorptive mechanisms are not affected.

Osmotic diarrhoea

As discussed earlier, the barriers of the small intestine allow a flux of water and electrolytes to maintain the osmotic balance. The presence of hypertonic fluid, poorly absorbed substances or osmotically active substances in the intestinal lumen can cause osmotic diarrhoea due to the movement of water from the extracellular fluid into the gut lumen. High concentrations of salts such as SO_4^{2-}, Mg^{2+} and PO_4^{3-}, which are only slowly absorbed in the intestine, can be responsible. Magnesium sulphate solution is commonly used as a laxative.

Absorption disorders can also give rise to osmotic diarrhoea. The presence of lactose or glucose in conditions associated with poor absorption can lead to secretion into the small intestine. Furthermore, when these nutrients enter the large intestine, they may be fermented by colonic bacteria so that each molecule is degraded to several products, thereby increasing the osmolarity even further. Consequently, the volume of water transported into the lumen may be too great for the colon to reabsorb it, leading to diarrhoea. Patients with chronic pancreatitis have insufficient enzyme release leading to malabsorption; this can often lead to diarrhoea. Stool characteristics typically change in response to malabsorption (due to lack of enzymatic breakdown) such as foul-smelling, bulky, pale stools. This is attributed to the incomplete breakdown of fats.

Rotavirus, a diarrhoea-causing virus, can damage the epithelium, resulting in blunting of the villi. Consequently, some enzymatic activity can be impaired and there is some loss of absorptive area. This can thus lead to osmotic diarrhoea. The intestinal morphology and absorptive capacity return to normal within 2–3 weeks.

Invasive diarrhoea

Invasive diarrhoea is caused by pathogenic infection. Infectious agents such as *Campylobacter*, *Shigella* and *Salmonella* can directly invade the mucosa, resulting in an inflammatory response. This increases intestinal permeability. Inflammatory mediators such as histamine and prostaglandins released from cells of the gastro-immune system can inhibit Na^+ absorption, once again disrupting the osmotic balance in the small intestine. This can lead to diarrhoea and potential ulceration of the mucosa, leading to dysentery. Norovirus is associated with approximately one-fifth of all infectious diarrhoea cases; despite this, the mechanisms of how this virus causes diarrhoea is still not fully understood.

Hypermotility of the intestines

Where hypermotility of the intestines is present, water and electrolytes may be delivered to the colon at a rate that is too fast for the water to be absorbed in the colon. In lipid malabsorption, lipids become fermented to produce hydroxylated fatty acids that increase motility in the colon (as well as inhibiting Na^+ transport, see above). Parasitic infection by *Giardia* is thought to increase motility in the intestines which leads to diarrhoea.

Treatment of diarrhoea

In addition to oral replacement therapy regimens discussed above, there are other treatments for diarrhoea:

Antibiotics

Antibiotics can be useful in the treatment of diarrhoea in enteric conditions such as amoebic dysentery, typhoid and cholera, which are caused by bacteria and protozoa. Milder types of bacterial and viral enteritis generally resolve without being treated. *Campylobacter* is a common infection that causes diarrhoea in developed countries and this can be treated with erythromycin. However, enteritis is usually caused by viruses in many underdeveloped regions of the world.

Antimotility drugs

Antimotility drugs, including opiates, codeine and loperamide, can be used to treat diarrhoea. These increase the tone and rhythmic activity of the intestine but decrease its propulsive activity. They also inhibit secretion in the intestine. They are not usually used in infective diarrhoea.

Absorbents

Absorbents such as kaolin, chalk and charcoal are also used to decrease diarrhoea, but their mechanism of action is not entirely clear. They may act by adsorbing microorganisms and toxins, by altering the intestinal flora in some way or by coating and protecting the intestinal mucosa.

Motility in the small intestine

The smooth muscle of the small intestine performs three major functions. First, it is responsible for a thorough mixing of the digestive juices arriving from the liver and pancreas with the chyme received from the stomach. Second, it foresees the dispersion of food molecules across the epithelium to enable maximum contact and absorption. Lastly, it is responsible for moving the contents, usually slowly but sometimes rapidly, towards the colon. It is important that the food is retained in each location for sufficient time to allow mixing, digestion and absorption of food substances.

Smooth muscle contracts spontaneously, even during fasting, although the contractions increase in strength and frequency after food has been ingested. The fine local and temporal control of intestinal motility in the different segments of the intestine is integrated by nervous and hormonal mechanisms.

Types of motility

Spontaneous contractions

The smooth muscle of small intestine displays spontaneous activity even when a meal is not present in the GI tract. This phase of contractions is often referred to as the interdigestive period. Spontaneous contractions of smooth muscle occur in the absence of stretch, hormones or nervous activity due to the uneven amplitude of the oscillating membrane potential. The inherent mechanisms of tone and rhythmicity may be augmented by a background of transmitters such as acetylcholine released from nerves in the vicinity. This slow-wave activity of the smooth muscle in the duodenum is influenced by that in the stomach. Some longitudinal muscle fibres from the stomach cross the pyloric sphincter region to the duodenum. The frequency of contractions in the duodenum is higher than in the stomach. Every fifth contraction of the muscle in the duodenal bulb is augmented by a contraction of the antrum due to the transmission of the slow waves via the fibres crossing the sphincter. This acts to prevent the duodenal contents flowing back into the stomach.

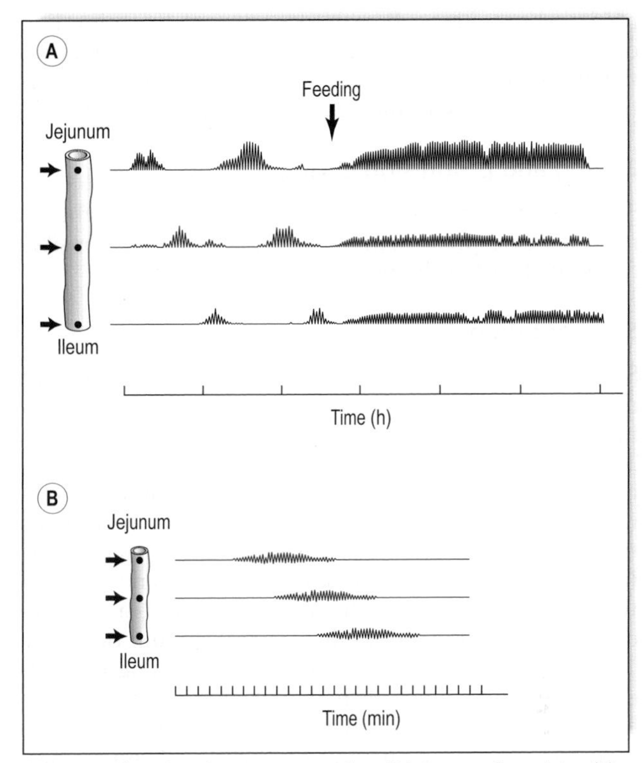

Fig. 5.11 The migrating motor complex. (A) Contractile activity. (B) Electrical activity.

There is also a regular type of spontaneous contraction, known as the migrating motor complex (MMC, see below), which moves distally down the intestine. Transmitters released during the progression of the MMC may be responsible for augmenting other types of spontaneous muscle activity. In addition, noradrenaline released from sympathetic nerves and adrenaline released into the blood, during fasting, and in times of stress can reduce the tone of the smooth muscle.

Migrating motor complex (MMC)

In fasting individuals, there are cycles of smooth muscle contractions with an average frequency of approximately 1.5 hours. These are the MMCs. Each cycle involves contraction of several adjacent segments of the small intestine, and it lasts approximately 10 minutes. The contractions occur sequentially in adjacent groups of segments. They begin in the stomach and migrate via the proximal small intestine towards the colon (Fig. 5.11). In the fasting state, the periodic sweeping of the contents towards the colon may cleanse the intestine of residual food and secretions. It may also prevent the migration of colonic bacteria into the ileum. As one sweep reaches the terminal ileum, another starts in the duodenum. This type of motility is terminated upon entering the fed state.

Mixing and propulsion during a meal

Segmentation mixes the contents of the lumen when a meal is being processed, while peristalsis is responsible for propelling the chyme along towards the colon.

Segmentation

Segmentation involves contraction of rings of circular muscle situated at intervals along a region of the small intestine (Fig. 5.12A). The contractions remain stationary. These rings of muscle then relax, and then adjacent segments contract. The overall effect is a continuous rhythmic division and subdivision of the intestinal contents that results in a thorough mixing of the chyme in the lumen. Segmentation increases in frequency and strength when chyme enters the duodenum. It occurs more frequently in the duodenum than in the jejunum or ileum. This is appropriate because the need for mixing is greatest in the duodenum, where the alkaline pancreatic juice and bile mix with acid chyme from the stomach to provide the appropriate neutral or slightly alkaline conditions necessary for digestion and micelle formation. At any one time, a group of segments contract and this is followed by a period of rest. This pattern is known as the minute rhythm.

Contraction of a ring of smooth muscle forces the chyme forwards and backwards, but because segmentation is more frequent in the proximal regions, the chances of the material being pushed towards the colon are greater than it being pushed towards the stomach. Thus, although segmentation is responsible for mixing the chyme, it also aids propulsion of the chyme towards the colon.

Peristalsis

Peristalsis involves the sequential contraction of adjacent rings of smooth muscle in the aboral direction, followed by relaxation of these rings of muscle, causing a wave of contraction that propels the chyme towards the colon (Fig. 5.12B). In humans, after a meal has been eaten, peristaltic activity in the small intestine is infrequent and of low strength. Furthermore, each wave of contraction travels only about 10 cm. However, there are occasional waves of intense contraction, known as peristaltic rushes, which travel the entire length of the small intestine. Both the short and the long waves are responsible for moving the chyme along the intestine towards the colon.

Contraction of the muscularis mucosae

In addition to the above types of motility due to contractions in the circular and longitudinal layers of muscle, sections of the muscularis mucosae undergo irregular

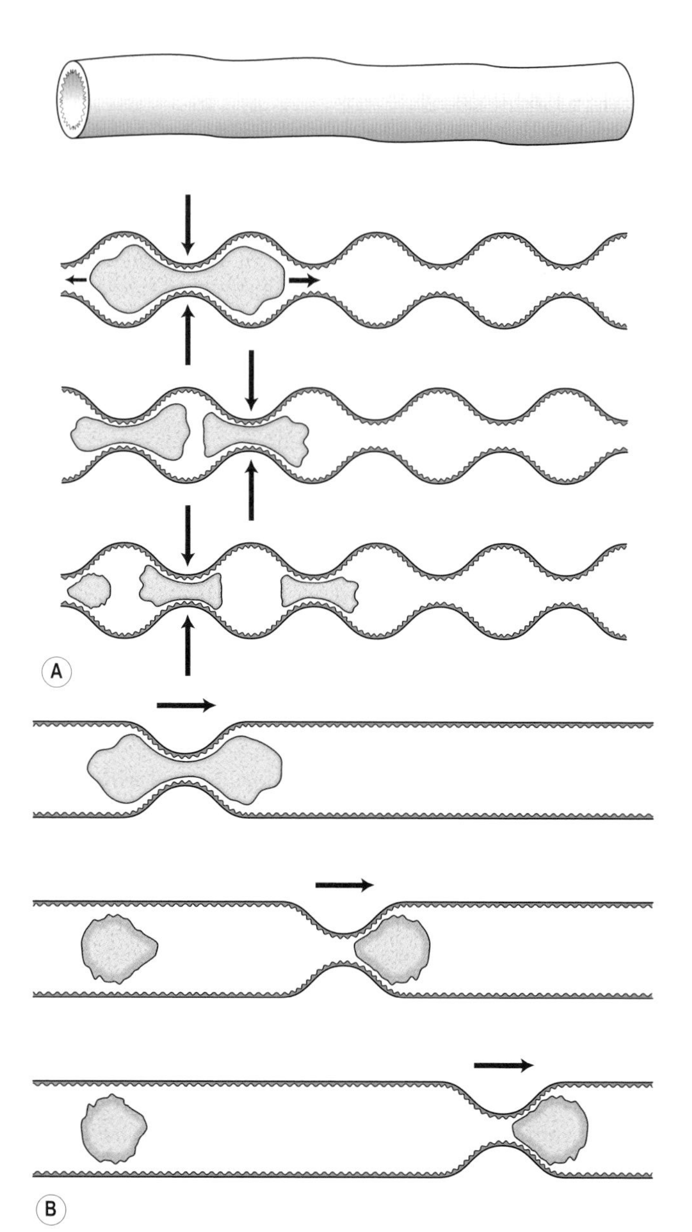

Fig. 5.12 Motility in the small intestine. (A) Segmentation. (B) Peristalsis.

contractions. These contractions assist in the mixing of the chyme. In addition, the villi contract in an irregular fashion. Contractions of the villi are most frequent in the proximal small intestine. They squeeze the lacteals in the centre of the villi, thereby emptying them of lymph and enhancing intestinal lymph flow.

Control of motility

Certain basic patterns of contractile activity may be programmed into the neural circuitry of the intrinsic nerve plexi. However, motility in the small intestine is under physiological control by various factors, including stretch, intrinsic nerves of the intramural plexi, extrinsic autonomic nerves, paracrine factors and circulating hormones.

An intrinsic property of smooth muscle is reflex contraction in response to stretch of the muscle, without the involvement of nerves or hormones. This is known as the myenteric reflex. However, reflex contractile activity due to activation of pressure receptors and chemoreceptors in the walls of the intestine is probably more important when a meal is being processed by the small intestine.

Nervous control

Activation of the intrinsic nerves in the intramural plexi can control segmentation and short peristaltic waves by influencing the basal electrical rhythm in the absence of extrinsic nerves and hormones. However, extrinsic parasympathetic and sympathetic nerves synapse with intrinsic nerves in the nerve plexi. The extrinsic nerves mediate long-range reflexes and both extrinsic nerves and hormones modulate the activity in intrinsic nerves. Segmentation and peristalsis are increased by activation of parasympathetic nerves and inhibited by stimulation of sympathetic nerves. Activation of the sympathetic nervous system, during stress for example, results in release of adrenaline into the circulation and this also inhibits motility. Sympathetic activation also causes marked vasoconstriction of the GI blood vessels.

Many transmitters, in addition to acetylcholine and the catecholamines, can influence intestinal motility. These include peptides, amines and nucleotides. The peptides include VIP, somatostatin, substance P and opioids. Peptides may be released from nerves and endocrine cells to influence GI contractility.

The initiation and propagation of the MMC depends largely on enteric neural activity. If the enteric neurones are blocked at a particular level, the MMC does not propagate past the block.

Hormonal control

Many peptide hormones are secreted by the stomach and small intestine in response to activation of pressure receptors and chemoreceptors to control motility.

- CCK stimulates contractions and increases the speed of small intestinal transit.
- Gastrin also stimulates contractions.
- Motilin increases motility by encouraging the MMC. This peptide is released from the walls of the duodenum and jejunum into the blood when the intestinal chyme becomes alkaline. It seems likely that when the acid in the chyme has been neutralised and the nutrients in the chyme have been digested that chyme becomes more alkaline, because alkaline juices are still being produced.
- VIP can both relax and contract smooth muscle; this effect is dependent on the specific VIP receptor present.
- Enteroglucagon is released into the small intestine in response to glucose and fat in the chyme. This hormone inhibits stimulated contractions but again slows transit.

Reflex control

Activation of pressure receptors by distension of the walls is involved in the reflex control of intestinal motility. A bolus of food placed in the small intestine will cause the smooth muscle behind it (in the orad direction) to contract, and that in front of it to relax. Furthermore, over-distension of the walls of one part of the intestine by food results in relaxation of the rest of the intestine (the intestino-intestine reflex). The pressure receptors are probably near the longitudinal muscle layer. The afferent and efferent limbs of this reflex involve activation of extrinsic autonomic nerves and would therefore be absent in a patient with a bowel transplant.

Trauma of other organs outside the GI tract, such as the kidneys and gonads, leads to inhibition of intestinal motility (atonic bowel or paralytic ileus). This inhibition ultimately involves activity in the sympathetic splanchnic nerve. Various regions of the central nervous system have been implicated in the control of intestinal motility in such conditions.

Gastro-ileal reflex

When food is present in the stomach, motility increases in the ileum, and the ileocaecal sphincter relaxes. This is known as the gastro-ileal reflex. Conversely, distension of the ileum decreases gastric motility (emptying) in the stomach (the ileogastric reflex). The gastro-ileal reflex appears to be mainly under the control of external nerves to the intestinal mucosa, but gastrin, released into the blood in response to food in the stomach, may augment the response.

Ileocaecal sphincter

The last portion of the ileum is separated from the colon by a ring of smooth muscle known as the ileocaecal sphincter. It is approximately 4 cm long in the adult human. Relaxation and contraction of the sphincter controls the rate of entry of material into the colon. It may have a role in preventing the movement of bacteria from the colon to the ileum. This sphincter is normally closed, but when peristalsis occurs in the last portion of the ileum in response to food in the stomach (the ileogastric reflex), distension of the ileum causes reflex relaxation of the sphincter muscle. This allows a small amount of chyme to enter the large intestine. The rate of entry is appropriately slow as it enables salt and water absorption from the chyme in the colon to take place before the next portion of chyme enters. Relaxation of the smooth muscle of the sphincter is coordinated by activity in the nerves in the intramural plexi.

Drugs that affect intestinal motility

Drugs that increase intestinal motility include purgatives, which accelerate the movement of chyme through the GI tract, and drugs that increase segmentation but not peristalsis. Laxatives can be used to treat constipation. The treatment of constipation is discussed below.

Secretory laxatives

Secretory laxatives cause an increased secretion of fluid and electrolytes by the mucosa into the lumen of the intestines. This results in fluid accumulation and watery chyme that flows rapidly through the intestines. They include castor oil, the active ingredient of which is ricinoleic acid. Others are cascara, aloe, senna and fig syrup, all of which are naturally occurring anthraquinone derivatives, and phenolphthalein, bisacodyl and danthron, which are synthetic agents. Senna and cascara contain derivatives of anthracene (such as emodin) bound to sugars to form glycosides. Hydrolysis of these glycosides by bacteria in the colon releases the active anthracene derivatives. These are absorbed to act on the myenteric plexus. This results in stimulation of secretion and motility. These agents can cause abdominal cramps due to excessive stimulation of smooth muscle. Prolonged usage can result in dependence, loss of normal intestinal function, and even an atonic colon.

Osmotic laxatives

Osmotic laxatives are poorly absorbed solutes that cause the volume of chyme to increase by transport of water down the osmotic gradient into the lumen. Salts such as Epsom's salts ($MgSO_4$ or $Mg(OH)_2$) which act in this way can be used to treat constipation. They have a rapid onset laxative effect, within a few hours of administration.

The concept of osmotic diarrhoea consequent to carbohydrate malabsorption in brush border diseases, such as lactase deficiency, has been exploited by the pharmaceutical industry in the development of lactulose that is now commonly used to treat constipation. Lactulose, a disaccharide composed of fructose and galactose, is not digested in the small intestine. It is digested to its component monosaccharides by bacteria in the colon. These are then fermented to lactic and acetic acid that act as osmotic laxatives.

Emollients

Emollients are non-absorbable substances that coat and lubricate the faeces. This accelerates their movement through the intestines and softens the rectal contents. Examples of emollients are didactyl sodium sulphosuccinate and liquid paraffin. Liquid paraffin can interfere with the absorption of fat-soluble vitamins, and for this reason, it is now seldom used.

Bulk-forming agents

Bulk-forming agents, such as bran and methylcellulose, are generally the preferred treatment for constipation as they are free from side effects, inexpensive and probably the most acceptable and natural of the alternatives. They consist of non-digestible cellulose fibres that become hydrated in the intestines. This alters the viscosity of the luminal contents to increase their flow through the intestines. Hydration causes them to swell, providing bulk, with consequent activation of the defaecation reflex.

Drugs that increase motility

Drugs that increase intestinal motility include serotonin 5-HT_4 receptor agonists such as prucalopride, muscarinic receptor agonists such as bethanechol, macrolides such as erythromycin, and anticholinesterases such as neostigmine. Such drugs that increase segmentation without increasing propulsive activity can be used for disorders of motility in the GI tract and for chronic constipation. They can also be used as antiemetics (via their actions on the central nervous system) prior to procedures such as diagnostic radiography or duodenal intubation. Domperidone, a dopamine D_2 receptor antagonist, can also be used to increase intestinal motility. Some drugs, including metoclopramide, have prokinetic side effects, thus increasing motility and having a laxative effect.

DIGESTION AND ABSORPTION

6

Chapter objectives and clinical presentations

After reading this chapter, review your learning by considering the following:

1. Explain the mechanisms of digestion and absorption of (a) carbohydrates, (b) proteins, (c) lipids and (d) minerals and vitamins.
2. Understand how intestinal disease impacts the absorption of nutrients.

Also, you should be familiar with the following clinical presentations:

- Coeliac disease
- Lactase deficiency
- Hartnup's disease
- Cystinuria
- Crohn's disease
- Rickets
- Osteomalacia
- Iron-deficiency anaemia
- Anaemia of chronic disease
- Hereditary haemochromatosis
- Pernicious anaemia

Clinical outlook

Coeliac disease is by far the most common condition associated with malabsorption seen in the Western world. Patients often present with a variety of non-specific symptoms; however, many are diagnosed based on blood tests showing vitamin or mineral deficiencies. Lactase deficiency is also commonly seen at birth or acquired later in life. Crohn's disease, a form of inflammatory bowel disease, is another common chronic gastrointestinal (GI) condition that is increasing in its incidence and prevalence globally. Whilst malabsorption in Crohn's disease is less common and often associated with surgical removal of diseased bowel, patients usually present with abdominal pain, diarrhoea and weight loss.

Introduction

In this chapter, the digestion of complex nutrients, the absorption of the products of digestion, and the absorption of vitamins and minerals will be considered, as well as the impact of small intestinal disease on nutrition. As absorption of different nutrients can occur in different regions of the GI tract, the regions affected by the disease process determine which nutrients will be poorly absorbed. Coeliac disease, which usually affects the proximal small intestine, and Crohn's ileitis, which usually affects the terminal ileum, will be used to illustrate some of the general principles of absorption, as well as the specific problems encountered because of malabsorption of the nutrients that are normally absorbed in the affected regions.

Absorption

Most nutrients are absorbed at a slow rate by passive diffusion throughout the small intestine. However, many important nutrients are absorbed at a faster rate by processes which involve saturable mechanisms. The proximal small intestine (i.e., the duodenum and jejunum) is the location of most of these special mechanisms, as most substances are absorbed predominantly in these regions. Fig. 6.1 shows the approximate sites of absorption of many important nutrients.

The important divalent cations, Ca^{2+} and Fe^{2+}, are absorbed mainly in the duodenum and jejunum. Hexoses, including glucose, galactose and fructose, are also absorbed in the duodenum and jejunum, as are amino acids, small (di- and tri-) peptides and some water-soluble vitamins. Fatty acids, monoacylglycerols and fat-soluble vitamins are also absorbed in the duodenum and jejunum. Cholesterol is absorbed throughout the small intestine. Vitamin C is absorbed in the proximal ileum. Vitamin B_{12} and bile salts are absorbed predominantly in the terminal ileum. Water and monovalent ions are absorbed throughout the small and large intestines. The defects in absorption seen in coeliac disease and Crohn's disease affect different regions of the small intestine.

Absorption of important nutrients

Carbohydrates

The average daily intake of carbohydrate in the human adult is between 250 and 800 g/day. The most useful

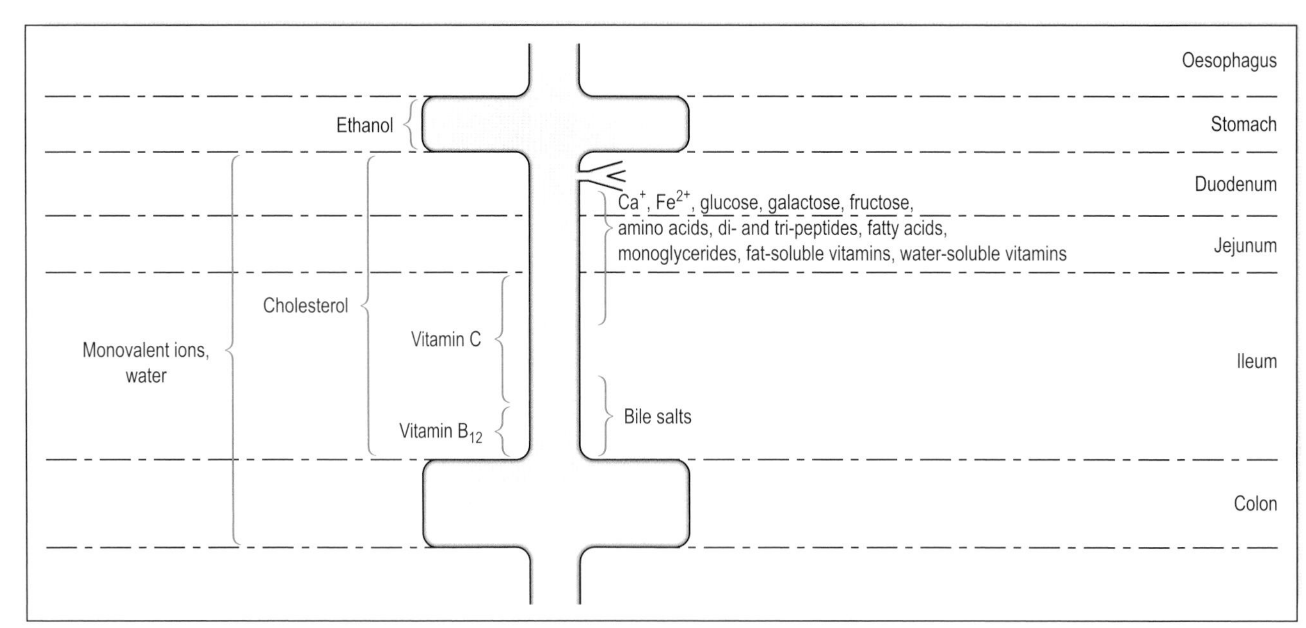

Fig. 6.1 Sites of absorption of important nutrients in the gastrointestinal tract.

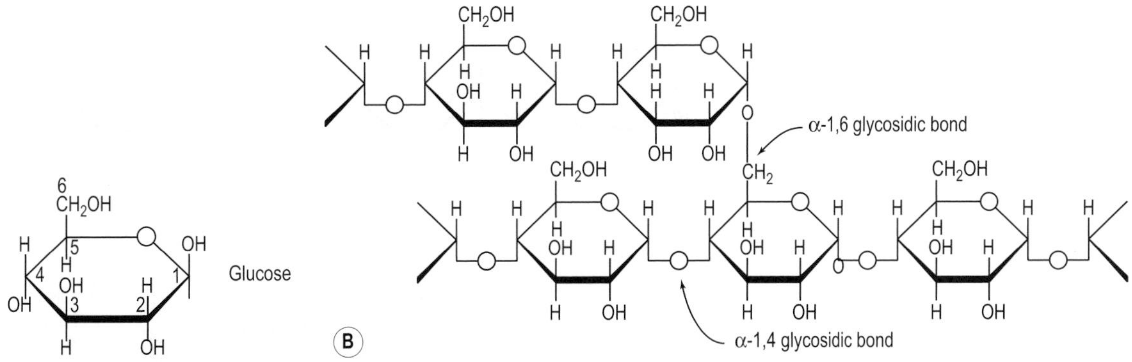

Fig. 6.2 (A) Structure of glucose showing the conventional numbering system for the carbon atoms. (B) Portion of an amylopectin molecule showing α-1,4 and α-1,6 glycosidic linkages.

carbohydrate in food is largely vegetable starch found in potatoes, bread, pasta, rice and to a lesser extent glycogen (animal starch) from meat and liver. These polysaccharides are composed entirely of D-glucose subunits linked together mainly by α-1,4 glycosidic linkages. In humans, over 90% of the starch in the diet is digested and absorbed. The remainder passes into the colon where it may be utilised by colonic bacteria.

Cellulose is another polysaccharide composed of glucose subunits present in the diet. However, it is not digestible in humans and other non-ruminants, because the subunits are linked by β-1,4 glycosidic bonds that cannot be hydrolysed by the enzymes in the digestive tract. Therefore, it passes into the colon. Nevertheless, cellulose is an important source of dietary fibre, providing bulk that stimulates intestinal motility and prevents constipation.

There are appreciable amounts of disaccharides within the diet, including sucrose, lactose, maltose and free monosaccharides like glucose, fructose and galactose (the latter are found in negligible amounts).

Structure of starch and glycogen

The molecular weight of vegetable starch ranges from a few thousand to 500,000 g/mol. It consists of two components:

1. Amylose in which the glucose subunits are linked together in straight unbranched chains via α-1,4 glycosidic linkages (Fig. 6.2A).
2. Amylopectin which consists of branched chains, with branches occurring at approximately every 30th glucose residue. α-1,4 Glycosidic linkages are present within the chains and α-1,6 glycosidic linkages occur at the branch points (Fig. 6.2B).

In general, starch consists of 20% amylose and 80% amylopectin by weight. Glycogen has a structure similar to amylopectin, but its molecular weight is usually greater (between 270,000 and 100,000,000 g/mol), and it has a more branched structure.

Digestion of carbohydrate

There are several enzymes that degrade starch and glycogen in the GI tract. These include the α-amylases secreted by the salivary glands and the pancreas, and isomaltase and glucoamylase, which are integral components of the intestinal absorptive cell membranes. Maltose, sucrose and lactose can also be degraded to their component monosaccharides by enzymes situated in the brush border of the upper small intestine (see below).

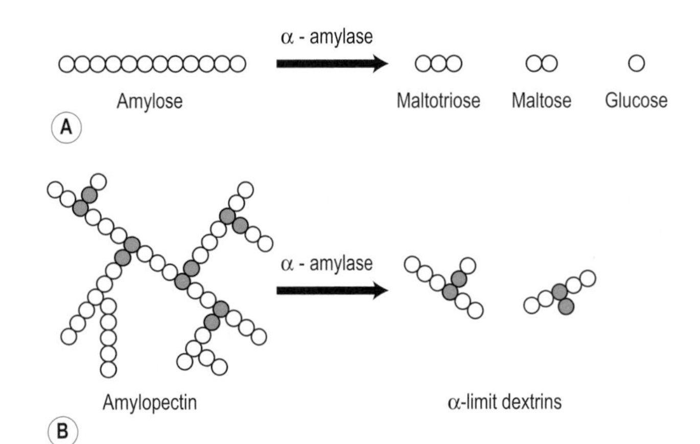

Fig. 6.3 Degradation of (A) amylose and (B) amylopectin by α-amylases. The filled circles indicate glucose subunits with α-1,6 glycosidic linkages.

α-Amylases

α-Amylases split the α-1,4 glycosidic linkages in amylose to yield maltose and glucose, but they do not act on maltose, a disaccharide composed of two glucose subunits linked by an α-1,4 linkage (Fig. 6.3). α-Amylases also act on amylopectin and glycogen at their α-1,4 linkages. Intermediate unbranched oligosaccharides and branched oligosaccharides (α-limit dextrins) are formed, the latter because α-amylase is unable to catalytically cleave close to an α-1, 6 linkage. Consequently, a mixture of products is produced (see Fig. 6.3).

Salivary amylase starts the digestion of starch. It continues to act for up to half an hour in the interior of the food bolus after it has arrived in the stomach. It is eventually inactivated at the low pH produced by the gastric acid when it penetrates the food bolus. It can digest up to 50% of the starch present in food. Pancreatic juice that contains a second α-amylase is released into the duodenum due to the presence of chyme in the digestive tract.

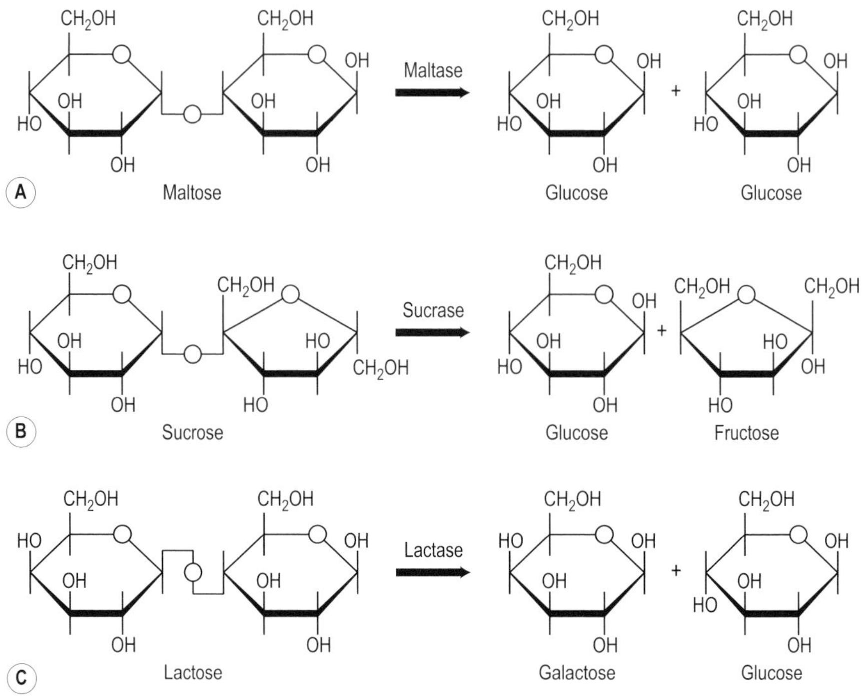

Fig. 6.4 Degradation of disaccharides by brush-border disaccharidases. (A) Maltose, (B) sucrose, (C) lactose.

Pancreatic amylase continues the digestion of starch and glycogen in the small intestine. Both salivary and pancreatic α-amylases are optimal at a neutral pH.

Role of brush-border enzymes

Isomaltase (α-1,6 glycosidase), a component of the sucrose-isomaltase glucoside enzyme, splits α-1,6 linkages in the branched poly- and oligosaccharides produced by amylase action in the small intestine. The combined action of α-amylase and α-1,6 glycosidase can degrade amylopectin and glycogen to a mixture of maltose and glucose, which both are further acted upon by maltase and isomaltase to liberate glucose. All these enzymes have access to the mixture of polysaccharides, oligosaccharides and disaccharides in the chyme during a meal.

The enzymes available to digest disaccharides are (summarised in Fig. 6.4):

- Maltase degrades maltose to glucose
- Sucrase degrades sucrose to glucose and fructose
- Lactase degrades lactose to galactose and glucose.

Thus, due to salivary and pancreatic amylases and then the action of the various brush-border enzymes, all carbohydrates are broken down to their constituent monosaccharides.

Brush-border diseases

Several brush-border diseases exist where the defect results in malabsorption of a specific carbohydrate. Intolerance of that carbohydrate in the diet develops. The unabsorbed sugar passes into the colon where some of it is fermented by bacteria. The remaining unaltered sugar and its bacterial fermentation products cause osmotic diarrhoea. The clinical symptoms of carbohydrate malabsorption are abdominal distension, gassiness, borborygmi, nausea, cramping, pain and diarrhoea. In some of these conditions, there is also a high incidence of ulceration of the mouth. Carbohydrate malabsorption is diagnosed by an oral tolerance test that involves administration of the suspected sugar by mouth and measurement of the sugar in the blood and faeces. If the individual is intolerant of the sugar, it appears in the faeces, but it (or its normal digestion products) cannot be detected in the blood. Confirmation is by examination of a jejunal biopsy to see if the appropriate enzyme or carrier protein is absent from the mucosa. Brush-border diseases include:

- *Lactase deficiency.* This is a common brush-border disorder that is usually expressed in adolescence or early adulthood. The enzyme, lactase, is induced by its substrate, lactose, in individuals who consume milk. There is generally a high incidence of lactase deficiency in Mediterranean and Asian races that do not normally consume milk after childhood, with the result that the enzyme is not present in their intestines. If milk is ingested in these individuals, they experience symptoms of lactose intolerance. A rare congenital form of lactase deficiency exists; feeding infants with this condition with normal milk causes diarrhoea. The problem can be overcome by feeding artificial milk in which lactose has been replaced by sucrose or fructose. There is a rise in H_2 elimination in the breath of affected individuals, which is the result of the metabolism of the unabsorbed lactose by bacteria in the colon.

- *Sucrase-isomaltase deficiency.* Individuals with this inherited brush-border enzyme disease are intolerant of sucrose and isomaltose.
- *Glucose/galactose malabsorption.* In this condition, there is a genetic defect in the Na^+-dependent glucose/galactose transporter, SGLT1. Ingestion of glucose or galactose produces the symptoms of brush-border disease. Treatment involves omitting these sugars, as well as lactose (which is degraded to glucose and galactose), from the diet. Fructose is absorbed normally via the GLUT5 transporter.

Case 6.1 Coeliac disease

A 25-year-old woman visited her doctor and complained of diarrhoea and flatulence. She had recently lost a considerable amount of weight, and she felt weak and exhausted most of the time. She also suffered from back pain. Upon questioning, she said her faeces were bulky, greasy and foul-smelling.

She recalled that she had had persistent diarrhoea throughout childhood, but the symptoms had disappeared during adolescence. She was referred to a gastroenterologist. The consultant arranged for blood and faecal analyses. The faecal tests confirmed the presence of steatorrhoea. The blood tests indicated that she had iron-deficiency anaemia (IDA), folate deficiency and Ca^{2+} deficiency. Her blood electrolyte concentrations and prothrombin clotting time were within the normal range. The consultant suspected coeliac disease and arranged for an endoscopy to be performed. A biopsy of the mucosa, taken at the examination, showed flattening of the villi and excessive plasma cells in the submucosa. A further blood test to measure the concentrations of transglutaminase antibodies was performed and this showed a high titre of antibodies. In view of these findings, the consultant told the patient to exclude wheat, rye, and barley flours (but not oat flour) from her diet, and to try to ensure that it was nutritionally balanced. She was prescribed iron, folate and vitamin D supplements. This diet was not easy to follow as so many food products contain these flours, but after a few weeks the patient had vastly improved. She had gained weight and was no longer feeling constantly tired.

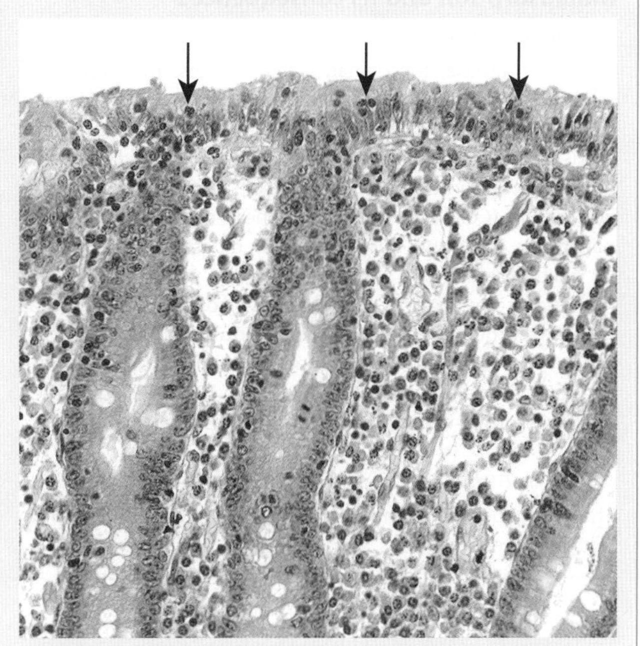

Fig. 6.5 Section of the jejunal mucosa in a patient with coeliac disease, showing flattened villi (as depicted by the arrows) and plasma cell infiltrates. (From Abbas AK, Kumar V, Deyrup AT et al. Robbins Essential Pathology. Courtesy ExpertPath: Elsevier; 2021.)

Defect and treatment

Coeliac disease is common in Northern Europe with an incidence of 1%. Genetic and environmental factors are involved.

Defect

The disease is due to an abnormal reaction to gluten, a constituent of wheat flour, which results in atrophy of the villi and malabsorption. The duodenum and proximal jejunum are usually more severely affected than the ileum. The damage is due to an abnormal immune response to gliadins (especially α-gliadin), which are components of gluten. It is a T-cell-mediated disease. Antibodies to the enzyme transglutaminase, which is released in tissues during inflammation, are present in 98% of affected individuals. The mechanisms involved in the damage have not yet been fully characterised but evidence suggests that both intestinal epithelial cells and local antigen-presenting cells along with CD4 T-cells trigger production of pro-inflammatory cytokines in response to the gliadin by transglutaminase. In addition, transglutaminase antibodies have been shown to affect the differentiation of epithelial cells, possibly by interfering with the action of the enzyme.

Diagnosis

Determination of the serum concentration of transglutaminase antibodies is a useful tool in the diagnosis of coeliac disease. The diagnosis of coeliac disease also requires a biopsy, usually of the duodenum, which would show flattened villi, crypt hyperplasia, infiltration with lymphocytes and plasma cells, as well as reduced cell differentiation. Fig. 6.5 shows a section through the jejunal mucosa in a patient with coeliac disease. The cells cannot be replaced quickly enough by stem cell division in the crypts, and many of the cells present are immature and therefore do not absorb nutrients effectively.

Continued

Case 6.1 Coeliac disease—cont'd

Treatment

Treatment of coeliac disease involves the individual following a gluten-free nutritious diet. The gliadin peptides that cause the abnormal reactions are present in wheat, rye and barley but not oats. The latter is therefore safe for individuals with coeliac disease.

Malabsorption and its consequences

Malabsorption

In coeliac disease, the damaged villi and loss of enterocytes leads to a reduced surface area for absorption of fat and other nutrients that are normally absorbed in the proximal small intestine. Malabsorption is exacerbated if damage to endocrine cells in the duodenum results in deficiency of cholecystokinin (CCK) and secretin, as these control secretion of pancreatic juice and bile, the major digestive juices in the GI tract. Steatorrhoea was present in the patient due to fat malabsorption. IDA was present due to iron malabsorption as iron is absorbed in the proximal small intestine.

The absorption of hexoses, amino acids, fat, fat-soluble vitamins, folate and Ca^{2+} ions could also be impaired as they are all absorbed in the proximal small intestine.

Consequences

The consequences of malabsorption in this condition, if it is left untreated, are:

- Weight loss and fatigue due to malabsorption of fuels such as carbohydrates and fat, and malabsorption of amino acids required for synthetic reactions.
- Anaemia and fatigue due to iron and folate malabsorption.
- Osteomalacia due to vitamin D and Ca^{2+} malabsorption and the formation of Ca^{2+} soaps from fatty acids (which prevents their absorption).
- Bleeding from the nose, GI tract, vagina and ureters, as a result of increased clotting time due to vitamin K deficiency. The blood loss would exacerbate the IDA.

Diarrhoea

The patient's blood electrolyte concentrations were measured because there can be a severe loss of electrolytes in diarrhoea.

Diarrhoea in this condition is due to:

- High concentrations of unabsorbed nutrients in the chyme which cause osmotic diarrhoea.
- The delivery of large amounts of fat into the colon which results in the production of hydroxylated fatty acids by colonic bacteria. These can act as cathartics.
- Milk intolerance, due to lactase deficiency, as this enzyme is present in the enterocytes of the brush border in the proximal small intestine.

Monosaccharide absorption

The most abundant monosaccharides in dietary carbohydrates are the hexoses (D-glucose, D-galactose, and D-fructose) and the products of digestion of starch, sucrose and lactose. Both L- and D-hexoses are absorbed slowly by passive diffusion in the GI tract. However, the plasma membrane of cells is relatively impermeable to polar molecules such as monosaccharides and the transport of these sugars into the enterocyte by passive diffusion is therefore slow. Glucose, galactose and fructose are absorbed by saturable mechanisms, mainly in the duodenum and jejunum. This is accomplished by membrane-associated transporters located in the brush border and basolateral membranes of the mature enterocytes. These bind the sugars and transfer them across the cell membranes and deliver them to the interstitial fluid in the lateral spaces, from where they are taken up into the adjacent capillaries to enter the portal blood. The transporters required to update these hexoses into the enterocyte are summarised in Table 6.1.

Pentoses are smaller than hexoses, but they are absorbed at a slower rate than glucose, galactose and fructose, indicating that they are probably absorbed by passive diffusion.

Table 6.1 Specificity of transporters for hexoses in the enterocyte

Transporter	*Glucose*	*Galactose*	*Fructose*
SGLT1	+	+	–
GLUT1	+	+	–
GLUT2	+	+	+
GLUT5	–	–	+

Hexose transporters

There are two types of hexose transporter in mammalian cells: Na^+/glucose-linked transporters (SGLTs) which are involved in the secondary active transport of glucose and Na^+-independent facilitative-diffusion hexose transporters. Six forms of SGLTs have been identified. However, only SGLT1, 3, 4 and 6 are present in the small intestine. There are currently at least 14 functional isoforms of linked transporters (GLUT1 to 14). All mammalian cells express at least one of these transporters. The most studied is GLUT4, an insulin-sensitive glucose transporter present in muscle and adipose tissue. GLUT1, 2 and 5 are all present in enterocytes. The specificity of the transporters is shown in Table 6.1. An inherited disorder where SGLT1 is absent from the brush border has been described.

Hexose transport

The uptake of glucose across the enterocyte plasma membrane involves the binding of glucose to SGLT1. SGLT1 is present only in mature enterocytes in the upper regions of the villi. Galactose also binds to this carrier but fructose does not. Glucose and galactose transport into the epithelial cell is via secondary active transport. The energy required is derived from the coupling of sugar transport to the transport of Na^+ down the concentration and electrical gradients from the lumen into the cell. Both Na^+ ions and the sugar are transported into the cell by SGLT1. This represents a major route for the uptake of both the sugar and Na^+ into the enterocyte. Thus, the uptake of glucose is stimulated by the presence of Na^+ in the intestinal chyme. The absorption of glucose is illustrated schematically in Fig. 6.6. Each carrier molecule binds two Na^+ ions and one glucose molecule. The glucose concentration in the cell may be higher than that in the lumen but the coupling of the transport of glucose with that of Na^+ enables glucose to be transported into the cell against a concentration gradient.

Fructose does not bind to SGLT1 in the brush border. It is transported into enterocytes down its concentration gradient by GLUT5 (which does not transport glucose; Fig. 6.6). The separate pathways for glucose and fructose transport into the enterocyte can be inferred from the fact that normal fructose absorption is present in patients with inherited glucose-galactose malabsorption, and this provides the rationale for the treatment of this condition with fructose. GLUT5 is present only in mature enterocytes on the tips and sides of the villi in the jejunum. In addition, when D-glucose is at a high concentration in the lumen of the small intestine, GLUT2 is also able to support uptake of D-glucose and D-galactose across the brush-border membrane. Glucose, galactose and fructose are all then effluxed across the basolateral membrane via GLUT2. Malabsorption of carbohydrate is a feature of coeliac disease; a condition associated with villus atrophy.

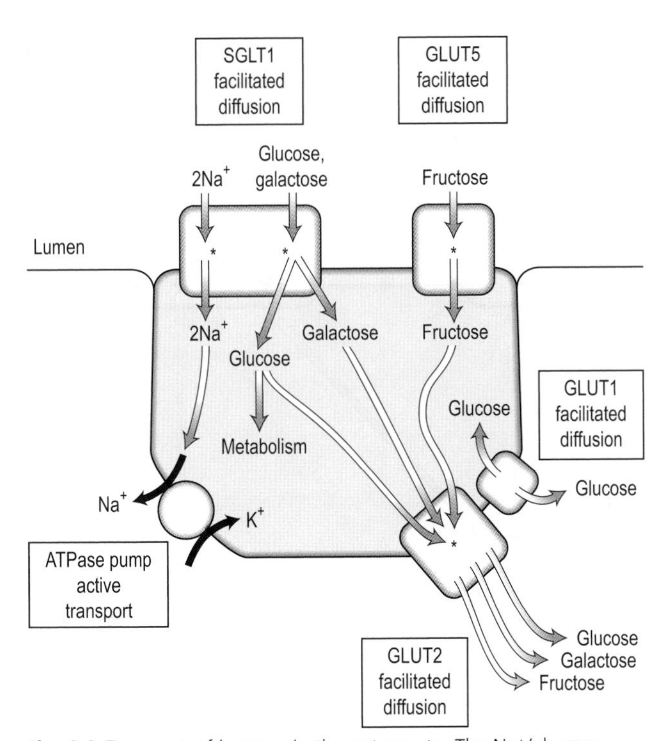

Fig. 6.6 Transport of hexoses in the enterocyte. The Na^+/glucose cotransporter (SGLT1) and the facilitative GLUT5 fructose membrane transporter reside in the brush-border membrane. GLUT1, GLUT2 and the ATPase pump reside in the basolateral membrane.

Protein

In the Western world, the amount of protein in the average diet exceeds that required for nutritional balance. The dietary requirement for protein in human adults is between 30 and 50 g/day. Protein is required to supply the eight 'essential amino acids' which the body cannot synthesise or cannot synthesise rapidly enough, and to replace nitrogen lost in the urine. In addition to that which is ingested, 10–30 g of protein (enzymes, mucins, etc.) are secreted into the digestive tract each day. An additional 25 g or so is derived from epithelial cells that have been shed into the lumen. Most of this protein is digested and absorbed. Approximately 10–20 g, derived from cell debris and colonic microorganisms, is eliminated in the faeces each day.

Digestion

Proteins are high-molecular-weight substances composed of up to 20 different amino acids, joined together in peptide linkages (Fig. 6.7). In adults, most proteins are degraded in the digestive tract to small peptides and amino acids. This is accomplished by a variety of proteolytic enzymes. These can be divided into two categories: endopeptidases and exopeptidases. Endopeptidases cleave peptide bonds in the centre of the peptide chains, the initial products being mostly large peptides, which are subsequently degraded to oligopeptides. Exopeptidases cleave bonds at the ends of the peptide chain, cleaving off amino acids one by one, in a stepwise manner: carboxypeptidases act at the C-terminus and

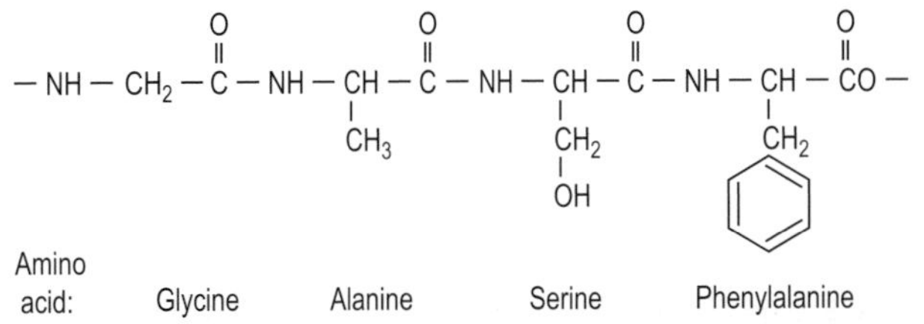

$$-NH-CH_2-\overset{O}{\overset{\|}{C}}-NH-\underset{\underset{CH_3}{|}}{CH}-\overset{O}{\overset{\|}{C}}-NH-\underset{\underset{\underset{OH}{|}}{CH_2}}{\underset{|}{CH}}-\overset{O}{\overset{\|}{C}}-NH-\underset{\underset{C_6H_5}{\underset{|}{CH_2}}}{\underset{|}{CH}}-\overset{O}{\overset{\|}{CO}}-$$

Amino acid: Glycine, Alanine, Serine, Phenylalanine

Fig. 6.7 Part of a peptide chain showing three peptide linkages.

aminopeptidases at the N-terminus. Enzymes that specifically attack dipeptides and tripeptides are also present. The combined actions of these enzymes digest proteins to small peptides and amino acids.

Digestion in the stomach

Pepsin is an endopeptidase which is secreted by the stomach as an inactive precursor, pepsinogen, which is activated by gastric juice. It favours peptide linkages where aromatic amino acids are present. It is responsible for the digestion of only approximately 15% of dietary protein. Protein digestion is not impaired in the absence of pepsin because other proteases are available.

Digestion in the small intestine

Pancreatic juice contains three endopeptidases (Fig. 6.8):

1. Trypsin, which prefers peptide linkages where the carboxylic acid group is provided by a basic amino acid.
2. Chymotrypsin, which prefers linkages where the carboxylic group is provided by an aromatic amino acid.
3. Elastase, which degrades elastin.

Pancreatic juice also contains two carboxypeptidases (A and B). Carboxypeptidase A has the highest specificity for bonds where the C-terminal amino acid is basic, such as lysine or arginine. The pancreatic enzymes are secreted as inactive precursors that are converted to the active enzymes in the duodenum. They all have slightly alkaline pH optima. At least 50% of the protein ingested is normally degraded in the duodenum.

Several peptidases reside in the brush border or the cytosol of the enterocyte. They are most abundant in the cells in the jejunum. The active sites of these enzymes face the intestinal lumen, acting in situ upon contact with the protein in the chyme. These include oligopeptidases, which degrade small peptides such as tetrapeptides, as well as dipeptidyl aminopeptidases that remove dipeptides from the N-termini of proteins.

The products of proteolytic digestion are tetrapeptides, tripeptides, dipeptides and some amino acids. Tripeptides, dipeptides and amino acids are transported into the epithelial cells via PepT1. In fact, it has been proposed that PepT1 can transport up to 400 different dipeptides and 8000 tripeptides. The transport of these small peptides into intestinal epithelial cells is via an inwardly directed proton electrochemical gradient mediated by PepT1. The internalised dipeptides and tripeptides are subsequently enzymatically cleaved to amino acids by cytosolic tripeptidases and dipeptidases and/or effluxed out across the basolateral membrane intact. These relationships are represented in Fig. 6.8.

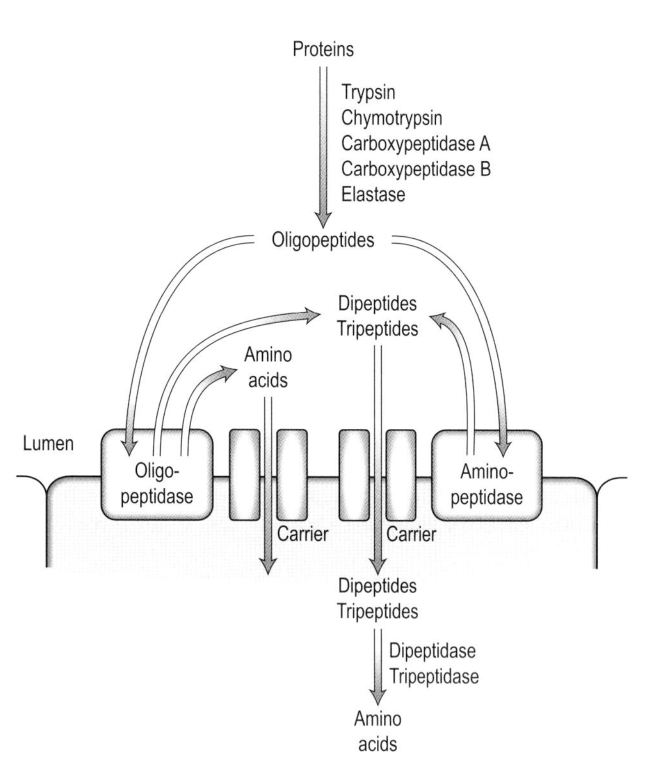

Fig. 6.8 Digestion of proteins and peptides, and absorption of di- and tripeptides and amino acids in the enterocyte.

Absorption of amino acids

The transport of amino acids across the membranes of the enterocytes into the blood can occur via passive diffusion, facilitated diffusion or active transport (Fig. 6.9). Relatively hydrophobic amino acids, such as tryptophan, are transported to an appreciable extent by passive diffusion. Only the L-isomers of amino acids are absorbed by facilitated diffusion and active transport. They are absorbed in the jejunum and the upper ileum. Carrier

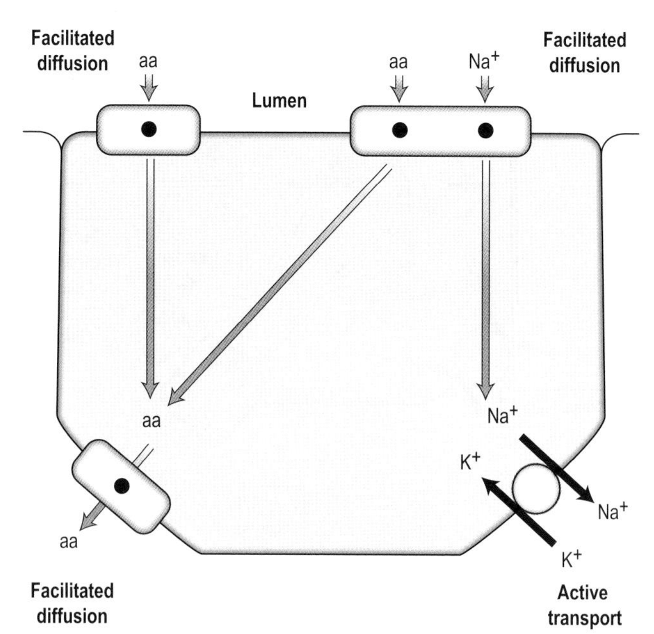

Fig. 6.9 Amino-acid carrier mechanisms in the brush border and basolateral border of the enterocyte. aa, amino acid.

Table 6.2 Carriers involved in amino-acid absorption in the enterocyte

		Apical	
System	***Solute carrier***	***Na^+ dependence***	***Amino-acid specificity***
ASC	SLC1A5	+	A, S, C, T, Q, N
B^0	SLC6A19	+	AA^0
B^{0+}	SLC6A14	+	AA^0, AA^+, β-alanine
b^{0+}	SLC3A1/ SLC7A9	-	R, K, O, cysteine
B	SLC6A6	+	Taurine, β-alanine
Imino	SLC6A20	+	P, HOP
Imino/Glycine	SLC36A1	-	P, G, A, GABA, β-alanine
X^-_{AG}	SLC1A1	+	E, D
		Intestinal basement membrane	
System	***Solute carrier***	***Na^+ dependence***	***Amino-acid specificity***
B	SLC6A6	+	Taurine, β-alanine
Gly	SLC6A9	+	G
L	SLC3A2/ SLC7A8 SLC43A2	- -	AA^0 (except P) L, M, I, F
T	SLC16A10	-	F, Y, W
y^+L	SLC3A2/ SLC7A7 SLC2A2/ SLC7A6	+ +	K, R, Q, H, M, L K, R, Q, H, M, L, A, C

HOP, hydroxyproline; GABA, γ-aminobutyric acid; AA^0, neutral amino acids; AA^+, cationic amino acids.

systems for amino acids exist in the brush border and the basolateral border (Table 6.2). Two terminologies are used to describe the different transporters.

1. The *systems*: This is the older terminology, where transporters are classified into systems or groups that transport amino acids with similar chemical and physical properties.
2. The *solute carriers*: This is the more modern terminology, where transporters are catalogued according to gene sequences.

The transport of most amino acids occurs against a concentration gradient and, therefore, depends on active mechanisms. Those that share the same transport mechanism compete for a binding site on the carrier protein. Table 6.2 shows the membrane locations of the transporters that have been characterised.

To date, six of the known amino-acid transport systems in the brush border are Na^+-dependent cotransporters, which operate in a manner resembling that of the SGLT1 glucose transporter. The pumping of Na^+ ions across the basolateral membrane produces concentration and electrical gradients that favour Na^+ transport into the cell. This provides the driving force for the operation of the cotransporters in the brush border. These are therefore secondary active transport mechanisms. The other two brush-border transporters do not require the presence of Na^+ ions in the lumen. The specificities of the transporters are shown in Table 6.2.

There are currently five recognised transporters in the basolateral border. These transporters are present in many different cell types. Acidic amino acids such as glutamate and aspartate are utilised by enterocytes as energy substrates and do not appear to be transported out of the cell by specific carrier mechanisms. The basolateral membrane also expresses carriers that transport amino acids from the fluid in the lateral spaces into the enterocyte, where they are used for protein synthesis. These systems require the presence of Na^+ ions in the intercellular fluid. Malabsorption of amino acids is a feature of coeliac disease due to damaged mucosa and the consequent loss of transporters from the epithelial cells.

However, of note, not all protein is digested into amino acids, and this is best exemplified in neonates where there is evidence of intestinal macromolecular transfer of intact proteins. This is particularly pertinent in the context of antibodies present in the maternal colostrum or milk which may contribute to the passive immunity of neonates.

Amino-acid malabsorption diseases

The existence of different transport systems for amino acids was first deduced from the study of rare amino-acid malabsorption diseases. In these autosomal recessive diseases, a group of amino acids is either poorly absorbed or not absorbed at all, while amino acids not in that group are well absorbed. In these conditions, there is an absence or deficiency of a specific amino-acid transporter. The defect is usually present in both the small intestine and the proximal tubules of the kidney, and the amino acids that cannot be transported can appear in the urine.

- *Hartnup's disease.* In this condition, the transport of neutral amino acids via SLC6A19 is defective, and neutral amino acids appear in the urine. Children with this condition exhibit skin changes, cerebellar ataxia and mental disturbances.
- *Cystinuria.* In this condition, the defect can be in either SLC3A1 or SLC7A9, both of which transport basic amino acids (arginine, lysine, ornithine) and cystine. In cystinuria, these amino acids appear in the urine. There is a tendency for kidney stones to develop in this condition, probably because the dipeptide cystine is poorly soluble.
- *Familial iminoglycinuria.* In this condition, there is a defect in the imino transport system leading to impaired absorption of the imino acids, proline and hydroxyproline.

In the above diseases, amino acids that are not absorbed via the amino-acid transporters can still be absorbed as components of small peptides. Therefore, supplements of dipeptides and tripeptides that contain the essential amino acids that cannot be absorbed as the free amino acids can be provided in the diet. This also explains why the amino acids can appear in the urine (due to similar defects in the kidney tubules), even though they cannot be absorbed as free molecules.

Minerals and trace elements

Chemical analysis of the human body has revealed the presence of over 20 elements. Some, such as oxygen, carbon, hydrogen and nitrogen, are abundant as constituents of organic molecules, or, in the case of oxygen and hydrogen, as components of water. Some elements are present in only trace amounts. Many enzymatic reactions will only take place if minute quantities of a particular ion are present. Therefore, these substances are required in the diet.

The cations required by the body are sodium, potassium, calcium, iron, magnesium, manganese, copper, molybdenum and zinc, and the anions are chloride, iodide, fluoride, phosphate and selenate.

The body requires Ca^{2+} for several physiological processes, including bone and teeth formation, synaptic transmission in the nervous system and glandular secretion. PO_4^{3-} is required for bone and teeth formation, acid-base balance, and many other functions. Iron is required for the synthesis of respiratory pigments such as haemoglobin, the respiratory pigment of red blood cells that transports oxygen to the tissues of the body. Mg^{2+} is required for nerve function and as a cofactor for many enzyme reactions. Copper and zinc ions, and many others are essential co-factors for enzyme reactions and are required in trace amounts.

Many ions, including Mg^{2+}, SO_4^{2-} and PO_4^{3-} are absorbed slowly in the small intestine by passive diffusion, although there also appears to be an additional active transport mechanism for Mg^{2+} in the ileum. Special mechanisms exist for the transport of Ca^{2+} and Fe^{2+}. Moreover, the absorption of these two ions is regulated according to the needs of the body. Deficiencies of Ca^{2+} and Fe^{2+} can occur in coeliac disease in which the proximal small intestine is damaged.

Calcium

The average adult diet contains 1–6 g of Ca^{2+}. In addition, approximately 0.6 g enters the tract as a component of secretions. Of this 2.2 g total, only 0.7 g is absorbed. Thus, after subtracting the amount entering the tract from non-dietary sources, the net amount entering the body per day is only approximately 100 mg.

Ca^{2+} ions can be absorbed along the entire length of the small intestine. Its absorption is via both passive and active mechanisms. When its concentration in the chyme is low (less than 5 mM), most absorption of Ca^{2+} ions is via active transport, but when its concentration is high, an appreciable proportion is absorbed by passive diffusion. This is a consequence of the rate-limiting property of active transport. Ca^{2+} can be absorbed against a 10-fold concentration gradient.

Cellular calcium uptake is mediated predominantly by the epithelial Ca^{2+} channel transient receptor potential vanilloid 6 (TRPV6; previously named ECaC2 and CaT1). There is also evidence that Cav1.3, an L-type channel located on the brush border, can mediate active transcellular Ca^{2+} absorption in the intestine. TRPV6 is thought to be particularly pertinent during the fasted state and/or starvation, and it is activated by apical membrane repolarisation and upregulated by vitamin D. In contrast, Cav1.3 is thought to be most relevant during digestion, mainly when diet and Ca^{2+} are plentiful. Calbindins (CB9k) are responsible for binding and trafficking the calcium once inside the cell. In addition, calbindin acts as a buffer ensuring that the free intracellular calcium levels remain low so as not to trigger apoptosis. Ca^{2+} efflux from enterocytes involves predominantly PMCA1b and to a lesser extent (20% of total cellular efflux) NCX1.

The process of calcium absorption in the small intestine is stimulated by a derivative of vitamin D_3. This vitamin can be ingested in the food (see below), or it can be formed in the skin from 7-dehydrocholesterol under the influence of sunlight. Vitamin D_3 is converted to 1,25-dihydroxyvitamin D_3 via reactions that occur in the liver and kidneys. This vitamin behaves as a hormone in the body and circulates via the blood to control

Ca^{2+} metabolism and homeostasis in various tissues. 1,25-Dihydroxyvitamin D_3 acts as a nuclear transcription factor for the vitamin D receptor and mediates the cellular effects of vitamin D by binding the vitamin D response elements of target genes involved in calcium import, calcium binding and efflux proteins. Vitamin D deficiency leads to calcium malabsorption that can cause rickets in children and osteomalacia in adults.

Absorption of Ca^{2+} ions is also stimulated by parathyroid hormone, another hormone that is intricately involved with Ca^{2+} homeostasis in the body. Parathyroid hormone is likely to indirectly modulate intestinal Ca^{2+} absorption through stimulation of renal 1α-hydroxylase, which is responsible for conversion of 25-hydroxycholecalciferol to the active form of vitamin D (1,25-dihydroxyhydroxycholecalciferol). This active form of vitamin D acts a nuclear transcription factor to regulate several calcium transport and binding proteins described above.

Bile salts indirectly facilitate the absorption of Ca^{2+} ions by promoting the formation of micelles in the lumen of the small intestine. This is partly because vitamin D is fat-soluble and its absorption depends on micelle formation, and partly because bile salts help to hold fatty acids in the micelles, thereby preventing them from forming insoluble Ca^{2+} soaps which cannot be absorbed. Thus, bile-salt deficiency can result in negative Ca^{2+} balance.

Calcium absorption is facultatively regulated to meet the needs of the body. The ability to absorb Ca^{2+} ions via secondary active transport is increased by calcium deprivation. Young and growing people absorb Ca^{2+} more rapidly than do mature and elderly people. Lactating women require Ca^{2+} for milk production, and they absorb Ca^{2+} avidly.

Rickets and osteomalacia

Calcium deficiency is usually due to vitamin D deficiency, either through dietary deficiency or lack of exposure to sunlight. It can also be due to a diet low in calcium. Malabsorption of vitamin D can potentially also occur in Crohn's and coeliac diseases. The deficiency leads to rickets in children and osteomalacia in adults. The main defect is inadequate mineralisation of bone matrix. Affected individuals tend to experience fractures, muscle and bone tenderness and occasionally tetany. In children with rickets, lower-limb deformities may occur. Treatment of the diseases is via supplementation of the diet with vitamin D and increased exposure to sunlight (which increases the synthesis of the active form of the vitamin, 1,25-dihydroxyvitamin D_3).

Iron

Iron is required by the body for a plethora of processes including erythropoiesis, oxidative phosphorylation and enzyme activity. Most notably, iron is essential for ribonucleotide reductase, which is the rate-limiting step in DNA synthesis. Thus, it is unsurprising that it is essential for life. Most of the iron within the body is implicated in the process of red blood cell synthesis and breakdown. The systemic circulating labile iron pool is utilised by the bone marrow for erythropoiesis and specifically the synthesis of haemoglobin. Red blood cells at the end of their life span (approximately 120 days) are then mostly engulfed by splenic macrophages and the iron is liberated from the haem moiety releasing iron and ultimately bilirubin, which is directed to the liver. The iron can then be effluxed by macrophages and reenter the labile iron pool to be recycled. In addition, the liver is a major iron-storage organ, and when the labile iron pool is in excess, iron can be directed to the liver to be stored. Conversely, when labile iron levels are low, iron stored in the liver can be mobilised to supplement the systemic iron pool. Since there is no active excretory mechanism for iron, the amount of iron absorbed in the small intestine must be tightly regulated. There is approximately only 2 mg/day of iron lost through the shedding of keratinocytes and enterocytes, which contain small amounts of iron. Thus, only approximately 2 mg of iron needs to be acquired through the diet daily.

Iron is acquired in the diet in the form of inorganic iron, predominantly in the ferric (Fe^{3+}) form and/or in the form of haem. Ferric iron is mostly found in vegetables and is poorly bioavailable, and this is mostly attributed to iron being complexed with other molecules such as phenolic compounds and because ferric iron must be reduced to ferrous (Fe^{2+}) iron to be imported by duodenal enterocytes. This reduction in ferric to ferrous iron can be mediated by stomach acid but also by a ferrireductase known as duodenal cytochrome B found on the brush border. Once reduced ferrous iron is transported into the enterocyte by the divalent metal transporter 1 (DMT1), the iron then has one of three fates: it is utilised by the cell, stored bound to a protein known as ferritin or effluxed out of the enterocyte via an efflux protein termed ferroportin. The cellular protein ferritin is particularly important since it binds to any free iron and prevents iron-mediated reactive oxygen species being generated through Fenton reaction chemistry within the cell. Without ferritin, cellular damage would occur including lipid peroxidation and DNA adducts. Thus, unsurprisingly, ferritin expression is indirectly regulated by iron levels through a mechanism involving iron-regulatory proteins. Once iron is effluxed across the basolateral membrane, ferrous iron is re-oxidised by a ferroxidase known as hephaestin and then becomes bound to transferrin, which ensures that the iron remains non-reactive. The circulating transferrin-bound iron can then be captured by cells expressing transferrin receptors on their surface. Like ferritin, transferrin receptors are also indirectly regulated by iron levels. In this instance, they are negatively regulated; when cellular iron levels are high, transferrin receptor expression is decreased whilst ferritin expression is increased. In the instance of intestinal haem transport, this is likely to be a carrier-mediated mechanism, although the carrier protein remains elusive. Previous studies have identified a carrier

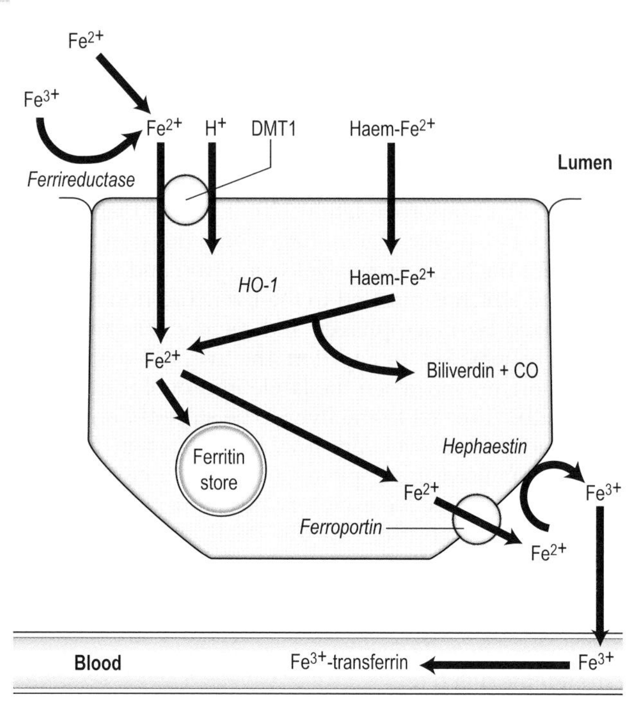

Fig. 6.10 Iron transport in the enterocyte. HO-1, haemoxidase-1.

termed haem carrier protein 1 (HCP1), although this was also later described to be a high-affinity folate transporter. Irrespective of the mechanism, the internalised haem is likely to be broken down by haem oxygenase-1 (HO-1) to liberate biliverdin, carbon monoxide and iron. The iron is then likely to be indistinguishable from the iron acquired through inorganic iron transport and thus has the same fate. The cellular metabolism of iron is summarised in Fig. 6.10.

While haem is more bioavailable than inorganic iron, half of the absorbed iron in the standard diet comes from haem whilst the other half comes from inorganic iron. On average, adults consume approximately 20 mg of total dietary iron, but since only approximately 10% is absorbed in the small intestine, the remainder transitions to the colon. Several studies have highlighted that excess colonic iron could be detrimental to colonic health through a few mechanisms, including dysbiosis of the colonic microbiome.

Regulation of iron absorption

Since iron is a prerequisite to so many processes, its metabolism is tightly regulated and mediated through the liver-derived hormone hepcidin. In instances of high iron, the liver is stimulated to release hepcidin (through a variety of proteins, including transferrin receptor 2 [TFR2], haemojuvelin and homeostatic iron regulator [HFE]) and this binds to the efflux protein ferroportin on a variety of cell types. In the context of enterocytes, iron binds to ferroportin, causing it to be internalised and degraded, resulting in a loss of cellular iron transport which aids in decreasing body iron levels. In instances of low iron, the liver hepcidin expression is suppressed, allowing for maximal iron absorption to remedy the iron deficiency. In instances of inflammation and infection, hepcidin is induced through the cytokine IL-6, which causes not only a loss of cellular iron absorption in the small intestine but leads to hepcidin binding to ferroportin on macrophages, thus preventing the efflux of iron out of the macrophages into the labile iron pool. In the long term, this causes anaemia of chronic disease (ACD), and the physiological relevance in the context of bacterial infection is that it limits how much iron the bacteria can acquire to fuel their proliferation. Presumably in the context of inflammation, hepcidin limits iron-mediated reactive oxygen species formation and further exacerbation of inflammation. Thus, ACD differs from IDA in that there is plenty of iron within the body, but much of the iron is locked within the reticuloendothelial system, thus resulting in an anaemia. Clearly, the gold standard for discriminating between ACD and IDA would be hepcidin since one would expect this to be high in ACD and low in IDA.

Iron-deficiency anaemia

Chronic iron deficiency results in IDA, a condition in which the synthesis of the respiratory pigment haemoglobin is reduced. In IDA, the red blood cells are characteristically small (microcytes) and contain a low concentration of haemoglobin (hypochromia). Males with IDA have a haemoglobin concentration below 130 g/L and females below 115 g/L. The prevalence is 2%–5% in adult males and postmenopausal females in the developed world. Tiredness is a prominent symptom of the condition because the reduced capacity of the red blood cells to carry oxygen results in the body's requirement for oxygen not being met. Treatment is by oral administration of iron salts such as ferrous sulphate.

The IDA may be due to a low-iron diet, menstrual blood loss, malabsorption of iron in conditions such as coeliac disease or chronic blood loss. 'Silent' chronic bleeding from the GI tract is also a feature of all GI cancers, and for this reason any adult with unexplained iron deficiency should be investigated for tumours of the large bowel, stomach and oesophagus.

Hereditary haemochromatosis

Haemochromatosis is a hereditary disease characterised by improper dietary iron metabolism which causes the accumulation of iron in several body tissues. Iron accumulation can eventually cause end-stage organ damage, most importantly in the liver and pancreas, manifesting as liver failure and diabetes mellitus, respectively. It is estimated that roughly one in every 300–400 people is affected by the disease, and primarily those of Celtic origin. However, it displays a very low penetrance. The organ damage is predominantly caused by the excessive iron which drives Fenton reactions, culminating in reactive oxygen species and cellular damage. By the time affected individuals develop the classic triad (diabetes mellitus, cirrhosis and skin pigmentation), the disease will have become advanced and potentially irreversible. Individuals with haemochromatosis absorb approximately 3–4 mg of iron per day and can accumulate between 500 mg to 1 g of iron per year. Clinical manifestations often occur after the age of 40 or when body iron stores are more than 15–40 g. In comparison, healthy individuals store approximately 3–4 g of iron. The crucial aspect to the treatment of hereditary haemochromatosis is to identify individuals early in their disease progression by assessing levels of transferrin saturation and serum ferritin, both of which are early signs of disease. By identifying these individuals, it allows for rapid treatment, which most commonly is phlebotomy. It can take up to 2–3 years to remove 20 g of iron from affected individuals based on weekly or biweekly phlebotomy. The genetics underpinning haemochromatosis can be explained by understanding how iron is regulated by hepcidin. High iron is sensed by hepatocytes and TFR2, HFE, and haemojuvelin proteins to induce hepcidin expression which then suppresses iron absorption through the interaction and degradation of ferroportin. Mutations in TFR2, HFE haemojuvelin, hepcidin and ferroportin can ultimately abrogate this axis and ultimately will allow for unabated iron absorption. Thus, haemochromatosis can be subclassified by mutation status.

Water-soluble vitamins

Water-soluble vitamins are essential for normal cellular functions, growth and development, and this is exemplified by the fact that deficiency results in a host of clinical conditions which range from growth retardation to neurological disorders. Except for some limited endogenous production of niacin, humans cannot synthesise water-soluble vitamins and, thus, must acquire them through dietary sources. It is well-recognised that the water-soluble vitamins ascorbate, biotin, folate, niacin, pantothenic acid, pyridoxine, riboflavin, and thiamine are transported via specific carrier-mediated processes. In addition, the gut microflora can also synthesise several water-soluble vitamins, which can be absorbed by the colon.

Ascorbic acid (AA) predominantly acts as a cofactor in an array of metabolic reactions which most notably include collagen synthesis. In addition, it acts as a scavenger of free radicals and keeps metal ions such as iron in their reduced state. AA deficiency leads to a variety of clinical abnormalities, including scurvy and poor wound healing. Also, AA can exist in an oxidised form, dehydroascorbic acid (DHAA), although this can be converted in enterocytes by DHAA reductase back into the reduced form. Intestinal absorption of AA involves sodium-dependent vitamin C transporter-1 (SVCT1) and SVCT2 but neither can transport DHAA. DHAA absorption is likely mediated by GLUT1, 3 and 4.

Biotin

Biotin (vitamin H) acts as a cofactor for carboxylases that are involved in a variety of metabolic reactions including gluconeogenesis and fatty acid metabolism. A deficiency in biotin can result in growth retardation and neurological disorders. In humans, biotin can be acquired through dietary sources and produced by the intestinal microbiome with the resultant biotin being absorbed by colonocytes. Biotin in the diet is either in a free form or bound to protein, and the latter can be digested to release biocytin and biotin–short peptide conjugates. These are then converted by biotinidase to biotin prior to absorption. Biotin is absorbed via Na^+-dependent carrier-mediated uptake mechanism involving the sodium-dependent multivitamin transporter (SMVT) localised on the apical brush-border membrane. The efflux of biotin across the basolateral membrane is likely to involve a specialised Na^+-independent carrier-mediated mechanism.

Folate

Folate or vitamin B9 refers to folic acid and all its derivative compounds. They predominantly act as coenzymes for an array of reactions, including cellular one-carbon metabolism and synthesis of purine, thymidine and homocysteine. A deficiency in folate can lead to a range of abnormalities, including megaloblastic anaemia and neurological disease. In addition to dietary folate, which is absorbed in the small intestine, the intestinal microbiome can also produce folate which is subsequently absorbed in the large intestine. Dietary folate consists of mono- and polyglutamates. Folate polyglutamates are hydrolysed to folate monoglutamates prior to absorption which involves the enzyme folylpoly-γ-glutamate carboxypeptidase. Bacterial-derived folate predominantly exists as folate monoglutamate. In both the small and large intestine, a pH-dependent, Na^+-independent carrier-mediated mechanism has been defined. Specifically, the reduced folate carrier (RFC) and the proton-coupled folate transporter (PCFT) are intricately involved. The latter has been formerly described as a haem transporter and termed HCP1. Both RFC and PCFT are expressed at the apical membrane of intestinal epithelial cells. Transport of the negatively charged folate by PCFT is acidic-pH-dependent (proton-coupled) and electrogenic. The PCFT system predominates in the proximal small intestine where the pH is more acidic, whereas the RFC system operates at neutral-pH as found in the distal small intestine and colon. It is unclear how folate is effluxed out of intestinal epithelial cells, but it is likely to involve multidrug resistance proteins.

Vitamin B_{12}

Deficiency of vitamin B_{12} also known as cobalamin (Cbl) manifests itself in a host of clinical, haematological and neuropathological disorders. Evidence suggests that approximately 6% of the Western population over the age of 60 years have low plasma Cbl, and this may underpin decreased cognitive function and dementia in the ageing population. This may in part be attributed to relatively low dietary intake. The process of dietary Cbl absorption is mediated by several proteins including haptocorrin in the saliva, intrinsic factor (IF) in gastric juice and the receptor for complexed IF–Cbl in the distal ileum. The IF produced by the parietal cells binds to Cbl, and there is always more IF in healthy individuals than Cbl. The IF–Cbl complex is then absorbed in the terminal ileum by a receptor-mediated process involving cubilin, a peripheral membrane-associated protein and the protein amnionless. Mutations in cubilin or amnionless have been demonstrated to lead to a Cbl malabsorption syndrome. Decreased absorption of Cbl can be attributed to many reasons, including a loss of IF in pernicious anaemia where there is autoimmune destruction of parietal cells. Once internalised, Cbl dissociates from IF and then becomes complexed to transcobalamin (TCB). More specifically, TCBII is synthesised by the liver and transports Cbl in serum. It is an essential protein in the delivery of Cbl to cells and tissues, although it only transports 20% of circulating cobalamins. Congenital deficiencies in TCBII result in an array of conditions, including neuropsychiatric disorders pancytopaenia-type haematological disorders, and megaloblastic anaemia. Cells ultimately can acquire TCB–Cbl through a receptor protein (TCblR), which belongs to the low-density lipoprotein receptor family. The vast majority of Cbl is ultimately stored in the liver and the kidney.

Pernicious anaemia

Deficiency of IF due to atrophy of the gastric mucosa is the most common cause of pernicious anaemia. Atrophy of the gastric mucosa also leads to the inability of the stomach to secrete HCl (achlorhydria) and pepsinogen. However, it is only the lack of IF that is serious, because pepsinogen and acid are not essential to life. Pernicious anaemia can also be an autoimmune disease and so patients can have high antibody titres in their blood even when foreign IF has not been ingested. Vitamin B_{12} can be injected intramuscularly, but this is usually only necessary once every three months, as it is stored in substantial amounts in the liver. Vitamin B_{12} is important for maturation of the red blood cells. Pernicious anaemia is characterised by a low red blood cell count but a high mean red blood cell volume, as the immature red blood cells present are larger than normal (macrocytic). If the condition is left untreated, patients can develop polyneuropathy, paraesthesia of fingers and toes, progressive weakness and ataxia, dementia and other psychiatric problems.

Lipids

Dietary lipids

The range of fat ingested by an individual varies enormously (25–160 per day). Most ingested fat is neutral lipids (triacylglycerols) present in butter, margarine, cooking oil and meat, among other sources. In addition, some phospholipids and cholesterol esters, and components of plant and animal cell membranes are present in food together with small amounts of other lipids.

Fat-soluble vitamins and essential fatty acids

Certain lipid molecules are essential in the diet, as they are required in the body but cannot be synthesised. These include the fat-soluble vitamins A, D, E and K, and, the essential fatty acids α-linolenic acid (omega-3) and linoleic acid (omega-6).

Deficiency of vitamin A results in hyperkeratosis of the skin and xerophthalmia or a disturbance of epithelial tissues. In humans, an early symptom of this condition is night blindness due to abnormal responses of the retinal rods.

Vitamin D is required for Ca^{2+} absorption (see below) and for normal calcium and phosphate metabolism. Vitamin D deficiency and the resultant Ca^{2+} deficiency lead to abnormalities in bones and teeth, paraesthesia (due to impaired nerve conduction), and skeletal pain and tetany (due to impaired muscle function).

Vitamin E is an important antioxidant. Deficiency in rodents causes sterility and muscle weakness, but its role in humans is not entirely clear.

Vitamin K deficiency causes bleeding diathesis due to defective blood coagulation because of failure to synthesise prothrombin, which is required for blood clotting. Part of the vitamin K requirement of an organism is supplied by bacteria that colonise the intestines.

Under normal circumstances, less than 6 g of fat is eliminated in the faeces per day and most of this arises from bacterial cells and cell debris. If larger amounts of fat are eliminated, the condition is known as steatorrhoea and indicates a deficiency in fat absorption.

Lipid solubility

Some lipids, like short-chain fatty acids (with a 10-carbon chain) and some polyunsaturated complex lipids containing short-chain fatty acids or polyunsaturated fatty acids, are soluble in water. These are absorbed by passive diffusion. They dissolve in the membrane and are transported down their concentration gradients into the cell and then into the portal blood. The transport of water-soluble lipids into the blood is a rapid process.

The digestion and absorption of most lipids are achieved by a variety of highly complex processes which enable the body to overcome the fact that although most lipid is insoluble in water, it must be transferred from the gut lumen to the lymph and eventually the blood via aqueous media, including:

- The chyme in the lumen,
- The cell's interior,
- The interstitial fluid,
- The lymph, and
- The blood.

A further problem is that the enzymes that catalyse the breakdown of the complex lipids (i.e., lipases, phospholipases and cholesterol esterases) are all water-soluble and insoluble in lipid, but obviously must gain access to the lipid molecules before they can hydrolyse them. The mechanisms that enable these problems to be overcome will be described after the reactions involved in the digestion of lipids have been outlined.

Digestion

The digestion of triacylglycerol is catalysed by lipases (glycerol ester hydrolases). The major lipase in the digestive tract is secreted by the pancreas. Minor lipases are present in saliva (lingual lipase) and gastric juice, but these are probably only important when the pancreatic enzyme is absent or inactive. The pancreatic enzyme cleaves the ester bonds at positions 1 and 3 in the triacylglycerol molecule, in a stepwise manner, with the formation of 1,2-diacylglycerol and 2,3-diacylglycerol intermediates. The ultimate products are 2-monoacylglycerol, which is absorbed without further degradation and fatty acids. The overall reaction is given in Fig. 6.11.

Cholesterol esterase is secreted in pancreatic juice. In intestinal chyme, it forms dimers that are resistant to proteolytic digestion. It cleaves the ester bond in cholesterol ester to form free cholesterol and fatty acid (Fig. 6.11). It also acts more slowly to hydrolyse triacylglycerol, lysophospholipids, monoacylglycerols and esters of fat-soluble vitamins.

Phospholipase A_2 is secreted in pancreatic juice as an inactive precursor. It is activated in the small intestine. It cleaves the ester bond at position 2 in many phospholipids, including phosphatidylcholine (lecithin), phosphatidylserine and phosphatidylethanolamine, to give a fatty acid and a lysophospholipid. The hydrolysis of phosphatidylcholine is shown in Fig. 6.11.

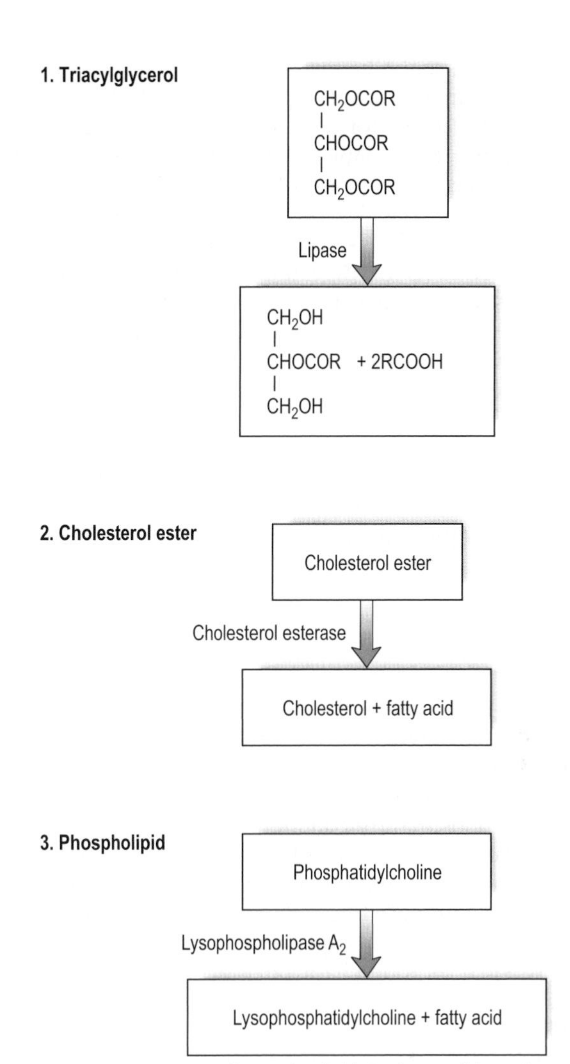

Fig. 6.11 Digestion of complex lipids in the small intestine.

Emulsification

Emulsification is essential for the efficient digestion of lipids. It enables the enzymes involved to gain access to their lipid substrates. If oil is added to water, it forms a layer on top of the water because it is insoluble and less dense than water. If some lipase is added, it dissolves in the water layer and will only attack the lipid at the lipid–water interface. Therefore, the rate of lipid hydrolysis is proportional to the surface area of the lipid–water interface. In the small intestine, the surface area of the lipid–water interface is increased by the process of emulsification, whereby the large droplets of lipid are broken down into tiny droplets that can be held in a stable suspension. The lipid–water interface is consequently increased enormously, enabling lipid digestion to proceed at a rapid rate.

The process of emulsification requires conjugated bile acids, which coat the lipid droplets and prevent them coalescing together. These substances are secreted in bile. Within 20 min of the beginning of a meal, the gallbladder contracts and empties concentrated bile into the duodenum. The emulsified droplets are 0.5–1.0 mm in diameter. A neutral or slightly alkaline environment is required for emulsification. This is normally provided by the intestinal chyme in which the alkaline secretions mix with the acid from the stomach and neutralise it.

Lipase is essentially inactive in the presence of bile acids, but colipase, a small protein (10,000 Da) present in pancreatic juice, forms a complex with lipase and bile acid, and this enables the colipase–lipase complex to spread over the surface of the minute droplets and hydrolyse the triacylglycerol present. Triacylglycerol is hydrolysed on the surface of the emulsion droplets and the products of digestion, monoacylglycerol and fatty acids are liberated from the droplets into the aqueous medium. The hydrolysis of triacylglycerol under these circumstances is more rapid than the absorption of its products. A small proportion of the fatty acids released from the droplets are water-soluble, which can be absorbed directly into the blood. However, most free fatty acids and monoacylglycerols are insoluble in water. They would soon saturate the chyme and separate out into large droplets again if it were not for the process of micelle formation.

Micelle formation

A micelle is a lipid particle 4–6 nm in diameter, which consists of an aggregate of approximately 20 lipid molecules. Bile acids are required for micelle formation. Bile itself contains micelles composed of bile salts, cholesterol, and phosphatidylcholine but in the small intestine the micelles have a more heterogeneous composition. In the small intestine, the initial constituents of the micelles in the duodenum are bile salts and 2-monoacylglycerols. These micelles then sequester other fat-soluble substances, such as long-chain fatty acids, cholesterol, fat-soluble vitamins and phospholipids. An individual micelle may contain several or all of these molecules, although fatty acids are quantitatively the most important. Cholesterol, long-chain fatty acids, and fat-soluble vitamins, which are highly insoluble in water, are maintained in the core region of the micelle. Monoacylglycerol and lysophospholipids orientate themselves so that their acyl chains are in the core region, and their more polar regions project towards the aqueous phase (i.e., in the shell region). Bile salts are present in the shell region. The polar groups on the bile salt impart a negative charge to the surface of the micelles. This causes mutual repulsion between different micelles, keeping them in stable suspension in the chyme. The negatively charged shell collects cations such as Na^+ that form an outer shell around the micelle. When the bile acid concentration is at or above its critical micellar concentration, the bile acid and insoluble lipids such as monoacylglycerol aggregate as micelles. With increasing bile acid concentration, more monoacylglycerol molecules are carried as micelles. In healthy humans, the critical micellar concentration is usually well below the concentration actually present, and micelles easily form. However, there are certain disease states where the concentration is too low, such as obstructive jaundice. The critical micellar concentration is higher for unconjugated bile acids than for conjugated bile acids. Consequently, if a considerable fraction of the bile acids is deconjugated in the intestinal lumen by bacterial action, micelle formation may be impaired.

Most fatty acids and monoacylglycerol are absorbed in the duodenum and upper jejunum, while the bile acids are absorbed more distally in the ileum. Cholesterol can be absorbed throughout the length of the small intestine, although a considerable proportion of it escapes into the colon. Thus, the composition of the micelles changes as they move down the small intestine; their content of fatty acids and monoacylglycerol diminishes while their proportional content of bile acids increases.

The constituent lipid molecules of micelles move back and forth between the micelles and the aqueous solution with great rapidity. The aqueous chyme is kept saturated with lipid molecules by the movement of fatty acids and monoacylglycerol from the micelles into the solution. Thus, the micelles serve as a reservoir of these products so that the aqueous phase in contact with the enterocyte brush border is always saturated with lipid molecules, and a dynamic equilibrium between the micelle and the solution is established. The dissolved fatty acids can be absorbed. However, the micelles first must diffuse across the 'unstirred layer' to the enterocyte cell membrane.

The unstirred layer

The unstirred layer is a layer of fluid in contact with the epithelial surface, which does not readily mix with the bulk of the chyme. Micelles and nutrients must diffuse through this layer to the surface membrane of the enterocyte. Thus, there is a concentration gradient of nutrients across the unstirred layer with the lowest concentration at the epithelial surface. A pH gradient also exists across the unstirred layer, with the fluid in contact with the brush border being slightly more acidic than the bulk of the chyme. This promotes the absorption of fatty acids as they tend to be less ionised and therefore more easily absorbed across the lipid membrane.

Fate of lipid in the epithelial cell

Lipids can dissolve in the lipid of the brush-border membrane and easily diffuse across it. The transported lipids are metabolised within the cell and used in the resynthesis of complex lipids (Fig. 6.12). The free fatty acids react with coenzyme A to form acetyl-CoA (Fig. 6.13A). Triacylglycerol is synthesised via both the α-glycerol-phosphate pathway (that also operates in liver and other tissues) and via the monoacylglycerol pathway, which involves direct esterification of monoacylglycerol by fatty acyl-S-CoA, a pathway which is restricted to mucosal cells (Fig. 6.13B,C). Phospholipids are synthesised by esterification of lysophospholipids with fatty acyl-S-CoA (Fig. 6.13D) and cholesterol ester by esterification of free cholesterol with fatty acyl-S-CoA (Fig. 6.13E).

Complex lipids are formed in the smooth endoplasmic reticulum of enterocytes. The complex lipid molecules

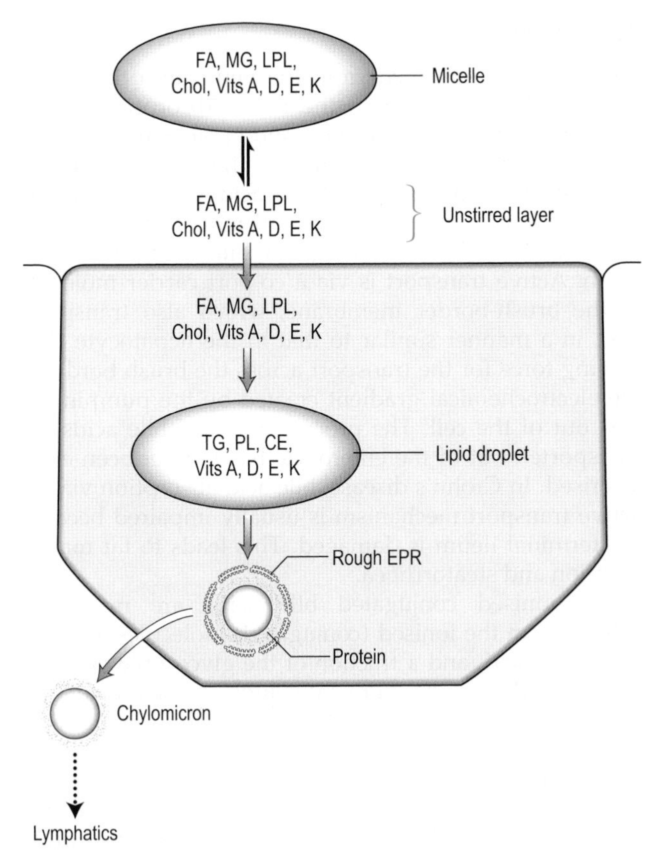

Fig. 6.12 Transport of lipids in the enterocyte. *Chol, cholesterol; FA, fatty acids; LPL, lysophospholipid; MG, monoacylglycerol; PL, phospholipid; TG, triacylglycerol; Vits, vitamins.*

aggregate together to form droplets within the cell. The phospholipids form at the surface of the droplets, with their polar heads orientated towards the exterior of the droplets. The droplets become surrounded with rough endoplasmic reticulum and the ribosomes synthesise a β-lipoprotein, which, together with the phospholipid, forms a coat around the droplets (see Fig. 6.12). The droplet with its protein and phospholipid coat is known as a chylomicron. Chylomicrons vary in size from a few nm to 750 nm in diameter. The different lipids, including the fat-soluble vitamins, are sequestered together in the same chylomicrons.

The chylomicrons are extruded from the lateral surface of the cell and taken up into the lymph in the lacteals. After a meal, the intestinal lymph becomes milky due to the presence of chylomicrons. The uptake of chylomicrons into the lymph is stimulated by adrenocorticoid hormones. Furthermore, fat malabsorption and steatorrhoea are features of both coeliac disease and Crohn's disease.

Defects in fat digestion and absorption

Disease of various organs can lead to fat malabsorption and steatorrhoea. This is a reflection of the complexity of

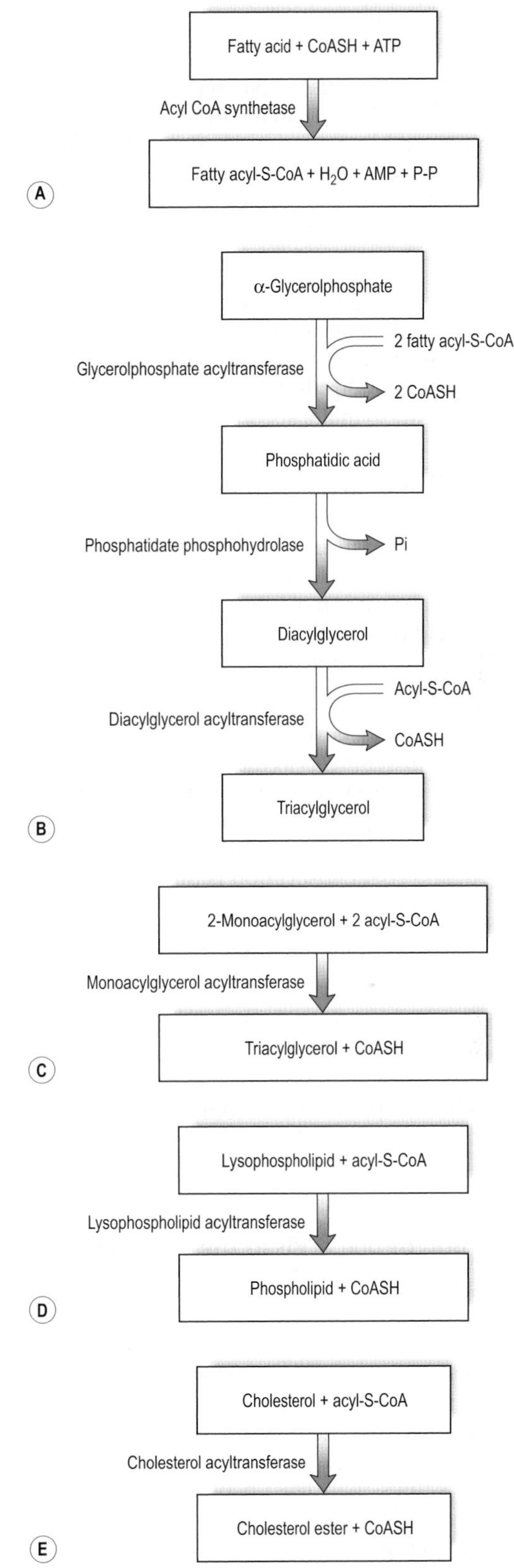

Fig. 6.13 Synthesis of complex lipids in the small intestine. (A) Formation of acetyl-S-CoA. (B) Synthesis of triacylglycerol via the glycerol phosphate pathway. (C) Synthesis of triacylglycerol via the monoacylglycerol pathway. (D) Synthesis of phospholipid from lysophospholipid. (E) Synthesis of cholesterol ester from cholesterol.

fat digestion and absorption. Some of these diseases are described below:

- *Liver or biliary tract disease* (such as gallstone disease and cirrhosis) can result in a deficiency of conjugated bile acids and HCO_3^- resulting in impaired emulsification of lipids and impaired micelle formation. *Note*: Some drugs, like cholestyramine, a resin used to treat diarrhoea caused by bile acids, bind bile salts and prevent them from forming micelles.
- *Pancreatic disease* (such as chronic pancreatitis) can result in deficiency of enzymes such as lipase, which digest fats, and reduced HCO_3^-, leading to malabsorption of lipids. Other pancreatic enzymes are also deficient, so malabsorption of other nutrients also occurs.
- *Intestinal disease.* In coeliac disease, where the villi are flattened, there is a reduced surface area available for absorption of nutrients such as fats in the affected regions. In Crohn's disease that commonly affects the ileum, the absorption of bile acids is defective, and the bile acid pool is reduced. This leads to reduced emulsification and micelle formation and therefore reduced fat digestion and absorption.
- *β-Lipoproteinaemia* is an inherited disorder where β-lipoprotein synthesis in the enterocytes and elsewhere is defective. Thus, in this condition, the synthesis of the protein coat of chylomicrons is inadequate and only large chylomicrons, if any, are formed, and so fat absorption is impaired.
- *Lymphatic disease* (obstruction by a tumour, for example) can lead to impaired transport of lipids from the lymph to the blood.
- *Adrenal disease,* where there is a deficiency of adrenocorticoid hormones, can lead to impaired transport of lipids to the lymph as these hormones stimulate the uptake of chylomicrons into the lymph.

Bile acids

Modification of bile acids in the small intestine

Bile acids are modified by intestinal bacteria. Primary bile acids are converted to secondary bile acids by dehydroxylation. Therefore, excessive bacterial action can lead to a greater proportion of secondary bile acids in the bile acid pool. In addition, a portion of the bile acids can be deconjugated by bacterial enzymes with the release of the amino-acid moieties. Conjugated bile acids have lower pKa values than the unconjugated acids and are therefore more ionised and more water-soluble at the slightly alkaline pH of the intestinal chyme. As they are ionised, they exist as salts with Na^+ and other cations.

Absorption

Bile acids are absorbed from the ileum into the portal blood and transported to the liver. Absorption in the small intestine is by both active and passive mechanisms. Active transport occurs only in the terminal ileum, and only ionised conjugated bile acids are absorbed by this active process. It is very efficient; normally, only approximately 5% of conjugated bile acids reach the colon. Active transport is via a co-port carrier molecule in the brush-border membrane, which also transports Na^+, in a manner similar to that in the hepatocyte. The driving force for the transport across the brush border is the electrochemical gradient created by the pumping of Na^+ out of the cell. The process whereby bile acids are transported out of the enterocyte has not yet been characterised. In Crohn's disease, bile acid absorption via the active transport mechanism is usually impaired because the terminal ileum is damaged. This leads to fat malabsorption and steatorrhoea.

Non-ionised conjugated bile acids are more fat-soluble than the ionised (conjugated) molecules. Glycine is a weak acid, and a fraction of the glycoconjugates are non-ionised and therefore fat-soluble. A small amount of it is absorbed passively through the lipid membrane. Taurine conjugates are almost completely ionised at the pH of the small intestine and are therefore not absorbed in this way. Excessive deconjugation of conjugated bile acids by intestinal bacteria leads to decreased absorption and a greater loss to the colon with a resulting decrease in the size of the bile acid pool. However, unconjugated bile acids are more fat-soluble than conjugated bile acids and a proportion is absorbed by passive transport in the intestines.

Bile pigments

Bile pigments are lipid substances with limited solubility in aqueous solution. Unconjugated bilirubin is more lipid-soluble than conjugated bilirubin, and it can be absorbed by diffusion across the lipid membrane of the enterocyte. Bacterial action in the intestines deconjugates some of the conjugated bile pigments, with the result that some bile pigment is reabsorbed into the portal blood.

Fat malabsorption

Fat digestion and absorption is a very complicated process necessitating the proper functioning of many organs including the liver, the pancreas and the small intestine. For this reason, many different defects of digestion and absorption can result in malabsorption of fats and steatorrhoea. Diseases where fat malabsorption is a prominent feature include coeliac disease and Crohn's disease.

Case 6.2 Crohn's disease

A 22-year-old man presented to the gastroenterology department with a 4-month history of progressive abdominal pain, loose stools and 3-stone weight loss. He reported the pain as being localised to his right lower quadrant and could wake him up at night. He opened his bowels 6–8 times a day and several times at night. He denied any past medical history and did not take regular medications. He reported that two of his distant cousins suffer from Crohn's disease. He smoked 20 cigarettes a day and worked as a builder. On examination, he had clubbing of his fingers and conjunctival pallor. He was tender in his right iliac fossa and a palpable distinct mass could be felt. Routine blood tests revealed significant anaemia with elevated markers of inflammation, including white cell count, C-reactive protein and erythrocyte sedimentation rate, along with low albumin. His faecal calprotectin test (biomarker of intestinal inflammation) was also significantly elevated.

Diagnosis and treatment

He underwent an urgent colonoscopy. This revealed patchy ulcers limited to his ascending colon with severe inflammation and ulceration of his terminal ileum (as shown in Figs 6.14 and 6.15). He underwent magnetic resonance imaging (MRI) of his small bowel which demonstrated inflammatory stricturing of 10 cm in his terminal ileum (Fig. 6.16). In addition, there was evidence of fistulation between the terminal ileum and a further segment of the small bowel (entero-enteric fistulation). He was given a course of steroids, following which he was commenced on a biological therapy called infliximab which resulted in resolution of his symptoms and disease activity.

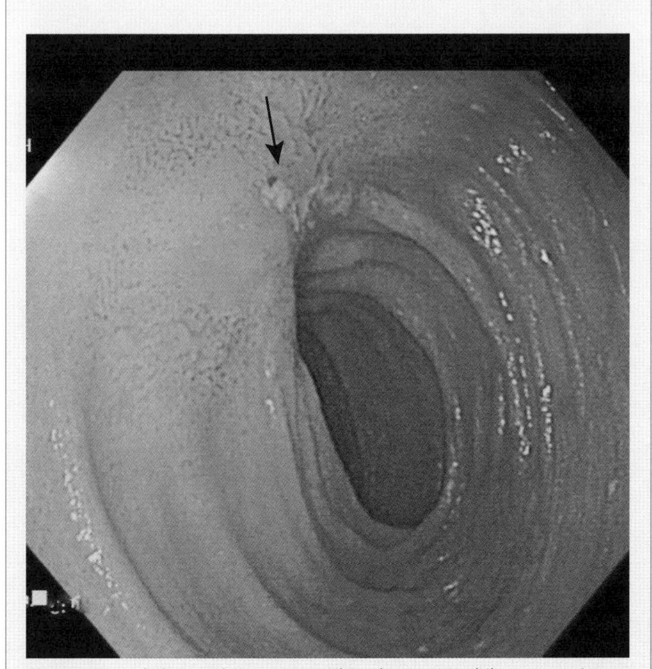

Fig. 6.14 Aphthous ulcers seen within the terminal ileum consistent with a diagnosis of Crohn's disease.

Crohn's disease is a form of immune-mediated inflammatory bowel disease that is characterised by transmural (across all the layers of the bowel wall) inflammation and may involve any part of the GI tract – from the oral cavity to peri-

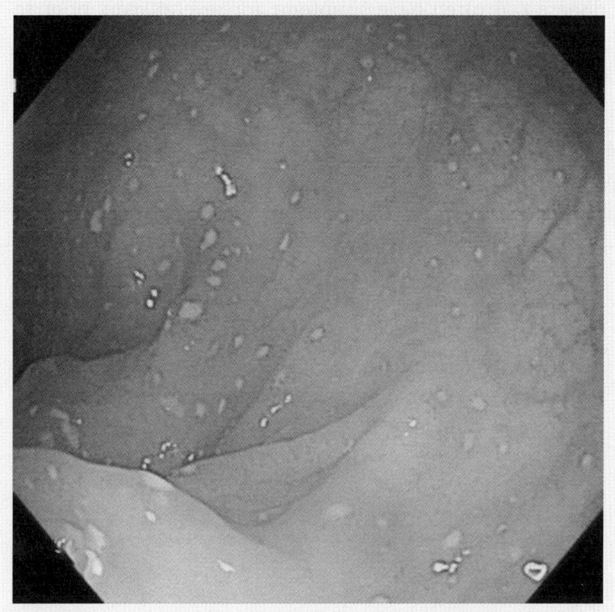

Fig. 6.15 Multiple aphthous ulcers (white patches) seen in the colon.

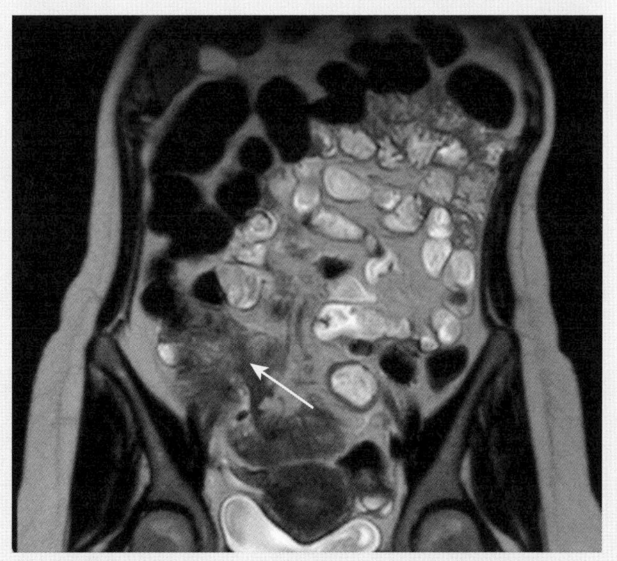

Fig. 6.16 Magnetic resonance imaging of the small bowel demonstrating significant inflammation and stricturing of the terminal ileum (red arrow).

Continued

Case 6.2 Crohn's disease—cont'd

anal region. The exact cause of inflammatory bowel disease is as yet unknown; however, it is thought to be a result of an interplay between genetics, a dysregulated immune response and environmental factors, including diet and gut microbiota. It affects the small bowel in nearly 80% of patients and is often localised to the distal ileum. Approximately one-third of patients will also suffer from perianal disease in the form of fistulas and abscesses. Patients with Crohn's disease can often have symptoms for several years prior to their presentation. These may include abdominal pain, diarrhoea with or without bleeding and significant weight loss. Identification of these red-flag symptoms are critical in differentiating this diagnosis from other functional causes of abdominal pain. Due to the transmural nature of the disease, patients with Crohn's disease can develop complications such as fistulas (tracts or communications between two organs such as between two loops of bowel, between the bowel or bladder or bowel and skin), abscesses and perianal disease. As Crohn's often affects the terminal ileum, patients may develop impairment in the enterohepatic circulation of bile acids with resultant fat malabsorption and bile acid diarrhoea. Moreover, they may develop vitamin deficiencies (i.e., vitamin B_{12}) and protein calorie malnutrition.

The diagnosis of Crohn's disease is often made in conjunction with patients' clinical presentation with the help of endoscopy, radiological imaging (computed tomography or MRI scan) and histology. Treatment of Crohn's disease is primarily in the form of treating the inflammation with immunosuppressive drugs such as biological therapies and small molecules. Surgery also plays a major part in its management, both as a primary form of treatment, as well as management of medication-refractory or complicated Crohn's disease.

THE ABSORPTIVE AND POST-ABSORPTIVE STATES

7

Chapter objectives and clinical presentations

After reading this chapter, review your learning by considering the following:

1. Can you explain the differences between the absorptive and post-absorptive states?
2. Can you describe the role of the different hormones on glucose levels?
3. Do you understand the differences between type 1 and type 2 diabetes and their clinical management?

Also, you should be familiar with the following clinical presentations:

- Type 1 and 2 diabetes mellitus
- Starvation

Introduction

The nutrient state of the blood depends on whether a meal is being processed in the gastrointestinal (GI) tract. When nutrients such as glucose and lipid are being absorbed and their concentrations in the blood are high, the pattern of energy metabolism is known as the absorptive state. In this state, a fraction of the blood glucose is used by various tissues to meet their immediate energy needs. The excess glucose and the absorbed lipid are stored as glycogen and lipid that can be used to provide energy between meals or during fasting: a pattern of energy metabolism known as the post-absorptive state. The change from the absorptive state pattern to the post-absorptive state pattern is brought about by changes in the blood concentrations of insulin and other hormones. The importance of maintaining the appropriate patterns of metabolism can be illustrated by considering the metabolic defects present in insulin-dependent diabetes mellitus (or type 1 diabetes), in which the secretion of insulin is severely impaired. In this chapter, we shall consider the metabolic abnormalities present in this condition and the consequences of these defects.

The absorptive state

In the absorptive state, the nutrients entering the blood from the GI tract are hexose sugars and amino acids. The liver is the first port of call for these absorbed nutrients. It takes up a large fraction of the nutrients, thereby altering the composition of the blood before it circulates to the rest of the body. The nutrients remaining in the blood are taken up by adipose tissue, muscle and other tissues. Lipids are absorbed from the small intestines into the lymph as components of chylomicrons. They enter the venous blood at the thoracic duct and are then metabolised and stored in adipose tissue.

Fate of absorbed carbohydrate

Absorbed carbohydrate consists of glucose, galactose and fructose. However, the liver converts fructose and galactose to glucose and then releases glucose into the blood. It is expedient therefore, to consider absorbed carbohydrate as glucose. Fig. 7.1 illustrates the various fates of glucose during the absorptive state.

A large fraction of the absorbed glucose enters the various cells of the body, where it is used to produce energy. During the absorptive state, glucose is the main fuel for most tissues of the body, which utilise it by glycolysis, the citric acid cycle and other pathways. The rest of the absorbed glucose is used to provide stores of energy for later use during the post-absorptive (fasting) state (see below). The tissues that store most of the body's energy are liver, adipose tissue and muscle. Glucose is taken up by all these tissues in the absorptive state.

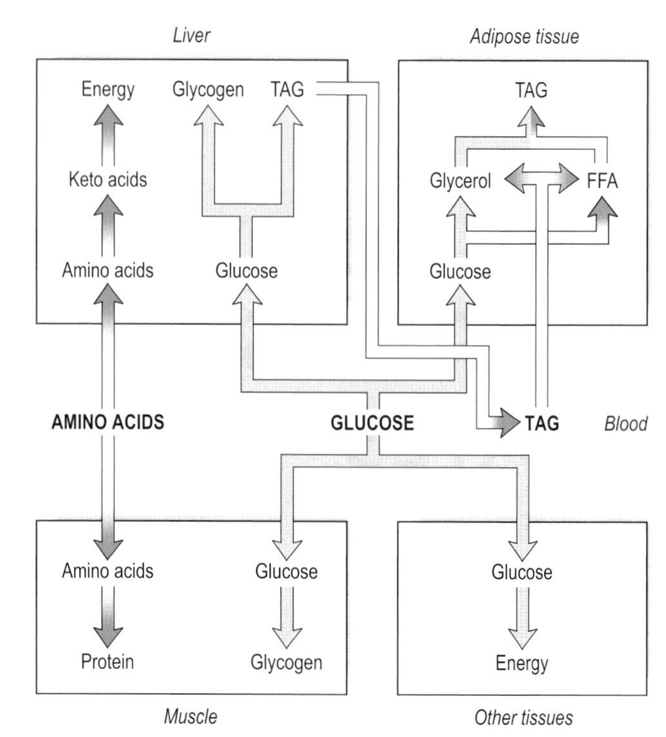

Fig. 7.1 Energy metabolism in the absorptive state. *FFA, free fatty acids; TAG, triacylglycerol.*

Some of the glucose taken up by the liver is converted to glycogen that is then stored in the liver, and some is converted to triacylglycerol. Glucose provides both the glycerol and the fatty acid moieties of triacylglycerol. Some of the triacylglycerol synthesised in the liver is stored there, but most is released into the blood as a component of very low-density lipoproteins (VLDLs). Very little glucose and fat is utilised for energy in the liver itself; the liver's main source of energy in the absorptive state is amino acids (see below.)

Another fraction of the blood glucose enters skeletal muscle where it is converted to glycogen for storage in the muscle. A further fraction enters adipose tissue, where it is converted to fatty acids and α-glycerol-phosphate, which are used in the synthesis of triacylglycerol.

In summary, during the absorptive phase, glucose is used for energy production by most tissues of the body, and the excess is stored in muscle and liver as glycogen, and in adipose tissue as fat. These relationships are outlined in Fig. 7.1.

Various inherited disorders of carbohydrate metabolism have been characterised, where either glycogen storage is excessive, or abnormal glycogen is produced. These conditions are due to defects in enzymes involved in glycogen metabolism.

Glycogen storage disorders

Most glycogen storage diseases are autosomal recessive disorders. They are caused by enzyme defects that lead either to accumulation of glycogen, or to an abnormality in the structure of glycogen. Glycogen is synthesised in liver or muscle.

Defects in liver enzymes

- *Phosphorylase or phosphorylase kinase.* A defect in either of these enzymes leads to hepatomegaly and hypoglycaemia; the prognosis is good.
- *Phosphorylase 6 kinase.* The defect leads to hepatomegaly, hypoglycaemia and fatiguability.
- *Debranching enzyme.* The defect leads to an abnormal structure of liver and muscle glycogen. The clinical features are similar to those for glucose-6-phosphatase deficiency (see below).
- *Branching enzyme.* A defect in this enzyme results in abnormal structure in liver glycogen. The clinical features are hepatomegaly and cirrhosis, and death in the first 5 years of life.
- *Glucose 6-phosphatase* (Von Gierke's disease, see Fig. 7.7). In this disease, the defect leads to hepatomegaly, ketototic hypoglycaemia, stunted growth, obesity and hypotonia. The liver, intestine, and kidney are affected. There is a high mortality rate.

Defects in muscle enzymes

- *Phosphorylase (McArdle's disease).* The symptoms are muscle cramps and myoglobinuria after exercise. The lifespan is normal.
- *Phosphofructokinase (see Fig. 7.7).* The clinical features are similar to those seen in phosphorylase deficiency (see above).
- *Lysosomal acid α-glucosidase.* A defect in this enzyme leads to cardiomyopathy and heart failure, and death in infancy. Liver, muscle and heart tissues are affected.

Fate of blood triacylglycerol

Absorbed triacylglycerol is carried in the lymph as droplets partially coated with protein, known as chylomicrons. The triacylglycerol synthesised from glucose in the liver is released to circulate in the blood, but as components of VLDLs. The blood enters the adipose tissue where the lipids, present in both VLDLs and chylomicrons, are hydrolysed to fatty acids and glycerol by a lipoprotein lipase present in the endothelial surfaces of the capillaries. Most of the fatty acids produced are taken up into the adipose cells (adipocytes) by passive diffusion, although a small fraction circulates to other tissues. The glycerol produced is either taken up by the adipose tissue cells or transported to other tissues. In adipocytes, the fatty acids and glycerol are reconstituted to triacylglycerol via the α-glycerol-phosphate pathway and stored in the cells. Thus, during the absorptive state, triacylglycerol in adipose tissue arises from three sources; absorbed glucose, VLDLs released from the liver and dietary triacylglycerol present in chylomicrons. These relationships are summarised in Fig. 7.1.

Adipose tissue is abundant in the body and widely distributed in subcutaneous, perirenal, mesenteric and other regions. An adipocyte contains a small amount of cytoplasm, which surrounds a large lipid droplet. There is very little water present in adipose cells. Lipid has a very low density. It provides a very efficient storage form of energy: 1 g of triacylglycerol contains more than twice as many calories as 1 g of glycogen or protein. Moreover, a 70-kg man has approximately 15 kg triacylglycerol that provides 135,000 kcal of energy, but only approximately 0.2 kg of glycogen, providing only 800 kcal of energy.

Fate of absorbed amino acids

In the absorptive state, a fraction of the absorbed amino acids is taken up by the liver (see Fig. 7.1) and converted to keto acids that are oxidised via the citric acid cycle and other pathways. Ketoacids are the liver's main source of energy in the absorptive state. Excess ketoacids can be converted to triacylglycerol in the liver. The conversion of amino acids to ketoacids involves deamination, with the formation of ammonia that is converted to urea in the liver. The urea is released from the liver into the blood and subsequently secreted by the kidneys.

Amino acids that are not taken up by the liver enter other tissues, such as muscle, where they are utilised for protein synthesis. Muscle is quantitatively the most important tissue in this respect. Protein is not a particularly labile source of energy, but it is broken down and used for energy during prolonged fasting.

Insulin

Insulin has a central role in the control of metabolism. If it is injected, the absorptive state is duplicated, and if its plasma concentration is very low, as in untreated type 1 diabetes, the pattern of metabolism that predominates is an exaggerated version of that seen in the post-absorptive state. Insulin is a polypeptide (MW 6000 Da), consisting of two peptide chains that are connected by two disulphide bridges (Fig. 7.2).

The prohormone precursor of insulin is a single peptide chain (MW 9000 Da) known as proinsulin, which is converted to insulin by proteolytic cleavage. This results in the removal of a peptide, known as C-peptide. In the prohormone, C-peptide connects the two peptide chains of insulin (see Fig. 7.2). Both insulin and C-peptide are stored in granules in the β-cells of the pancreas. C-peptide is secreted with insulin in a ratio of 1:1 but is excreted in the urine, unlike insulin that is removed from the blood by the liver. Its concentration in the urine can

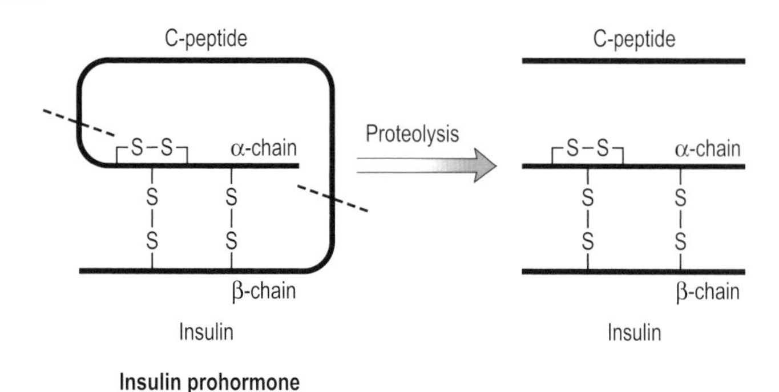

Fig. 7.2 Proteolytic processing of the insulin prohormone to insulin and C-peptide.

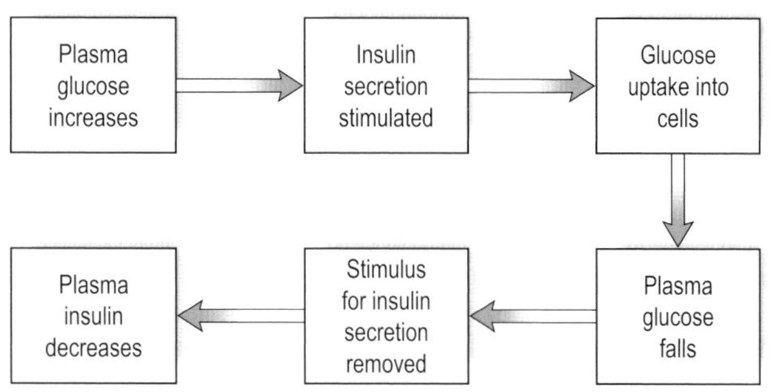

Fig. 7.3 Feedback control of insulin release.

be used to assess an individual's ability to secrete insulin. It has no established biological function.

The release of insulin into the blood is stimulated by eating and inhibited by fasting, and insulin is largely responsible for promoting the pattern of metabolism seen in the absorptive state. High levels of glucose and amino acids in the blood (as when a meal is being processed) are the primary stimuli for insulin secretion. The hormone acts on most tissues of the body, but muscle, adipose tissue and liver are quantitatively the most important. However, some tissues, such as brain and erythrocytes, which are obligatory utilisers of glucose for fuel, are not sensitive to insulin.

Control of insulin secretion

Insulin is a protein hormone secreted by the islets of Langerhans in the pancreas. It is released by exocytosis in response to raised intracellular Ca^{2+} concentrations. The release of insulin from the pancreas is controlled to a large extent by the concentration of glucose and amino acids in the blood perfusing the pancreas. Other factors, such as hormones and neurotransmitters, potentiate or inhibit the effects of the blood nutrients on insulin secretion.

Control by glucose

The secretion of insulin in response to an increase in blood glucose is under feedback control (Fig. 7.3). After a meal, the blood glucose increases as it is absorbed from

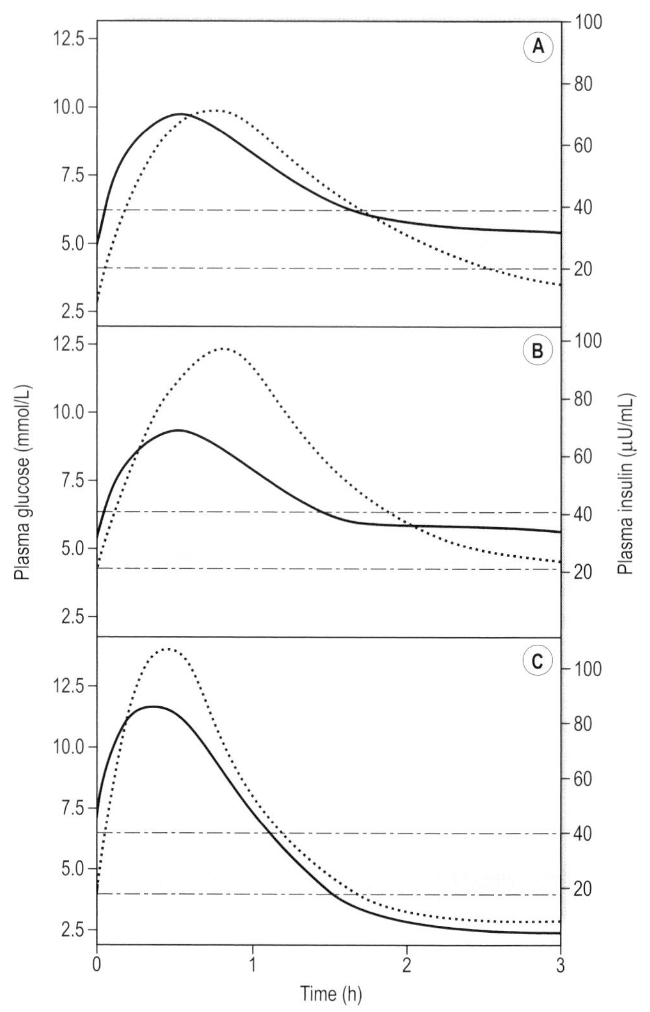

Fig. 7.4 Glucose (solid line) and insulin (dotted line) responses to a carbohydrate meal in (A) a normal individual, (B) an obese individual, and (C) an individual with reactive hypoglycaemia. The shaded areas show the normal range for fasting plasma glucose concentration.

the GI tract. This results in stimulation of insulin secretion from the β-cells of the islets of Langerhans. These cells respond to both the actual glucose concentration, and the rate of change of glucose concentration in the blood. The effect is due to the uptake and intracellular metabolism of glucose in the β-cells. Glucose is transported into these cells via the GLUT2 transporter which ultimately leads to ATP generation, elevated intracellular Ca^{2+} and insulin exocytosis.

Insulin lowers blood glucose by promoting its uptake into cells, predominantly by GLUT-4 (see below). Thus, as the concentration of insulin in the blood rises, the concentration of glucose falls and the stimulus for insulin secretion is removed. Consequently, the concentration of insulin falls. The feedback control of insulin secretion by plasma glucose is summarised in Fig. 7.3.

The concentration of plasma insulin normally parallels the rise and fall in the levels of plasma glucose. This is illustrated in Fig. 7.4A, which shows the results of a glucose drink in a fasting individual. Concentrations of glucose above 5 mmol/L are effective in increasing insulin release. The response to an oral glucose load (glucose tolerance test) is used to diagnose diabetic states, where the fasting glucose concentration is not sufficiently raised to give a clear diagnosis on its own. In obese individuals, there is a slower uptake of glucose into cells after a meal and an exaggerated insulin response to the increase in plasma glucose (Fig. 7.4B). The plasma insulin concentration rises to a higher level than in people of normal weight.

The glucose tolerance test may also be used to diagnose hypoglycaemic states. After a high carbohydrate meal, the concentration of plasma glucose may rise rapidly. This causes a rapid secretion of insulin from the β-cells, with an earlier and higher peak than after a more balanced meal. This results in a rapid fall in plasma glucose to levels that may be lower than normal (hypoglycaemia). This effect is exaggerated in some individuals, whose β-cells produce an excessive insulin response to the rise in plasma glucose. They are said to have 'reactive hypoglycaemia' (Fig. 7.4C). Various symptoms result from hypoglycaemia, including tremor, hunger, weakness, uncoordinated movements, blurred vision and impaired mental ability. Such people need to control their blood glucose levels by limiting their intake of carbohydrates and eating small meals at frequent intervals. Patients who have undergone gastrectomy can have similar symptoms due to rapid entry of food into the small intestine.

Control by amino acids

Insulin secretion is also controlled by the levels of amino acids in the blood. Thus, after a high protein meal, which results in a high level of amino acids, insulin secretion is increased. The most potent amino acids in this respect are arginine, leucine and alanine. The mechanism whereby these amino acids exert this effect first involves their transport into the β-cells. The anionic amino acids depolarise the membrane and open voltage-gated Ca^{2+} channels. The resulting Ca^{2+} influx then stimulates insulin secretion.

Control by other hormones

Glucagon stimulates insulin release and somatostatin inhibits it. Glucagon is produced by the α-cells and somatostatin by the D cells in the pancreas. The actions of these hormones on insulin release from the pancreatic β-cells may be local paracrine effects, or they may act locally via the blood in the islet capillaries.

Oral administration of glucose causes a greater increase in blood insulin levels than the same glucose load injected into the blood. The mere presence of food in the GI tract elicits an increase in insulin secretion (known as the 'incretin effect'). This indicates that insulin secretion is controlled by factors originating in the GI tract (the enteroinsular axis). The duodenal hormones cholecystokinin (CCK), gastric inhibitory peptide (GIP), and glucagon-like peptide 1 (GLP-1) have all been reported to induce insulin secretion. These hormones are all secreted when a meal is being processed in the GI tract.

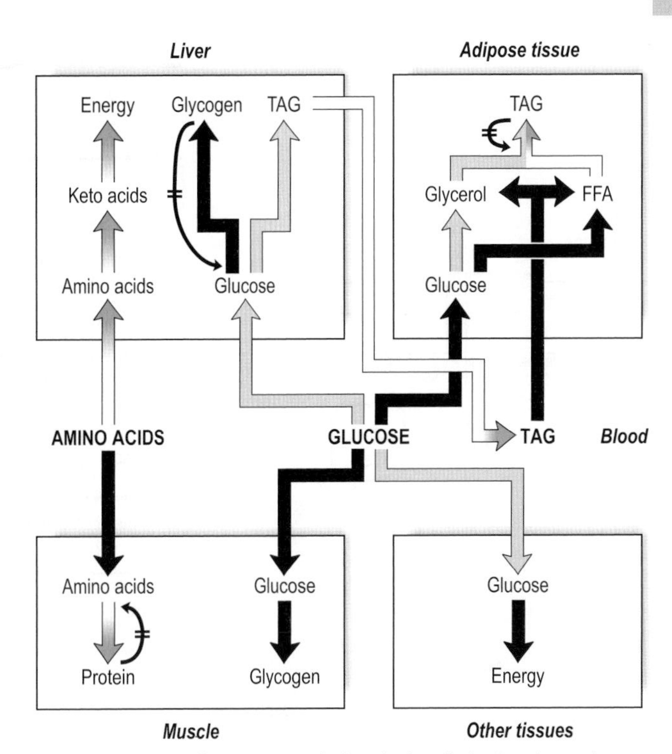

Fig. 7.5 Control of energy metabolism by insulin in the absorptive state. The bold arrows indicate the pathways and uptake mechanisms stimulated by insulin, and the arrows crossed out indicate the pathways inhibited by insulin. *FFA, free fatty acids; TAG, triacylglycerol.*

Control by nerves

The islets of Langerhans are innervated by both parasympathetic and sympathetic nerves. Stimulation of the vagus (parasympathetic) nerve fibres that innervate the β-cells potentiates insulin release via acetylcholine acting on muscarinic receptors. It is phospholipase C-mediated and involves Ca^{2+} uptake into the β-cells. Stimulation of the sympathetic nerves inhibits insulin release via noradrenaline acting on β_2-adrenergic receptors on the islet β-cells.

Actions of insulin in the absorptive state

The actions of insulin during the absorptive state are indicated in Fig. 7.5. It acts on membrane receptors in many cells to promote the uptake of glucose, amino acids, K^+, Mg^{2+} and PO_4^{3-}. In addition, it stimulates or inhibits rate-limiting steps in many pathways involved in energy metabolism. It directly stimulates the entry of glucose into muscle and adipose tissue, but not liver. This is a primary action of insulin. However, an increase in intracellular glucose speeds up the reactions in which it is utilised, via the mass-action effect due to

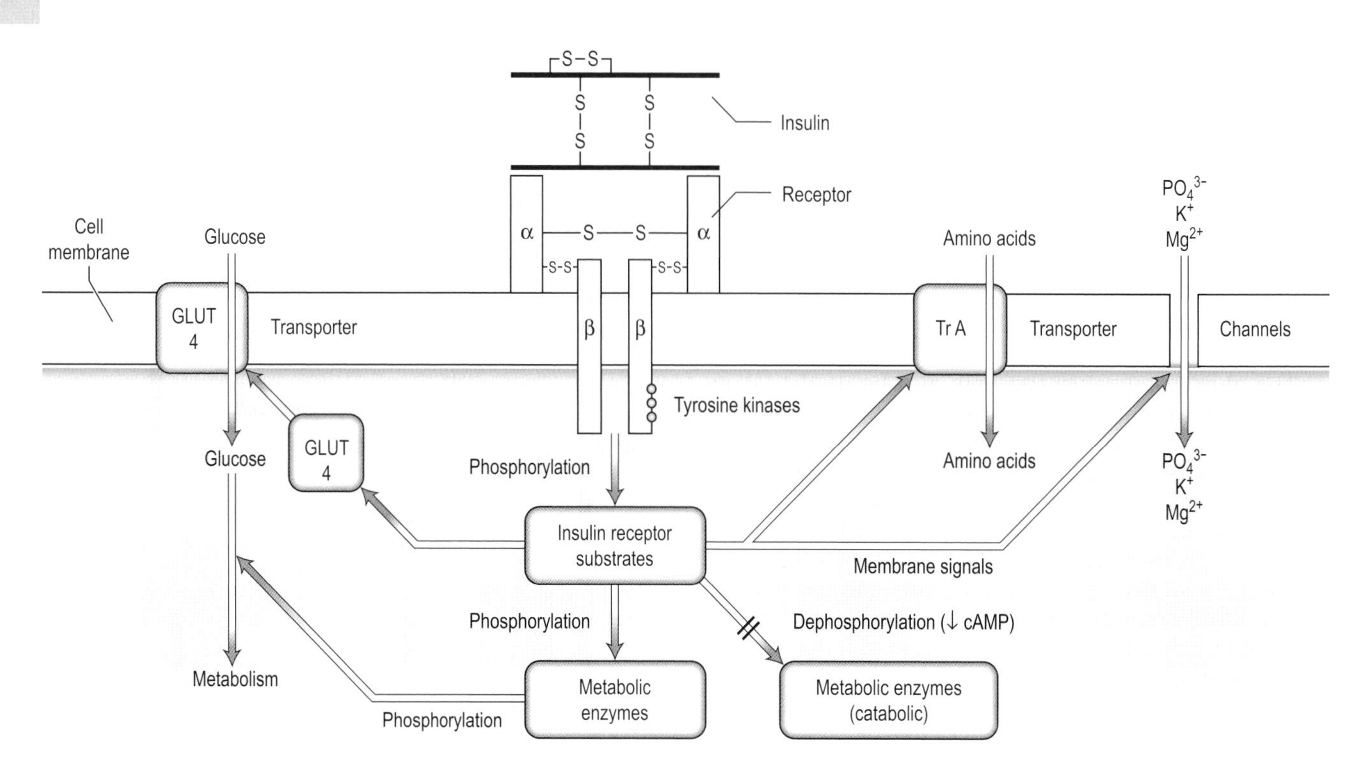

Fig. 7.6 Downstream effects of insulin receptor activation. *GLUT4, hormone-sensitive glucose transporter; Tr A, amino acid transporter A.*

the increased supply of the reactant. These are secondary effects of insulin. Thus, glucose oxidation and lipid and glycogen synthesis are all stimulated in insulin-sensitive tissues when blood insulin concentration increases because more glucose enters the cells.

In addition to the secondary effects of insulin on metabolism, it also exerts primary effects on metabolism by directly stimulating rate-limiting reactions in a variety of pathways. It stimulates key reactions involved in the utilisation of glucose for energy production via the citric acid cycle, and in its utilisation for the synthesis of glycogen and triacylglycerol. At the same time, it inhibits glycogenolysis, gluconeogenesis and lipolysis.

Insulin also directly stimulates the uptake of amino acids into muscle and other tissues. This results in increased synthesis of protein by a mass-action effect. In addition, it directly inhibits the breakdown of protein.

The overall effect of insulin in the absorptive state is to provide glucose for utilisation as energy, to promote the storage of excess carbohydrate and fat in forms which can be used later to provide calories in the post-absorptive state, and to increase protein synthesis (see Fig. 7.5).

The insulin receptor

Insulin binds to a receptor in the cell membrane of insulin-responsive tissues. The receptor is a transmembrane glycoprotein with both extracellular and cytoplasmic faces. Fig. 7.6 shows the effects of activation of the receptor by insulin.

The receptor is a tyrosine kinase. When it is not bound to insulin, it is enzymatically inactive, but when it combines with insulin, a conformational change occurs, which results in the exposure of three intracellular phosphorylation sites on the β-subunit tail. These sites can be autophosphorylated, using ATP as the substrate, activating the enzyme. The phosphorylated receptor kinase can then activate tyrosine residues on various intracellular proteins, known as insulin receptor substrate (IRS) proteins. When these proteins become phosphorylated, they in turn phosphorylate several intracellular kinases and phosphatases. These activated enzymes then stimulate glucose and amino acid uptake and several rate-limiting reactions in various metabolic pathways. However, activation of the receptor also suppresses the levels of intracellular cAMP, which results in suppression of various catabolic processes as well as gluconeogenesis (see below). After activation of the receptor, it is endocytosed and either degraded or recycled.

Glucose entry into cells

Basal glucose uptake in muscle and adipose tissue is via the GLUT1 transporter. However, facilitated glucose transport involves GLUT4, which is an insulin-sensitive transporter. This transporter is bound to endosomes in the cytosol, and it cycles between the cytosol (predominantly in transport vesicles) and the cell membrane (see Fig. 7.6). When insulin concentration in the blood is low, most of the transporters reside in the cytosol, bound to the endosomes. Activation of the insulin receptor by insulin stimulates the translocation of the transporters from the cytosol into the membrane and increases the synthesis of the GLUT4 transporter. At low insulin concentrations, glucose transport is the rate-limiting step in

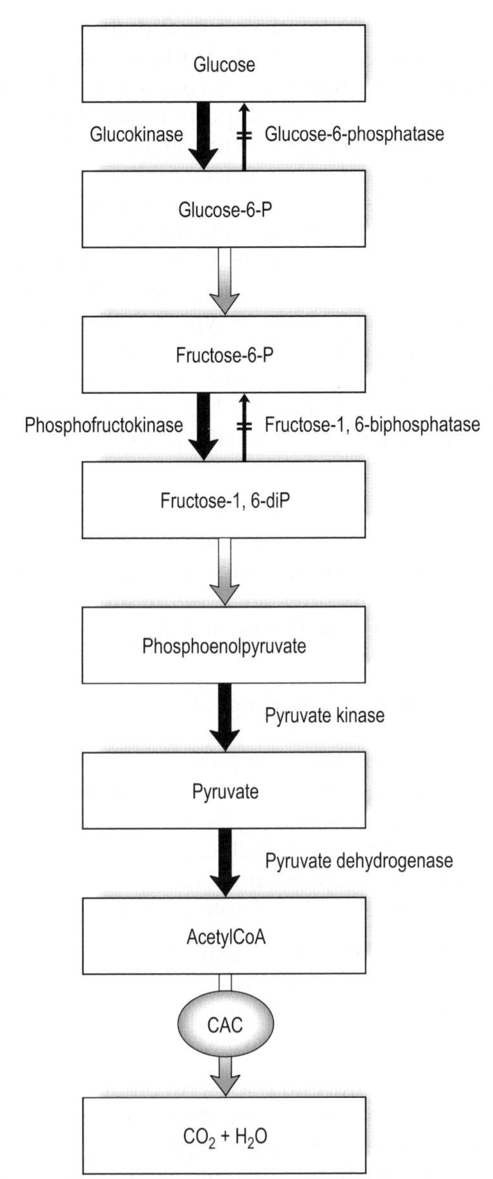

Fig. 7.7 Control of glycolysis by insulin. The bold arrows indicate the enzymes stimulated by insulin, and the crossed arrows indicate those inhibited by insulin.

the utilisation of glucose. After a meal, when high concentrations of insulin are present, glucose transport into cells can be stimulated up to 20-fold.

Glycolysis

Insulin increases the utilisation of glucose via glycolysis by increasing the synthesis of several enzymes involved (Fig. 7.7).

It increases the synthesis of liver glucokinase, phosphofructokinase and pyruvate kinase, which catalyse key steps in the pathway. In addition, it inhibits the synthesis of glucose-6-phosphatase and fructose-1,6-bisphosphatase which catalyse reactions which oppose the utilisation of glucose via glycolysis.

Glycogen synthesis

An increase in glucose in cells stimulates glycogen synthesis by a mass-action effect, but insulin also stimulates glycogen synthesis directly by stimulating the activity of glycogen synthase, the rate-determining enzyme of the pathway. In addition, insulin promotes the synthesis of glucokinase in liver (but not muscle), which catalyses the formation of glucose-6-phosphate. These actions enable more glucose to enter the glycogenic pathway in liver. In addition, insulin inhibits hepatic glucose-6-phosphatase, thereby inhibiting the release of free glucose into the blood.

Triacylglycerol synthesis

The effect of insulin on the synthesis of triacylglycerol from glucose in adipose tissue is summarised in Fig. 7.5. Insulin stimulates fatty acid synthesis from glucose by activating several of the enzymes involved in the pathway, including pyruvate dehydrogenase which catalyses the conversion of pyruvate to acetyl CoA in the mitochondrion. Acetyl CoA is then directed to fatty acid synthesis because insulin activates acetyl CoA carboxylase that diverts acetyl CoA to the synthesis of fatty acid in the cytosol.

Inhibition of glycogenolysis, lipolysis and gluconeogenesis

Insulin suppresses the mobilisation of body energy stores. It inhibits glycogen and triacylglycerol breakdown and gluconeogenesis.

Amino acid transport and protein synthesis

Insulin facilitates the uptake of amino acids through the amino acid transport system A. There is a wealth of evidence that several other amino acid transporters are equally able to modulate insulin synthesis. Specifically, insulin binding to its receptor triggers activation of the phosphatidylinositol-3-kinase (PI3K)-Akt pathway and subsequent activation of mTORC1, culminating in increased cellular protein synthesis.

Insulin sensitivity

The magnitude of the effects produced by insulin depends not only on its concentration in the plasma, but also on the sensitivity of the tissues to it. The responsiveness of tissues to insulin varies even in normal individuals. Thus, for example, habitual exercise increases tissue sensitivity to insulin. It is pertinent to note that, during exercise, muscle contraction induces GLUT4 translocation to the plasma membrane in an insulin-independent manner.

Insulin sensitivity is decreased in obese individuals, leading to abnormally slow uptake of glucose into tissues after a meal (see Fig. 7.4B). Relatively high amounts of insulin are secreted in response to the resulting elevated plasma glucose. The elevated insulin tends to maintain the fasting concentration of plasma glucose within the normal range. Recent reports suggest that visceral adiposity, which leads to inflammation and inflammatory cytokine production, and this may contribute to an impairment in insulin signalling observed in obese individuals.

Post-absorptive state

Some tissues, such as the brain and erythrocytes, can only survive if glucose is delivered to them for fuel. They cannot initially utilise other nutrients to any significant extent. Lack of glucose causes brain damage, coma and death within minutes. During the post-absorptive state when glucose is not being absorbed from the GI tract, the plasma levels of glucose are maintained within a physiological range. This is brought about in two ways. First, glucose is generated by glycogen breakdown, glycogenolysis and gluconeogenesis (glucose supplying reactions). Second, many tissues can utilise substrates other than glucose, such as fatty acids, for energy provision. This spares the available glucose for the tissues that are obligatory utilisers of it (glucose sparing reactions). However, in starvation, when the blood glucose falls slowly, the nervous system can adapt after a few days to use ketones as a source of energy. In type 1 diabetes, where insulin is deficient, and in type 2 diabetes where the tissues are insensitive to insulin, the metabolic state resembles the post-absorptive state.

Non-insulin-dependent diabetes mellitus (NIDDM)

In the Western world, the incidence of type 2 diabetes is approximately 7%–10%. It affects more men than women (ratio 3:2), and is much more prevalent in ethnic minority groups, especially those of African Caribbean, Black and South Asian origins, who are 2–4 times more likely to develop this type of diabetes. Obesity and lack of physical exercise are predisposing factors for type 2 diabetes. Thus, the incidence of type 2 diabetes is increasing in the Western world, as more people are becoming obese and more are following sedentary lifestyles. In both types of diabetes, there is a predisposition to vascular disease and hypertension, high cholesterol, high VLDLs, neuropathy, retinopathy and nephropathy. It may be pertinent that some of these problems, like hypertension, are associated with obesity even in non-diabetic individuals.

Defects

In type 2 diabetes, insulin secretion is eventually impaired, although the plasma concentration may be initially normal or even increased in response to the hyperglycaemia. As the disease progresses, the β-cells become less responsive to increases in plasma glucose, and the β-cell mass may eventually be diminished by up to 40% (whereas in type 1 diabetes these cells are destroyed).

A further serious defect in type 2 diabetes is that tissues such as liver, muscle and adipose develop insulin resistance. The resistance involves not only glucose uptake into muscle and adipose tissue, but also the metabolic actions of insulin, such as its effects to stimulate glycogen synthesis in muscle and liver and to inhibit lipolysis in adipose tissue. Consequently, circulating glucose and plasma free fatty acids are increased. In most cases, insulin binds normally to its receptor but insulin signalling in the cell is attenuated. The mechanism is unknown. In some cases of type 2 diabetes, there is a structural abnormality of the receptor or a known intracellular protein. The metabolic defects are similar to those seen in type 1 diabetes but they are usually less severe. Thus, ketosis is not usually present.

Treatment

Type 2 diabetes can often be controlled if the patient follows a healthy, calorie-restricted diet and a more active lifestyle. These measures increase tissue sensitivity to insulin. If they are insufficient, oral drugs are used. These include:

- Sulphonylureas. These drugs stimulate insulin secretion by binding to a component of the ATP-sensitive K^+ channel in the β-cell membrane and directly closing it. They are therefore only effective in patients with a functioning β-cell mass. A potentially serious side-effect is hypoglycaemia because the action of many sulphonylureas can persist for over 24 hours. They may also promote weight gain.
- Meglitinides. These drugs also stimulate insulin secretion by closing the ATP-sensitive K^+ channel in the β-cells. They are short-acting and promote insulin secretion in response to meals.
- Biguanides. Metformin is a useful biguanide drug that increases insulin sensitivity and reduces hepatic glucose output by suppressing gluconeogenesis. It does not induce hypoglycaemia or cause weight gain.
- Thiazolidinediones. These drugs promote insulin resistance by an unknown mechanism. They reduce hepatic glucose output and enhance glucose uptake into tissues.
- Intestinal enzyme inhibitors. Inhibitors of α-glucosidase, such as acarbose, suppress carbohydrate absorption, thereby reducing the rise in blood glucose that accompanies meal consumption. Side effects are osmotic diarrhoea and flatulence due to undigested carbohydrate passing into the colon.

Insulin-dependent diabetes mellitus (IDDM)

Type 1 diabetes affects mostly young people, with the most common age of onset being between 10 and 14 years. Type 1 diabetes is caused by reduced secretion of insulin due to necrosis of the pancreatic β-cells. Consequently, the metabolic derangement is more severe than type 2 diabetes and can lead to marked weight loss and ketoacidosis.

Type 1 diabetes affects both sexes equally, but there is a slightly earlier peak in age of onset in females than males. It is more prevalent in Caucasians than non-Caucasians, and more prevalent in people living in the northern hemisphere. There is also strong evidence that type 1 diabetes is a polygenic disease with a strong genetic component. The major susceptibility locus for type 1 diabetes maps to the HLA region on chromosome 6p21. This accounts for approximately 30%–50% of the genetic risk. Moreover, there are more than 40 non-HLA loci which have been implicated, including the insulin gene (*INS*), *CTLA4*, *PTNP22* and *IL2RA*.

Type 1 diabetes is an immune-mediated disease which is characterised by autoantibodies against islet β-cell components including insulin, glutamic acid decarboxylase and insulinoma-associated tyrosine phosphatase protein (IA-2). Ultimately, the destruction of the islet β-cell in type 1 diabetes is attributed to a complex interplay between the innate and adaptive immune system.

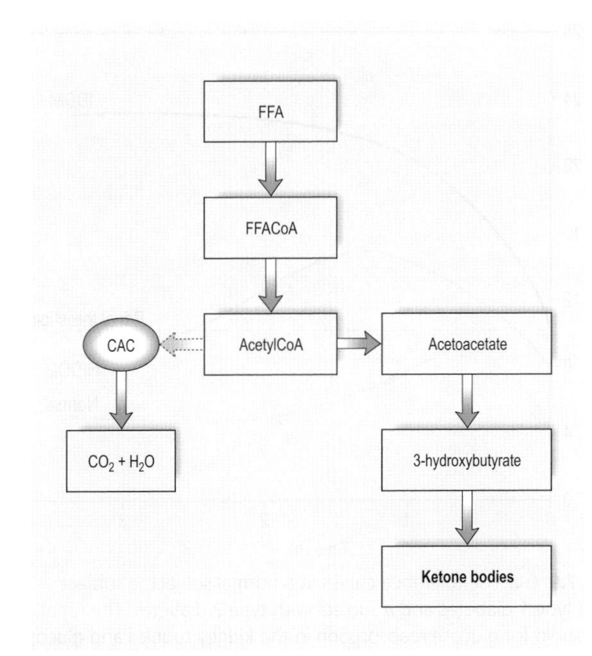

Fig. 7.8 Ketone body formation in the post-absorptive state. The dashed arrow indicates where the build-up of acetyl CoA diverts it away from the citric acid cycle in the mitochondrion towards ketone body formation in the cytosol.

Treatment of type 1 diabetes

Type 1 diabetes is treated by subcutaneous injections of insulin. If inadequate insulin is administered, the patient may become comatose because of ketoacidosis, electrolyte imbalance and dehydration. However, an overdose of insulin can also lead to coma due to hypoglycaemia. Therefore, the amount of insulin administered must be carefully adjusted to bring the blood glucose concentration back to normal. Fig. 7.4C shows the changes in plasma glucose following an oral glucose load in a person with reactive hypoglycaemia, a condition in which there is hypersecretion of insulin. The response resembles that seen in an individual who has been injected with too much insulin.

Metabolic state

In untreated type 1 diabetes, when insulin concentrations are very low, the plasma glucose concentration is high because the uptake of glucose into muscle, adipose tissue and other tissues is impaired, and the utilisation of glucose for energy provision and glycogen and fat synthesis is reduced. Insulin also inhibits glycogenolysis and lipolysis, so these catabolic processes occur at an increased rate in its absence. Increased glycogenolysis in liver results in glucose release into the blood. Increased glycogenolysis in muscles results in lactate release, which is used by the liver for glucose production by gluconeogenesis. Increased lipolysis results in fatty acids and glycerol being released into the blood. The glycerol is taken up and used to produce glucose via gluconeogenesis. Thus, these processes all result in further increases in blood glucose and exacerbate the hyperglycaemia.

Fatty acids formed in the adipose tissue are released into the blood and taken up by various tissues and oxidised to acetyl CoA. In type 1 diabetes, if the levels of fatty acids are excessive, acetyl CoA production in the liver exceeds the capacity of the citric acid cycle to oxidise it and the excess is converted to ketone bodies (Fig. 7.8). These are released into the blood, resulting in high concentrations of plasma ketone bodies and ketosis. Metabolic acidosis results from the high concentrations of (acidic) ketone bodies and fatty acids in the blood plasma.

Amino acid uptake into tissues is also reduced in type 1 diabetes, due to very low insulin levels and protein breakdown is increased. This results in an excessive conversion of amino acids to glucose via gluconeogenesis in the liver. Thus, the overall effect of these metabolic disturbances is elevated levels of glucose, ketone bodies and fatty acids in the plasma.

Glucose tolerance test in types 1 and 2 diabetes

Tests that may be performed to assess the diabetic status of an individual include plasma and urine glucose, plasma insulin and plasma and urine ketone bodies. Glucose and ketone bodies in blood and urine can be measured by automated colorimetric procedures and insulin by radioimmunoassay. In untreated type 1 diabetes, blood and urine glucose concentrations are high and plasma insulin concentration is very low or undetectable.

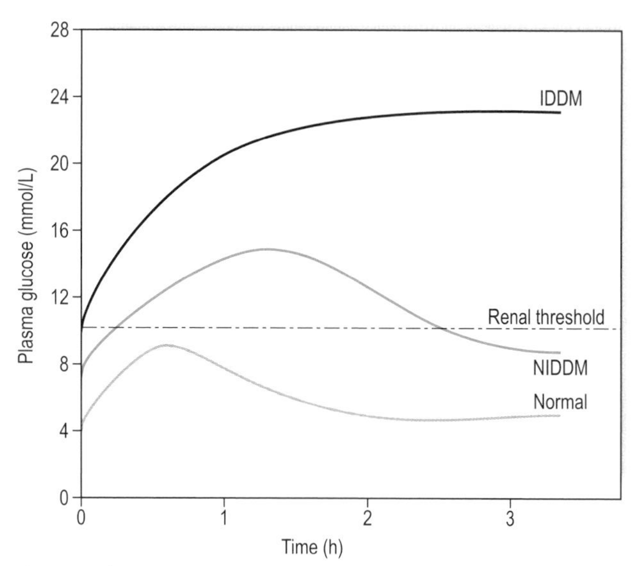

Fig. 7.9 Glucose tolerance curves in a normal subject, a subject with type 1 diabetes and a subject with type 2 diabetes. The renal threshold for glucose reabsorption in the kidney tubules and glucose excretion in the urine is indicated.

In severe cases, plasma and urine ketone concentrations are high.

The diabetic status of an individual can be assessed by an oral glucose tolerance test, although this is rarely necessary in type 1 diabetes because of the presence of a markedly raised blood glucose concentration and glucosuria. For the glucose tolerance test, the patient fasts overnight and then drinks a solution containing 75 g of glucose in 250–300 mL of water. A 'fasting' sample of blood is obtained immediately prior to the glucose load and then further blood samples are obtained at 30-min intervals thereafter, for 3 hours. Fig. 7.9 shows the results of such a test in a normal individual, a patient with type 1 diabetes and a patient with type 2 diabetes.

In a normal individual, the fasting plasma glucose concentration is usually within the range 3.5–7.0 mmol/L. After an oral glucose load, it increases to reach a peak between 30 and 60 min and returns to normal by 2 hours. In both diabetic patients, the fasting concentration of glucose was abnormally high, but it was highest in the patient with type 1 diabetes. After the glucose load, the plasma glucose concentration increased to a very high level in both patients, but it was highest in the patient with type 1 diabetes and remained higher for longer than in the patient with type 2 diabetes.

Comparison with post-absorptive state

The pattern of metabolism in untreated type 1 diabetes is an exaggeration of that seen in the post-absorptive state. Insulin levels are low, glucose and amino acid uptake into tissues is reduced, and glycogenolysis, lipolysis, gluconeogenesis and protein breakdown increase. These events result in increases in plasma glucose, plasma fatty acids and ketone bodies. Furthermore, in diabetes mellitus, despite the presence of hyperglycaemia, there are increases in many of the hormones associated with the post-absorptive state, including plasma catecholamines, glucagon, cortisol and adrenocorticotropic hormone (ACTH), and sometimes growth hormone. Increases in secretion of these hormones accompany various types of stress, and they are probably partly due to activation of the sympathetic nervous system. Thus, for example, stimulation of the preganglionic sympathetic nerves to the adrenal medulla causes the release of adrenaline into the blood, and stimulation of the sympathetic nerves to the α-cells of the pancreas causes release of glucagon. However, in type 1 diabetes, the predominating mechanism causing the release of these hormones (which are normally suppressed by hyperglycaemia) is largely unknown.

In non-diabetic subjects, in the post-absorptive state, the plasma glucose and ketone bodies do not normally exceed the threshold for reabsorption in the kidney, so metabolites do not appear in the urine.

Diabetic ketosis and fluid and electrolyte disturbances

Diabetic ketoacidosis is the first presentation of type 1 diabetes in 20%–30% of patients. In these individuals, insulin levels are usually below the levels of detection. Mortality from ketoacidosis is 2%–5% in developed countries. Ketoacidosis can be precipitated in patients with type 1 diabetes by several factors, including infections, neglect of insulin medication and myocardial infarction, but in many cases the precipitating factor is unknown.

Lipolysis increases in untreated type 1 diabetes. This is due to the absence of insulin, and the presence of elevated plasma glucagon, catecholamines, cortisol and growth hormone. Increased lipolysis leads to increased production of ketone bodies (hyperketonaemia). The consequent high plasma concentrations of the keto acids, α-hydroxybutyrate and acetoacetate, cause metabolic acidosis. The increase in plasma H^+ ions results in stimulation of the rate of breathing which partially readjusts the blood pH (see the companion volume *The Respiratory System*). The kidneys are also involved in compensatory adjustments for acidosis by excreting H^+ ions (see the companion volume *The Renal System*). In untreated clinical ketoacidosis, these compensatory mechanisms are not sufficient to maintain the pH within the normal physiological range (i.e., 7.25–7.45).

In ketoacidosis, ketones as well as glucose are lost in the urine as the threshold for reabsorption in the kidney proximal tubules is exceeded. The presence of these solutes in the urine causes an osmotic diuresis (polyuria). The increased flow of urine causes dehydration and thirst (polydipsia), which are exacerbated by increased water loss via the lungs (due to hyperventilation). Although vasopressin (antidiuretic hormone), the hormone which stimulates water reabsorption, is released from the posterior pituitary in response to the increased osmolarity of the blood and the reduced blood volume, the osmotic diuretic effect prevails.

Furthermore, the increased level of glucose and ketone bodies in the plasma causes water to pass out of the cells of the body, down the osmotic gradient, into the plasma. This helps to maintain the plasma volume. However, as the polyuria causes the plasma volume to become more severely decreased, renal perfusion declines. This results in further elevation of plasma glucose.

In ketoacidosis, the plasma Na^+ concentration is usually normal or low. This is partly because of the osmotic effect of plasma glucose drawing water out of the cells, but also because the hormone aldosterone is released from the adrenal cortex into the blood in response to the reduced extracellular fluid volume. This hormone decreases Na^+ excretion by increasing its reabsorption in the kidney tubules and opposes the effect of decreased insulin and elevated glucagon.

Total body K^+ also falls in diabetic ketoacidosis. Insulin normally increases K^+ uptake into cells (see above), and when the plasma concentration of insulin is low, the plasma concentration of K^+ increases. A net loss of K^+ from cells of the body occurs in ketoacidosis as intracellular K^+ is exchanged for H^+ from the blood, and K^+ is consequently lost in the urine. Treatment of ketoacidosis involves administration of insulin, fluid and electrolytes.

The causes of some of the symptoms in individuals with ketoacidosis are not entirely clear. The weight loss is partly due to loss of fluid in the urine and partly to loss of muscle and adipose tissue mass due to increased proteolysis and lipolysis, respectively. The mental confusion and coma are partly attributable to the acidosis and dehydration, but other factors such as cerebral hypoxia are probably also involved. The cause of the abdominal discomfort and vomiting is unclear.

Glucose-supplying reactions

The reactions that supply glucose to the blood during the post-absorptive state are outlined in Fig. 7.10.

During the post-absorptive state, glycogen stored in the liver is broken down to glucose, which is liberated into the blood. Muscle glycogen is also broken down in the absorptive state, but muscle lacks glucose-6-phosphatase (the enzyme which converts glucose-6-phosphate to free glucose), and so in muscle glucose-6-phosphate is broken down to lactate and pyruvate, which are released into the blood. These metabolites are taken up by the liver and then converted to glucose (via gluconeogenesis, see below), which is liberated into the blood. The stores of glycogen in liver and muscle can amount to 600–800 g in the post-absorptive state. This source of glucose is sufficient to meet the energy needs of the body for approximately only 4 hours.

In any prolonged period of fasting, the stored glycogen is used up and gluconeogenesis becomes the more

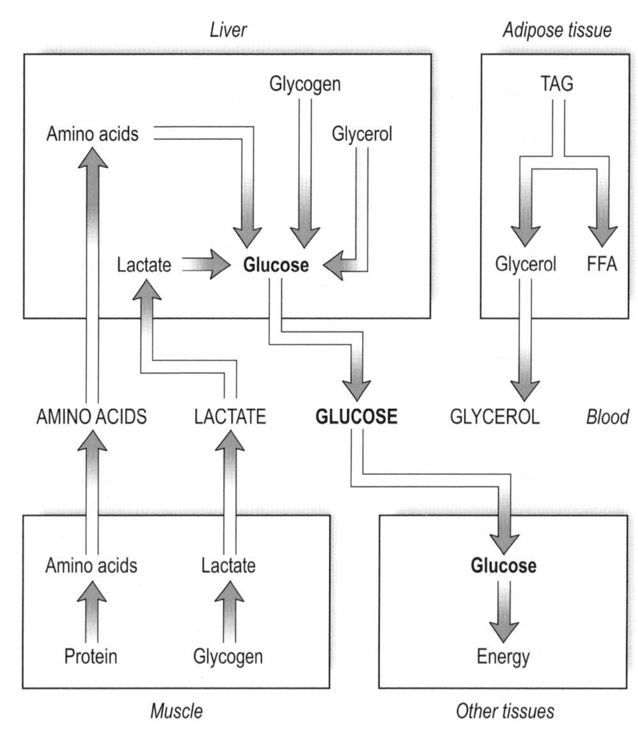

Fig. 7.10 Glucose-supplying reactions in the post-absorptive state. *FFA, free fatty acids; TAG, triacylglycerol.*

important process for generating glucose and maintaining the plasma glucose concentration. Lactate provides one substrate for gluconeogenesis, but in prolonged fasting, amino acids derived from protein in muscle and taken up by the liver are quantitatively the most important substrate for the generation of glucose via gluconeogenesis. Glycerol derived from triacylglycerol in adipose tissue and taken up by the liver is also converted to glucose via gluconeogenesis.

Glucose-sparing reactions

Most of the energy requirement of the body during the post-absorptive state is derived via glucose-sparing reactions that utilise the energy stored as triacylglycerol during the absorptive state. Fat is broken down in adipose tissue to glycerol and free fatty acids, which are released into the blood. The glycerol is used for gluconeogenesis in liver (see above), but the fatty acids are taken up by many other tissues and oxidised to CO_2 and water via the fatty acid oxidation pathway and the citric acid cycle.

In the post-absorptive state, the liver takes up a portion of the fatty acids from the blood. In the liver, fatty acids can be converted to acetyl CoA, which is degraded to CO_2 and water by fatty acid oxidation and the citric acid cycle with the production of energy. However, when large quantities of fatty acids are being produced, as in the post-absorptive state (or diabetes mellitus), the rate of acetyl CoA formation can exceed the capacity of the liver to utilise it via the citric acid cycle. The acetyl CoA is then converted to ketone bodies (Fig. 7.11).

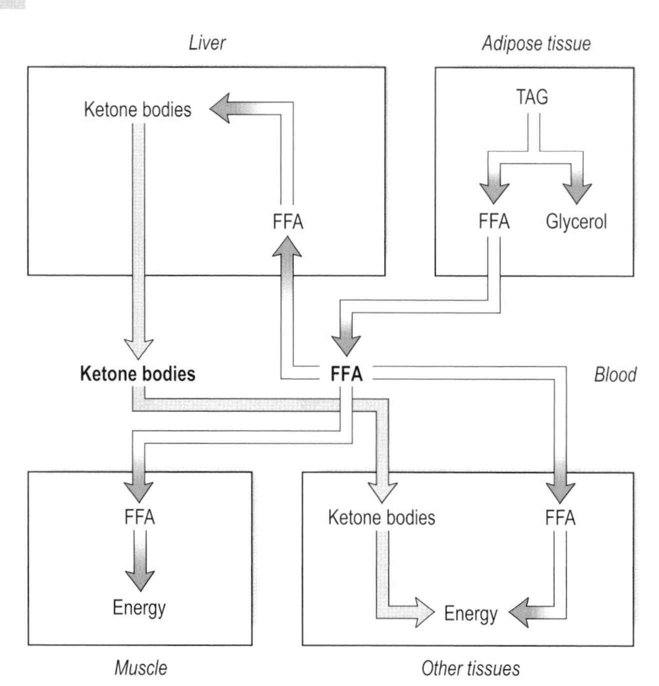

Fig. 7.11 Glucose-sparing reactions in the post-absorptive state. *FFA, free fatty acids; TAG, triacylglycerol.*

Some of the ketone bodies are used for energy purposes in the liver, and the rest are liberated into the blood, taken up by other tissues and utilised via the citric acid cycle (after conversion to acetyl CoA). The ketone bodies are acetone, acetoacetate and α-hydroxybutyrate. The production of acetone during the fasting state accounts for the distinctive breath odour of fasting people and patients with type 1 diabetes. Thus, the liver uses ketone bodies for energy production and ceases to use amino acids during the post-absorptive state, thereby sparing them for gluconeogenesis. Thus, ketone body production is also a means of supplying extrahepatic tissues with fuel during fasting. Some ketone bodies are weak acids, like acetoacetic acid and α-hydroxybutyric acid, and in pathological conditions such as diabetes mellitus, where there is excessive fat utilisation, excessive ketone body production can result in severe acidosis.

Thus, in the post-absorptive state, fatty acids and ketone bodies are provided to tissues which can utilise them for energy during fasting, sparing the glucose for tissues such as the nervous system, which is dependent on it. The energy provided during the post-absorptive state by glycogenolysis and gluconeogenesis provides about 800 kcal/day, which is the equivalent of approximately 180 g glucose/day. However, the average adult needs between 2000 and 3000 kcal/day. Thus, most energy is provided by substrates other than glucose (i.e., largely free fatty acids and ketone bodies). Most adults have enough energy stored in triacylglycerol in adipose tissue to supply sufficient fuel to enable them to survive without food for several weeks.

Control of the post-absorptive state

The onset of the pattern of metabolism in the post-absorptive state is due to both the decline in insulin concentration in the plasma and the increase in the concentrations of several other hormones. These hormones include adrenaline, glucagon, cortisol, growth hormone, thyroid-stimulating hormone and ACTH. They are all released either directly or indirectly in response to low blood glucose.

When the blood glucose concentration falls, the main stimulus for insulin release is removed and the insulin concentration falls. Thus, the major stimulus for glucose uptake into tissues and for synthesis of energy stores is abolished. The inhibitory effect of insulin on glycogenolysis and lipolysis is also abolished. Thus, the pattern of metabolism occurring in the absorptive state is effectively suppressed. The pattern of metabolism in untreated type 1 diabetes resembles the post-absorptive state.

The overall effect of the hormones that control metabolism in the post-absorptive state is to increase plasma levels of glucose, by inhibiting glucose uptake in tissues, and by stimulating glycogenolysis and gluconeogenesis. They also stimulate processes that lead to the provision of alternative energy substrates. Thus, they promote both glucose-supplying reactions and glucose-sparing reactions. These effects are summarised in Figs 7.12 and 7.13.

Thus, the effects of this group of hormones oppose the actions of insulin and facilitate the post-absorptive state. The plasma concentrations of many of these hormones are also increased in type 1 diabetes.

Release of hormones in the post-absorptive state

Adrenaline is released from the adrenal medulla by activity in the preganglionic sympathetic nerves that innervate it. Sympathetic nerves are stimulated by low blood glucose. For this reason, low blood glucose precipitates the symptoms associated with activation of the sympathetic nervous system, such as an increase in anxiety levels and palpitations. Many individuals experience these symptoms in the late afternoon when the blood sugar concentration tends to be low.

Glucagon is produced by the α-cells of the islets of Langerhans. Its release is regulated by the concentration of plasma glucose. Low plasma glucose stimulates glucagon release and high blood glucose inhibits it. Thus, blood glucagon concentrations are high during the post-absorptive period. The release of growth hormone from the pituitary is also stimulated by low blood glucose. Other pituitary hormones are also secreted in response to low blood glucose, including ACTH. Table 7.1 lists some of the hormones that are released in the post-absorptive state, in response to low blood glucose.

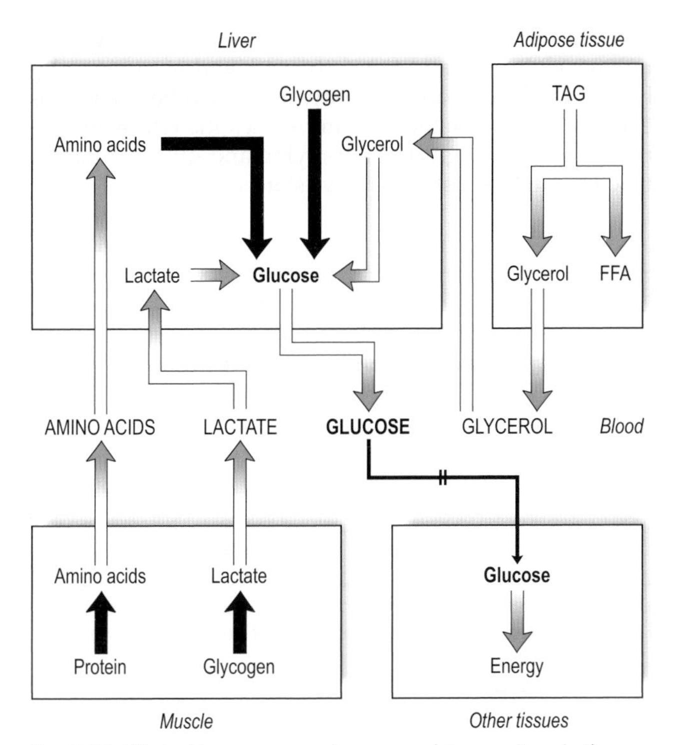

Fig. 7.12 Effect of hormones on glucose-supplying reactions in the post-absorptive state. The bold arrows indicate the pathways that are stimulated, and the crossed arrow indicates inhibition of glucose uptake by cortisol and growth hormone. In liver, glycogenolysis is stimulated by adrenaline and glucagon, and gluconeogenesis from amino acids is stimulated by glucagon and cortisol. In muscle, glycogenolysis is stimulated by adrenaline. *FFA, free fatty acids; TAG, triacylglycerol.*

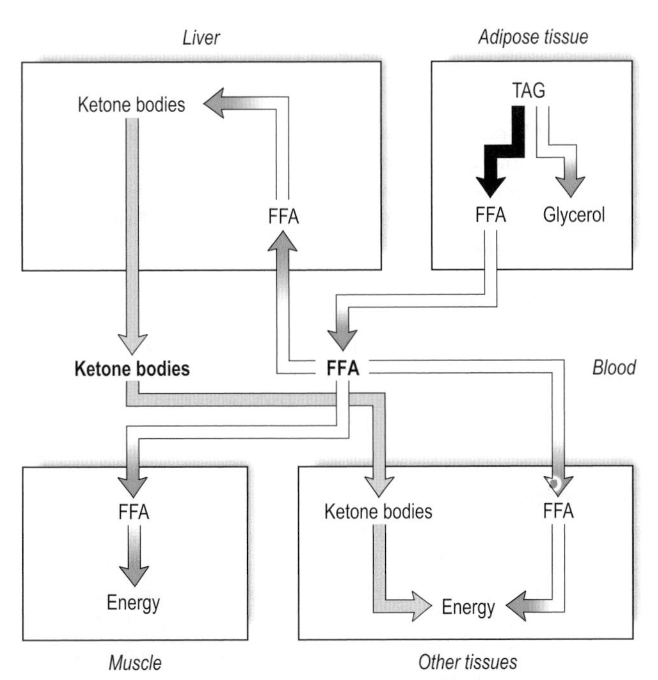

Fig. 7.13 Effect of hormones on glucose-sparing reactions in the post-absorptive state. The bold arrow indicates the stimulation of lipolysis by adrenaline, glucagon and growth hormone in the post-absorptive state. The effect of cortisol on lipolysis is permissive. *FFA, free fatty acids; TAG, triacylglycerol.*

Table 7.1 Hormones secreted in the post-absorptive state

Hormone	*Origin*
Glucagon	α-cells of the pancreas
Adrenaline	Adrenal medulla
Cortisol	Adrenal cortex
Growth hormone	Anterior pituitary
Adrenocorticotropin	Anterior pituitary
Thyroid-stimulating hormone	Anterior pituitary

The hormones listed are collectively responsible for the pattern of energy metabolism that pertains in the post-absorptive state. They are all secreted either directly, or indirectly, in response to low blood glucose.

Actions of hormones in the post-absorptive state

Effects on glucose-supplying reactions

The effects of hormones on glucose-supplying metabolic pathways in the post-absorptive state are shown in Fig. 7.12 and Table 7.2. Growth hormone and cortisol inhibit the uptake of glucose by reducing the number of GLUT4 transporters in the cell membrane. For this reason, patients with growth hormone-producing tumours can develop diabetes. Moreover, in diabetic animals, removal of the pituitary, which secretes growth hormone, reduces the severity of diabetes.

Adrenaline and glucagon stimulate glycogen breakdown to glucose in liver, with the liberation of glucose into the blood. In addition, adrenaline, but not glucagon, stimulates glycogen breakdown to lactate and pyruvate in muscle. These products are released into the blood, taken up by the liver, converted to glucose via gluconeogenesis and the glucose is then released into the blood. Cortisol also stimulates glucose-6-phosphatase resulting in increased release of glucose into the blood. Glucagon and cortisol also stimulate gluconeogenesis from amino acids in liver. Furthermore, cortisol also stimulates the breakdown of protein to amino acids in liver.

Effects on glucose-sparing reactions

The effects of hormones on glucose-sparing metabolic pathways in the post-absorptive state is summarised in Fig. 7.13 and Table 7.2. Adrenaline, glucagon and growth hormone stimulate lipolysis in adipose tissue, thereby increasing the free fatty acid concentration in the plasma. Cortisol has a permissive effect on lipolysis: it has no effect by itself, but it potentiates the effects of adrenaline, glucagon and growth hormone. The sympathetic nerves to adipose tissue are also stimulated by low blood glucose. These nerves release mainly noradrenaline that, like adrenaline, increases lipolysis in adipose tissue. The effects of adrenaline and noradrenaline are exerted on the rate-limiting step in the lipolysis pathway, i.e., the hydrolysis of triacylglycerol to diacylglycerol and free fatty acid which is catalysed by the 'hormone-sensitive' lipase. The effect of these hormones involves an increase in the intracellular concentration of cAMP that triggers an intracellular cascade of reactions (see Fig. 7.13) similar to that seen for the activation of phosphorylase (see above). The subsequent hydrolysis of diacylglycerol to monoacylglycerol and free fatty acid, and of monoacylglycerol to glycerol and free fatty acid, by other lipases, is extremely rapid. Table 7.2 summarises the effects of hormones to control glucose-supplying and glucose-sparing reactions in the post-absorptive state.

Table 7.2 Control of the post-absorptive state

Effect	*Adrenaline*	*Glucagon*	*Growth hormone*	*Cortisol*
Plasma glucose	↑	↑	↑	↑
Glucose uptake			↓	↓
Glycogenolysis	↑	↑	↑	
Gluconeogenesis		↑	↑	↑
Plasma FFA (Lipolysis)	↑	↑	↑	↑

Effects of some of the hormones, released in the post-absorptive state on aspects of energy metabolism, which result in either increases in blood glucose, or the provision of energy substrates (FFA, free fatty acids) that spare glucose for the tissues dependent on it for their energy requirements.

Case 7.1 Starvation

A young man recently became homeless and had lost a significant amount of weight as a consequence of starvation. He was recently found weak and emaciated and taken to a local walk-in centre.

Metabolism in starvation

Plasma glucose

It is important that the individual's plasma glucose concentration does not fall too far because the nervous system is an obligatory utiliser of glucose during the initial phase of fasting. Later, it can adapt to utilise keto acids.

The metabolic processes that would have been occurring to enable this man to maintain his plasma glucose concentration are:

- Glycogenolysis in liver,
- Glycogenolysis in muscle, which would provide glucose indirectly via lactate production and
- Gluconeogenesis in liver, which would provide glucose from amino acids, lactate and glycerol.

The rescued man's plasma insulin concentration would be at the basal level, as it is largely controlled by plasma glucose concentration, which would have been maintained within physiological limits.

Energy provision

The man's energy provision for tissues that are not obligatory users of glucose would be mostly from stores of body fat. Fatty acids derived from triacylglycerol in adipose tissue would provide a large part of the energy requirements of most other tissues. Ketone bodies derived from fatty acids would be utilised for energy in liver. He would be unlikely to be excreting glucose and ketone bodies in his urine, but acetone could probably be detected on his breath.

The man's plasma glucagon concentration would be high initially, as low glucose stimulates glucagon secretion from the pancreatic α-cells. However, after a few days of fasting it returns to normal. Thus, in this man, the levels of glucagon would not be elevated.

Acid–base status

The starving man would probably have metabolic acidosis due to the production of ketone bodies and fatty acids, but respiratory and renal compensation would be occurring.

Treatment

It would not be advisable for this man to drink a concentrated solution of glucose because it would pass too quickly into the small intestine and cause osmotic diarrhoea, and he could become dehydrated. The rapid absorption of glucose could cause him to suffer from rebound hypoglycaemia and possibly fainting. However, isotonic or hypotonic solutions would help. He should probably drink isotonic fluid containing glucose for a while.

8

THE COLON

Chapter objectives and clinical presentations

After reading this chapter, review your learning by considering the following:

1. Can you describe the anatomy of the colon including the arrangement of skeletal and smooth muscle?
2. Are you aware of the three key functions of the colon?
3. Can you describe the mechanisms by which water, ions and selected nutrients are absorbed in the colon?
4. Can you detail how the intestinal microbiome aids in digestion?
5. Are you aware of the importance of fibre in the diet?
6. Can you describe the motility observed in the colon and how it changes in some diseases?

Also, you should be familiar with the following clinical presentations:

- Hirschsprung's disease
- Constipation
- Ulcerative colitis
- Colorectal cancer

Clinical outlook

Examples of common conditions of the colon seen in a gastroenterology clinic are chronic constipation and ulcerative colitis. Patients with chronic severe constipation are managed medically and often require multiple classes of laxatives. Patients with ulcerative colitis usually present with bloody diarrhoea and require endoscopic examination of their bowel to confirm the diagnosis. They may develop flares (worsening of symptoms) intermittently that require appropriate escalation of treatment. These patients require long-term treatment and follow-up in gastroenterology clinics.

Introduction

The colon is the last 150 cm or so of the gastrointestinal (GI) tract. It is a tube of approximately 6 cm in diameter that extends from the ileum to the anus. Its main functions are absorbing water and electrolytes, producing and absorbing vitamins, and forming, storing and propelling faeces towards the rectum. Water is absorbed as the chyme (originating from the small intestinal) travels through the large intestine such that the faecal material becomes more solid as it passes through the colon. In addition, the colon produces a thick mucinous secretion, which lubricates the passage of the faecal material through it. The colon is also home to the intestinal microbiome, which has many important functions. Specific bacterial species found within the gut flora are responsible for the synthesis of vitamins which will be detailed in this chapter.

Disease of the colon can result in diarrhoea, constipation or both. In this chapter, Hirschsprung's disease (megacolon) will be used to illustrate the importance of the motor function of the colon. It is a condition in which there is an absence of intramural ganglion cells from the wall of the colon, usually in a distal region (see Case 8.1). Other diseases of the colon include colitis, diverticulitis and irritable bowel syndrome (IBS; not to be confused with inflammatory bowel disease, or IBD).

Anatomy

The arrangement of the large intestine and its associated structures is shown in Fig. 8.1.

It can be divided into various regions: the caecum, the ascending colon, the transverse colon, the descending colon, the sigmoid colon and the rectum. The rectum is the portion beyond the sigmoid colon. The lumen of the colon becomes narrower towards the rectum. The lumen of the rectum, which is wider, provides a reservoir for faecal material, prior to defecation.

The caecum forms a blind-ended pouch below the junctions of the small intestine and the large intestine.

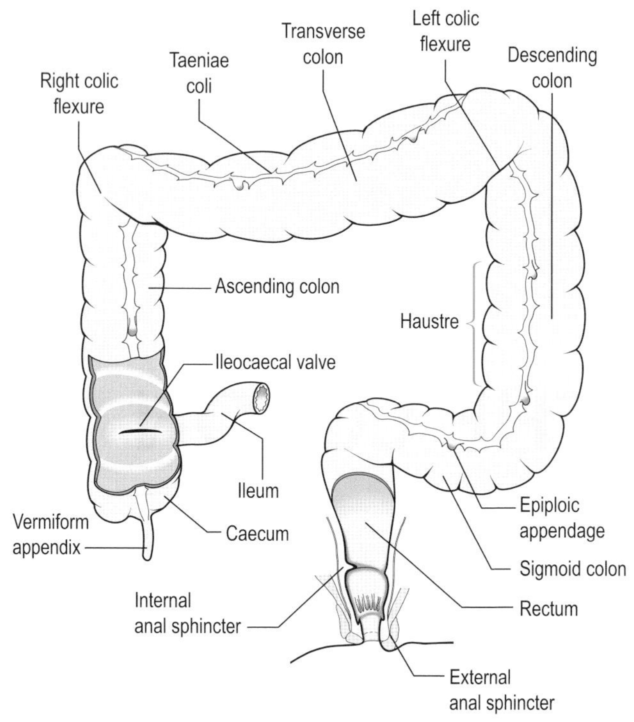

Fig. 8.1 Anatomical features of the large intestine.

The appendix is a small finger-like projection from the end of the caecum. It has a thick wall and a very narrow lumen that often collects debris.

In the large intestine, the outer longitudinal smooth muscle layer is arranged in three prominent bands, known as taeniae coli. There is also a segmental thickening of the circular smooth muscle. Together, these features impart a sacculated appearance to the organ. It has no villi, only projections. The mucosal surface is therefore smoother than that of the small intestine, and the consequence of this is that the surface area of the colon is much smaller than that of the small intestine.

The anal canal is the terminal portion of the rectum. It begins at a region where the rectum suddenly becomes narrower. The surface of the upper portion of the anal canal exhibits several vertical folds, known as anal (or rectal) columns (Fig. 8.2).

These folds are relatively more pronounced in children than in adults. The depressions between the anal columns are known as anal sinuses. The sinuses end abruptly at the lower ends of the columns (the dentate line) where there are small crescent-shaped folds of mucosa oriented around the wall. These folds are termed anal valves. The anal canal is surrounded by sphincter muscle that controls the release of faecal material. The internal sphincter is a thickening of the circular layer of the muscularis externa. The external sphincter, which consists of several parts, is composed of striated muscle. The arrangement of the sphincters is shown in Fig. 8.2.

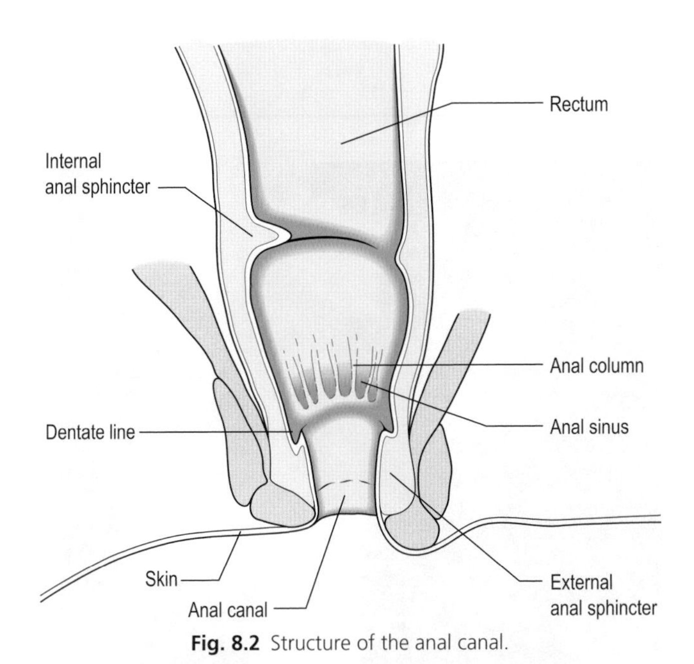

Fig. 8.2 Structure of the anal canal.

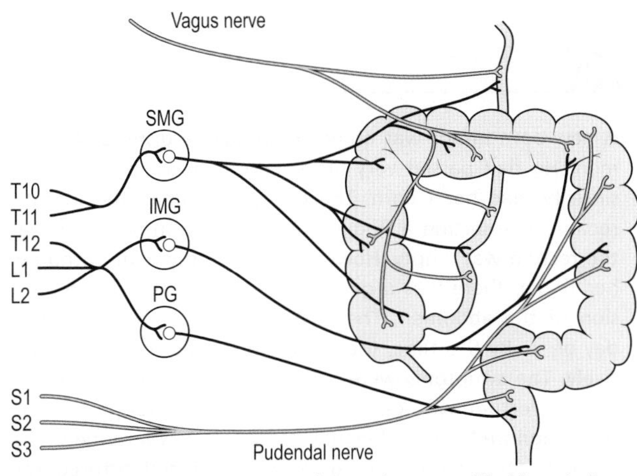

Fig. 8.3 Autonomic innervation of the colon. Grey-filled lines indicate parasympathetic nerves, and solid black lines indicate sympathetic nerves. L1, L2: lumbar segments. S1, S2, S3: sacral segments of the spinal cord. T10, T11, T12: thoracic segments. *IMG, inferior mesenteric ganglion; PG, pelvic ganglion; SMG, superior mesenteric ganglion*.

Innervation

Extrinsic parasympathetic innervation to the colon is shared between the vagus nerve and pelvic splanchnic nerves. The vagus nerve supplies the ascending and transverse colon up to the level of the splenic flexure, with the remainder of the colon then supplied by pelvic splanchnic nerves derived from spinal neural segments S2–S4. This parasympathetic outflow is illustrated in Fig. 8.3.

These cholinergic parasympathetic nerves exert their actions in three separate ways namely, by synapsing with neurones in the intramural plexi of the colon, direct innervation of the smooth muscle of the colon and influencing pressure of the internal anal sphincter. The importance of the excitatory cholinergic neurones of ganglia of the submucosal and myenteric intramural plexi is demonstrated by the fact that their absence is said to be responsible for Hirschsprung's disease.

The colon is also innervated by adrenergic sympathetic nerves from the lower thoracic and upper lumbar segments of the spinal cord. These nerves synapse with inhibitory nerves in the intramural plexi. They also synapse directly with the smooth muscle of the colon and have an opposite effect on pressure of the internal anal sphincter.

The external anal sphincter is different in that is it amenable to both involuntary and voluntary neuronal control. Its voluntary control is achieved via somatic motor fibres that form pudendal nerves and arise from ventral horns of spinal neuronal segments S2–S4, also known as the nucleus of Onuf.

The mechanisms of both voluntary and involuntary control of the anal sphincters depend largely on mechanical actions of muscles of the pelvic floor. In particular, the contraction of the levator ani, an external skeletal muscle, constricts the lower end of the rectum. Contraction of another external skeletal muscle, the puborectalis muscle that is attached to the external side of the wall of the anal canal, pulls the upper canal forward. This produces a sharp angle between the rectum and the anal canal, thereby preventing faeces from entering the anal canal until defecation is initiated. The levator ani and the puborectalis muscles are both innervated by somatic motor fibres of the pudendal nerve.

Terminals of afferent sensory nerve fibres are present in the mucosa, submucosa and muscle layers of the colon. Although the colon is fairly insensitive to painful stimuli, it is very sensitive to changes in pressure. Stretching of the colon because of overdistension results in abdominal pain, but removal of lesions, such as polyps, from the lining of the colon can be achieved painlessly without anaesthetic. There is a profusion of sensory nerve fibres in the wall of the anal canal. Some of these are sensitive to touch, some to cold, some to pressure and others to friction.

Histology

As in other regions of the GI tract, the wall of the large intestine is composed of four layers: the mucosa, the muscularis externa, the submucosa and the serosa (Fig. 8.5A).

The mucosa contains numerous straight tubular glands that extend through the full thickness of the mucosa (Fig. 8.5B). The surface epithelium of the mucosa and glands consists of simple columnar epithelial cells. The predominant cell type is the columnar absorptive cell which resembles the enterocytes of the small intestine. The simple columnar epithelium is folded to form invaginations, which are known as crypts. The cells

Case 8.1 Hirschsprung's disease

A new-born infant was observed to have a distended abdomen. He had passed very little meconium in the two days since he had been born. The doctor examined the infant's rectum by inserting a finger. The examination revealed that the rectum was empty. However, when the doctor withdrew her finger, there was a gush of meconium, and decompression of the abdomen. The obstruction reoccurred within a day or so. By this time, the child had started to vomit excessively. The symptoms were relieved by an enema. A biopsy of the rectum was performed and Hirschsprung's disease was diagnosed. An abdominal operation was arranged. The surgeon removed the distal large bowel and sutured the remaining colon to the lower rectum. The child made a good recovery, and his symptoms disappeared.

Defect, diagnosis and treatment

Defect

Hirschsprung's disease, also known as congenital megacolon (enlarged abdomen), is a familial disease that affects one in 5000 live births. It is more common in males and is associated with Down's syndrome. The genetic mechanism is not fully understood, but it involves multiple chromosomal deletions. A similar condition (acquired megacolon) can arise later in life, from a variety of causes (Fig. 8.4).

In Hirschsprung's disease, intramural ganglion cells are absent from the myenteric and submucosal plexi, usually in a segment of the distal colon. This is due to a defect in embryonic development, involving the arrest of the caudal migration from the neural crest, of the cells that are destined to become ganglion cells of the intramural plexi. Examination of biopsy specimens reveals an absence of ganglion cells from the affected segment. Excitatory and inhibitory neurones are missing. The segment involved is of variable length, in a region extending from the anal canal proximally up the colon. The lumen becomes narrowed in the aganglionic segment due to tonic contraction of the smooth muscle. The passage of faecal material is obstructed at this narrowed segment, and it accumulates in the region proximal to the aganglionic segment. Usually, the normal reflex relaxation of the internal anal sphincter in response to distension of the rectum cannot be elicited in this condition. Because the aganglionic segment creates an obstruction to faecal flow, the proximal large bowel becomes chronically distended, giving rise to the name 'megacolon'.

Diagnosis

The normal reflex relaxation of the internal anal sphincter in response to distension of the rectum usually cannot be elicited in this condition.

A well-known finding in Hirschsprung's disease is an elevated level of acetylcholinesterase in the narrowed segment. This is indicative of an abnormality of the cholinergic innervation. Diagnosis of Hirschsprung's disease is by barium enema and biopsy showing an absence of ganglion cells. In cases where the diagnosis is unclear, a histological frozen section of the region can be stained for the enzyme to see if the levels are elevated to aid the diagnosis.

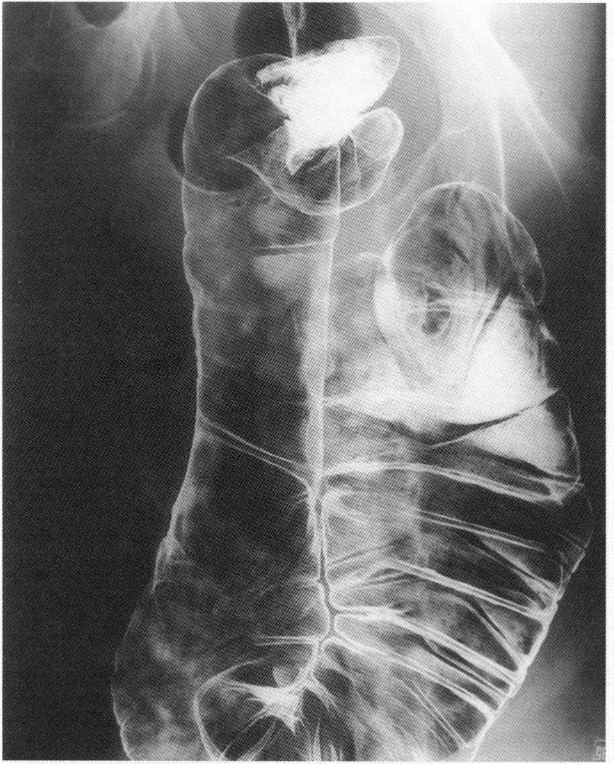

Fig. 8.4 An abdominal X-ray showing a grossly dilated colon filled with gas (megacolon). The mucosa has been coated with barium.

Treatment

Surgery is effective in correcting the disturbance of motility. Various procedures can be performed depending on the extent of involvement of the colon. They all involve removal of the aganglionic segment.

Motility

The importance of the intramural nerves in the control of motility in the colon becomes clear from the symptoms of Hirschsprung's disease. Loss of the ganglionic cells from a segment of the large bowel disrupts the coordinated propulsive activity of the organ, leading to severe constipation. Both excitatory and inhibitory neurones are affected.

An absence of excitatory cholinergic ganglion cells prevents segmental contractions and coordinated propulsion from taking place. However, the parasympathetic cholinergic fibres from the sacral spinal cord innervate the muscle directly and their activity results in sustained contraction

Case 8.1 Hirschsprung's disease—cont'd

because modification of the contractile activity by inhibitory interneurones in the plexi can no longer take place. Furthermore, the adrenergic sympathetic nerve fibres can no longer act via inhibitory interneurones to augment the inhibition of the cholinergic nerves in the plexi. Thus, effective relaxation of the circular muscle is lost. Moreover, extrinsic sympathetic nerves also synapse directly on smooth muscle, and activation of the α-receptors on the smooth muscle cells by these nerves produces excitation and increased muscle tone. Thus, both parasympathetic and sympathetic extrinsic influences lead to sustained tonic contraction of the smooth muscle in the aganglionic segment. The presence of the contracted segment results in blockage of the colon.

The defecation reflex

The loss of reflex inhibition of the internal anal sphincter in Hirschsprung's disease illustrates the importance of the intramural nerves in the reflex control of defecation. The innervation of the internal sphincter is defective in this condition and there is a fluctuating but continuous contraction of the sphincter, sometimes referred to as 'sampling'. The normal relaxation response of the sphincter muscle to distension of the rectum does not occur. This is because its relaxation normally depends on the presence of inhibitory fibres in the intramural plexi. Hence, secondary relaxation of the external sphincter does not occur, and defecation does not occur.

The basic defecation reflex in response to distension of the rectum depends on the transmission of afferent impulses to the intramural nerve plexi, and efferent impulses from these plexi to the muscle of the rectum and internal anal sphincter, to cause reflex contraction of the rectum and relaxation of the internal anal sphincter. This basic reflex is not operational if the ganglion cells are absent. Moreover, the anal sphincter is innervated directly by parasympathetic cholinergic and sympathetic α-adrenergic nerve fibres. The activity in the extrinsic nerves normally reinforces the basic reflex via synapses with neurones in the plexi. However, these influences cannot occur in Hirschsprung's disease, and both the direct parasympathetic and sympathetic innervation of the sphincter muscle cause contraction of the sphincter. In Hirschsprung's disease, the sphincter remains contracted.

The response of the external anal sphincter is normal in Hirschsprung's disease as the somatic motor innervation is not affected.

residing within the crypts are constantly renewed by the proliferation of stem cells residing within pockets (the depth of the crypt). Intestinal cells leave the crypt at a rate of 200–300 cells/day to replenish those lost to sloughing when chyme transits through the tract. Its main function is to absorb ions and water. However, some nutrients, such as short-chain fatty acids, are also absorbed within the large intestine (particularly in the proximal colon). There are also goblet cells within the colon that are more numerous than in the small intestine. They produce mucus, which lubricates the intestine and coats the faecal material, which becomes increasingly more solid enabling it to move along easily.

There are also undifferentiated cells and sparsely distributed endocrine cells of various types that secrete hormones into the blood. The lamina propria (containing mostly connective tissue, lymphocytes and other immune cells), muscularis mucosa of the colon, and submucosa are similar in the small and large intestines. Nodules of lymphatic tissue are present in the mucosa, and these usually extend into the submucosa. In the region of the junction between the rectum and the anal canal, the muscularis mucosa breaks up into bundles, and further down the anal canal it disappears.

The muscularis externa (the muscular wall of the tract surrounding the submucosa) consists of circular and longitudinal layers of smooth muscle, as elsewhere in the GI tract. However, in the large intestine (except for the rectum) the outer longitudinal layer appears to be incomplete. It is arranged in three bands, known as taeniae coli. However, between these bands there is a very thin sheet of longitudinal muscle. In the rectum, the outer longitudinal muscle is a uniformly thick layer (as in the small intestine), and this presumably aids defecation. The inner layer of the muscularis externa consists of circular rings of smooth muscle, which allows effective peristalsis as is the case in the small intestine. The submucosa is similar to that present elsewhere in the GI tract. The outer layer is a typical serosa, except where it is in direct contact with other structures (as on much of its posterior surface), when its outer layer is an adventitia.

The appendix

The appendix is a narrow, tube-like structure. Its wall resembles that of the colon, except that it has a complete layer of outer longitudinal muscle, and numerous lymph nodules in the mucosa and submucosa which disrupt the muscularis mucosa, giving it the appearance of isolated lengths of smooth muscle. It has long been considered a vestigial organ, or an organ that has lost its function during evolution. However, recent studies have identified potential immunological functions in addition to important processes associated with maintaining intestinal health. It is becoming widely accepted that the appendix

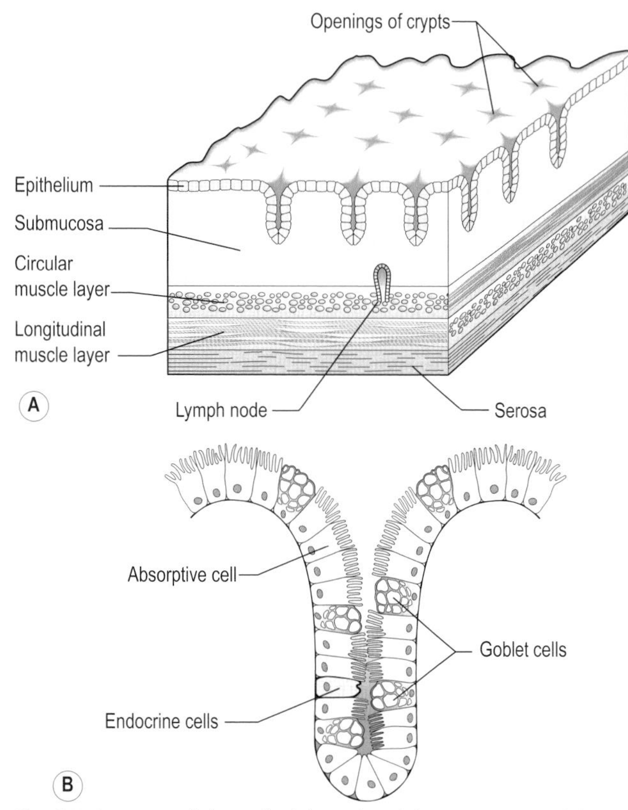

Fig. 8.5 Structure of the wall of the colon. (A) Layers present. (B) Cell types in the epithelium.

may be a backup reservoir of commensal gut flora that can rapidly be re-established if it is eradicated from the colon in specific diseases.

Acute appendicitis is the most common surgical emergency and the most common cause of intra-abdominal sepsis. Patients commonly present with vague, periumbilical abdominal pain which moves to the right iliac fossa. Appendicitis occurs when the appendix becomes obstructed. An abscess forms within it, resulting in a secondary inflammatory process within the wall. This inflammation can result in thrombosis of the blood vessels (appendicular artery and vein) supplying it. The loss of blood supply leads to gangrene and perforation of the appendix. It is the absence of any secondary blood supply to the appendix (that could prevent gangrene) that makes appendicitis such a dangerous condition.

The anal canal

The terminal ramifications of the superior rectal artery and veins are in the submucosa of the anal columns. The numerous veins in this region are longitudinal and thin-walled. They can become dilated and convoluted to produce a condition known as haemorrhoids or piles. The mucosa of the upper part of the anal canal is similar to that of the large intestine, with straight, tubular glands. Numerous goblet cells are found throughout the epithelium. Anal glands are in the region of the anal sinuses. Most of these extend into the submucosa, but some extend into the muscularis externa. They are branched, straight, tubular glands containing mucous cells. The duct of each gland consists of stratified columnar epithelium. It opens into the anal crypt, which is a small depression in the mucosa. If a duct becomes occluded, the glands can become infected, creating perianal abscesses.

The key function of the anal canal is that performed by the sphincter, which comprises an internal (smooth muscle) ring and an outer (striated muscle) ring. This sphincter, which is under both autonomic and somatic nerve control, enables defecation to occur (see below).

Functions of the colon

Secretion

The large intestine secretes a thick mucinous secretion, with a high content of K^+ and HCO_3^- ions. The electrical potential across the mucosa, set up by the entry of Na^+ into the cell, is partly responsible for driving the transport of K^+ ions into the lumen. As the colon is capable of such high K^+ ion secretion, it plays an important role in maintaining K^+ homeostasis. K^+ ion secretion is found to increase in a range of intestinal diseases and extra-intestinal diseases (such as renal disease and severe ulcerative colitis). Early studies demonstrated K^+ excretion could be explained by the lumen-negative transmucosal electrical potential difference, with K^+ likely travelling through tight junctions. However, it is now recognised that K^+ ion movement is also facilitated through BK channels. *In vivo* studies utilising BK-knockout models demonstrate that K^+ secretion is absent, suggesting such channels are the sole exit pathway into the lumen. HCO_3^- ions are secreted in exchange for Cl^- ions.

Secretion in the colon is stimulated by distension and by mechanical irritation of the walls. Secretomotor neurones are excitatory motor neurones that innervate the intestinal crypts from the submucosal and myenteric nerve plexi which stimulate secretion via the release of acetylcholine and vasoactive intestinal peptide (VIP). Stimulation of the parasympathetic pelvic nerves also elicits secretion. This is directly via synapses on the epithelial cells and indirectly via synapses with neurones in the intramural plexi. Stimulation of the sympathetic nerves suppresses secretion in the colon via adrenaline and somatostatin release. For this reason, somatostatin analogues can be administered to treat secretory diarrhoea.

Absorption and digestion

Ions and water

The absorption of ions and water occurs mainly in the proximal region of the colon. In the context of Na^+ transport, this is mediated via an electrogenic Na^+ channel which produces an electrical potential of about 30 mV (lumen-negative) across the mucosa which promotes the secretion of K^+ into the lumen. K^+ is also absorbed in the distal colon, where the transport is via exchange with H^+ ions. The latter is an active process, involving an anionic exchange mechanism similar to that for H^+/K^+ exchange in the stomach.

The electrical potential caused by Na^+ absorption, promotes the secretion of K^+ into the lumen, but K^+ is also absorbed in the distal colon, where the transport is via exchange with H^+ ions. The latter is an active process, involving an anionic exchange mechanism similar to that for H^+/K^+ exchange in the stomach.

The absorption of water and ions is under both neural control via the enteric nerve plexi and hormonal control. Aldosterone increases net water absorption in the colon by stimulating the synthesis of the electrogenic Na^+ channel in the luminal membrane of the epithelial cell and increasing the number of Na^+K^+-ATPase molecules in the basolateral membrane. Glucocorticoids also stimulate the transport of Na^+ ions by increasing the number of ATPase pumps (hence the fluid retention seen in patients taking prednisolone and other steroid medication), and angiotensin stimulates the absorption of water and Na^+ in the colon. Vasopressin (antidiuretic hormone, ADH) decreases water absorption.

Bacterial-derived nutrients

The intestinal microbiome is home to a diverse community of bacteria, viruses and fungi in symbiosis, a mutually beneficial relationship, with their host—humans. The intestinal microbiome is considered in greater detail in Chapter 9. Gastric acid in the stomach destroys most bacteria that are ingested, and the stomach and small intestines are only sparsely colonised by bacteria. Most of the flora that colonise the GI tract reside in the large intestine. Many bacteria are lost in the faeces. The colonic microflora population is so complex and diverse that we have yet to identify some species and strains.

The bacteria in the large intestine synthesise various vitamins that are required by the body. These are vitamins of the B complex, including thiamine, riboflavin, vitamin B_{12} and vitamin K. The synthesis of vitamin K is especially important because the standard diet does not contain enough to meet the body's demand, like for normal blood clotting. In fact, animals bred in germ-free conditions develop clotting defects. Intestinal absorption of the water-soluble vitamins takes place via specific carrier-mediated processes. Fat-soluble soluble vitamins are absorbed fairly readily.

Intestinal bacteria also facilitate digestive processes themselves, specifically through the conversion of primary bile acids to secondary bile acids, and the deconjugation of conjugated bile acids. The importance of bile salt recycling in the digestion of fat is discussed in Chapter 4. The lipid solubility of these substances is greater than that of primary bile acids, and a proportion of them are absorbed passively in the colon. Bile salt reabsorption takes place in the terminal ileum. This is important in the context of IBD which can commonly affect this intestinal section and thus impair a patient's reabsorption capacity, which will have downstream nutritional consequences. Colonic bacteria can also convert bilirubins to urobilinogens. The reactions involved are described in Chapter 4.

Absorption of drugs

Administration of drugs via the rectum is used clinically to treat local and systemic conditions. For example, anti-inflammatory drugs such as aminosalicylates can be used in this way to treat the rectal mucosa in patients with ulcerative colitis limited to the rectum. The local treatment of constipation and haemorrhoids can also be achieved using rectally administered drugs.

However, this route can also be used for drugs that produce systemic effects. It is used following abdominal surgery in patients suffering from vomiting or who require analgesia. In such patients, absorption from the small intestine can be unreliable. Rectal drug delivery can be useful for drugs that have poor stability, solubility or permeability following oral administration. Rectal administration can also partially bypass the hepatic first-pass effect, meaning that rectal formulations are useful for drugs with high levels of first-pass metabolism.

Motility of the colon

Within the colon there are predominantly two types of motility:

- Colonic rhythmic phasic contractions
- Giant migrating contractions

Colonic rhythmic phasic contractions

One of the main functions of the colon is to desiccate. Thus, the fluid contents of the ascending colon gradually become semi-solid to solid in the sigmoid colon as water is absorbed. To meet this challenge, the colon generates two types of rhythmic phasic contractions (RPCs): short-duration RPCs (2–3 seconds in duration) and long-duration RPCs (15–20 seconds).

The short-duration contractions have no propagation, and their amplitudes vary considerably. The long-duration contractions may propagate over short distances. The longer duration enables them to turn over and propel the semi-solid to solid contents more effectively. Colonic RPCs are highly disorganised in space and vary widely in amplitude and duration, making them effective in turning over of faecal material with a very slow rate of propulsion.

Colonic giant migrating contractions

Giant migrating contractions (GMCs) are large-amplitude lumen-occluding contractions that propagate very rapidly (about 1 cm/s) in the distal direction over appreciable distances to produce mass movements. Spontaneous GMCs occur randomly about 2–10 times a day in the proximal, middle, or descending segments of the colon. Colonic GMCs occur in both the fasting and fed states.

Effect of food and importance of fibre

The volume of faeces entering the colon can be increased if fibre is ingested. Fibre consists of polymeric substances (commonly polysaccharides) such as cellulose, hemicelluloses, pectins, gums and waxes. These substances are found in bran, fruit and vegetables. Foods that contain large amounts of indigestible material causes stimulation of mechanoreceptors in the walls of the colon, resulting in its rapid transit through the large intestine. Moreover, polysaccharides, such as cellulose, take up water and swell to form gels. This makes the faeces softer and more easily moved through the colon and anus. This is how fibre in the diet aids constipation. The same gel-forming properties of fibre are associated with their impact on slowing gastric emptying, and they hasten small intestinal transit and slow absorption of nutrients such as glucose from the small intestine.

Western diets are low in fibre compared with diets in many other parts of the world, such as rural Africa, and the relative lack of fibre in the diet may account for the higher prevalence of many diseases of the large intestine in Western populations than in other populations. Diseases such as constipation, diverticular disease, haemorrhoids and cancer are more prevalent in Western populations. However, as a Western diet is adopted more globally, the prevalence of such diseases are slowly normalising across the globe. Many systematic reviews have concluded that increased consumption of dietary fibre lowers the risk of developing colorectal cancer; however, there are inconsistencies in the evidence. Reasons for observing an apparent lack of benefit are (1) dietary fibre is highly heterogenous in nature and (2) dietary-type intervention/retrospective studies are themselves difficult to interpret based on inter-individual differences in defining fibre consumption.

Some fibres have variable capacities for being fermented by colonic bacteria. The ability for a bacterial community to ferment an indigestible fibre will result in their selective growth and expansion; these fibres are known as prebiotics. Not only can fermentation benefit the microbes, but the end-products (short-chain fatty acids, such as butyrate) are utilised by the colonic epithelium as an energy substrate. In addition, butyrate maintains the intestinal epithelium integrity and consequently has multiple health-promoting effects. The recommended daily consumption of fibre for adults is 25–30 g; the average consumption is only 15 g.

Intestinal gas

Intestinal gas can also stimulate motility in the colon, mainly via causing distension. The gases that can be present include carbon dioxide, hydrogen, oxygen, methane and nitrogen. These gases do not smell. The odour associated with expelled gas is due to traces of other substances, such as ammonia, hydrogen sulphide, indole, skatole, short-chain fatty acids and volatile amines. A normal individual releases approximately 500 mL of gas per day. The gases are partly swallowed air, but they can also be derived from substances in the food, produced in the lumen by neutralisation of gastric acid, or by bacterial fermentation processes. They can also arise via diffusion from the blood.

Laxatives

Some ingested substances stimulate motility in the colon via activation of chemoreceptors. An example of such a compound is senna bisacodyl. The formulation of this drug ensures it is not absorbed in the upper intestinal tract and protects it from destruction in the acidic stomach; the intact drug then reaches the colon where it can exert its effect. It is in fact a pro-drug, meaning the active form is not present until the inactive pro-drug is metabolised in some way. In this case, intestinal deacetylase and bacterial enzymes hydrolyse bisacodyl to a deacetylated active metabolite, which stimulates the intestinal mucosa. The increase in motility and peristalsis is mediated via the myenteric plexus. This plexus can be damaged by prolonged high doses of laxatives. Recent studies have demonstrated that 5% of patients using bisacodyl regularly (greater than 3 times per week) after a year demonstrated radiographic changes of colonic redundancy and dilation of colon, with loss of haustral markings.

Control of motility in the colon

The smooth muscle cells of both the longitudinal layer and the circular layer exhibit spontaneously oscillating membrane potentials. In the longitudinal layer, the amplitude of the oscillations sometimes reaches the threshold level for action potential generation, resulting in spontaneous contractions of the muscle. In the circular layer, however, contractions do not usually occur unless the muscle is stimulated by nerves, which release transmitters such as acetylcholine in the vicinity of the pacemaker cells. Acetylcholine increases the time course of the slow-wave oscillations, and these longer waves elicit contractions (Fig. 8.6).

Haustration and segmentation are occurring most of the time, although they are not perceived. However, the frequency of these movements diminishes during sleep. They are spontaneous contractions that are modified by various factors, such as stretch that increases the strength of the contractions. Other factors that control colonic motility include extrinsic autonomic nerves, intrinsic nerves in the intramural nerve plexi and hormones.

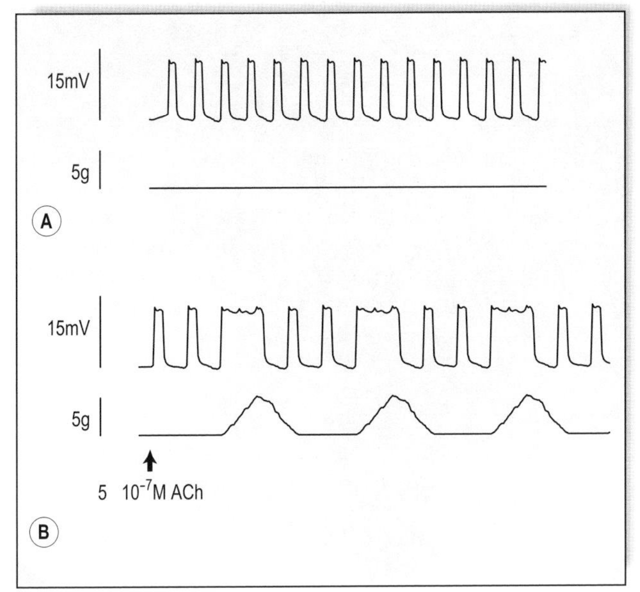

Fig. 8.6 Oscillating membrane potential (upper traces) and contractile activity (lower traces) in the circular smooth muscle of the colon. (A) Unstimulated muscle. (B) The effect of acetylcholine (ACh) (added at the arrow).

Nervous control

Motility in the colon is controlled by intrinsic nerves of the intramural plexi and by extrinsic autonomic nerves. Fig. 8.7 illustrates these pathways.

Intrinsic nerves that release acetylcholine or substance P stimulate motility, and intrinsic nerves that release purines, VIP and nitric oxide (NO) inhibit it. The importance of the intrinsic nerve plexi to the normal functioning of the colon is illustrated by the problems that occur in Hirschsprung's disease and Chagas disease (trypanosomiasis). Both conditions are characterised by an absence of intramural ganglion cells in a narrowed region of the colon. Hirschsprung's disease is a congenital abnormality, while the defect in Chagas disease is due to trypanosome parasites *(Trypanosoma cruzi)* which infest the wall of the intestines. The parasites produce a toxin that destroys the intramural ganglion cells, leading to symptoms similar to those seen in Hirschsprung's disease.

Extrinsic autonomic nerves are also involved in the control of the colon. They synapse with neurones in the plexi to modulate the effects of the intrinsic innervation, and they innervate the smooth muscle directly. Stimulation of the parasympathetic nerves increases motility, both via the interneurones and via their direct action on the muscle. Stimulation of the sympathetic nerves inhibits motility via the interneurones in the plexi, but their direct action on the muscle causes increased contraction (see Fig. 8.7). α-Adrenergic receptors are present at the synapses of sympathetic nerves, both in the plexi and on the muscle. The inhibitory interneurones in the plexi, with which the sympathetic nerves synapse, are not adrenergic (see above).

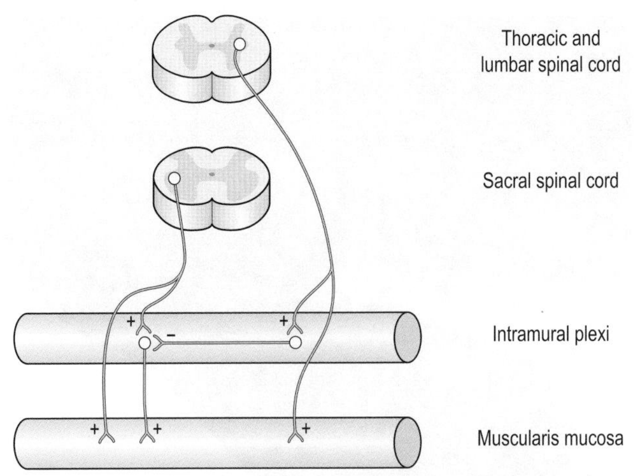

Fig. 8.7 A simplified scheme for the control of motility in the colon.

Reflex control

Distension of parts of the GI tract proximal to the colon can result in reflex motility of the colon itself. The best-known reflex is the gastrocolic reflex which is when an individual has eaten, and stomach distension induces motility in the colon; this is why individuals feel the urge to defecate soon after having eaten a meal. The gastrocolic reflex is multifactorial, involving neurological, mechanical and paracrine mediators. Several neuropeptides such as cholecystokinin, serotonin, neurotensin and gastrin mediate the reflex.

Defecation

Defecation (Fig. 8.8) is a reflex response to the sudden distension of the walls of the rectum resulting from mass movements in the colon moving the faecal material into it.

The reflex response has four components:

- Increased activity in the sigmoid colon
- Distension of the rectum
- Reflex contraction of the rectum
- Relaxation of the internal and external anal sphincters (which are normally closed).

Control of defecation

Defecation is an intrinsic reflex mediated by impulses in the internal nerve plexi, which is reinforced by an autonomic reflex that is transmitted in the spinal cord. The reflex is integrated via the defecation centre in the sacral spinal cord. However, defecation is also influenced by signals from higher centres. Fig. 8.9 illustrates the pathways involved in the neural control of defecation.

When faeces enter the rectum, distension of the wall activates pressure receptors. These send afferent signals that spread through the myenteric plexus to initiate peristaltic

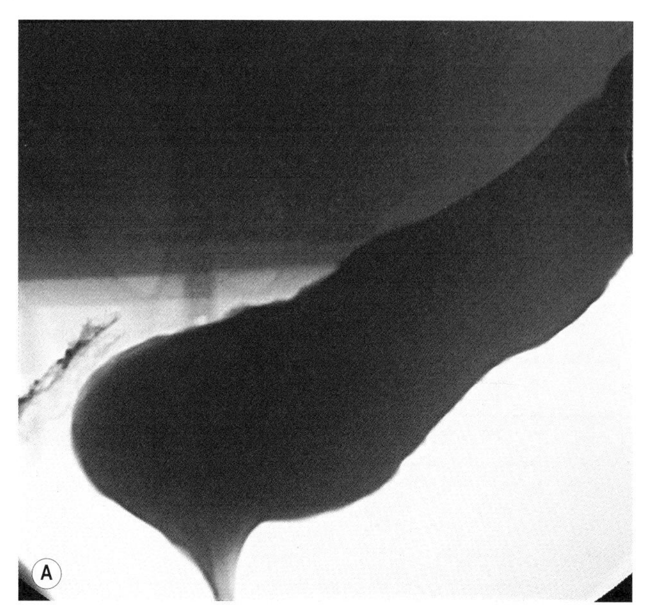

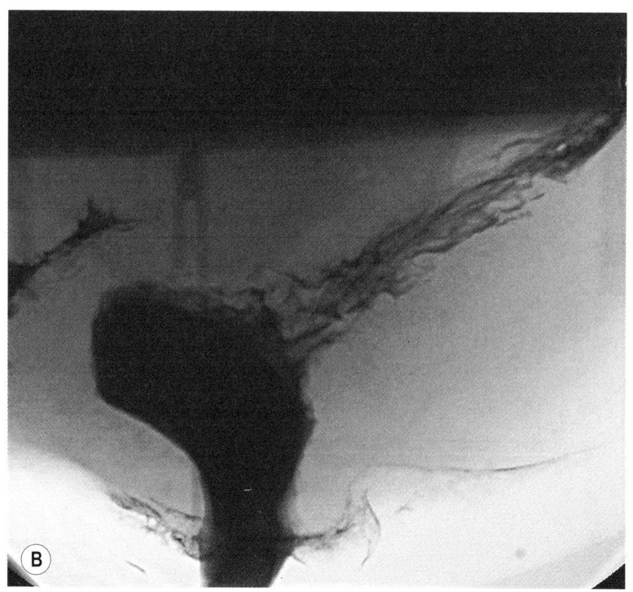

Fig. 8.8 An X-ray showing a rectum filled with contrast (barium) (A) before and (B) during contraction/defecation.

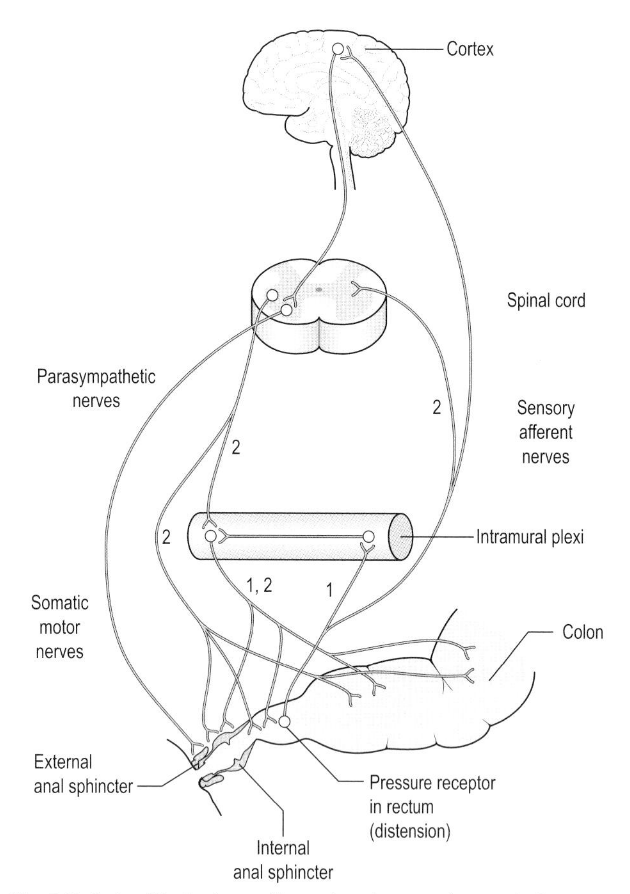

Fig. 8.9 A simplified scheme illustrating the neural control of defecation. The basic reflex operates via the intramural plexi, and the spinal parasympathetic reflex reinforces the basic reflex. Control is also exerted by the conscious brain. 1, components of the basic reflex; 2, components of the spinal sympathetic reflex.

waves in the descending and sigmoid regions of the colon and the rectum. These waves of contraction force the faeces towards the anus. As the wave approaches the anus, the sphincters are inhibited and they relax. The external sphincter that is innervated by somatic motor nerves is under voluntary control. If the external sphincter is relaxed voluntarily when the faeces are pushed towards it, defecation will occur.

This intrinsic reflex is augmented by an autonomic reflex. This involves parasympathetic nerve fibres in the pelvic nerves arising from the sacral spinal cord, which innervate the terminal colon. Thus, activation of pressure receptors by distension of the rectum sends afferent impulses to the spinal cord (as well as to nerves in the intramural plexi). This results in impulses being transmitted in the parasympathetic nerve fibres to the descending colon, the sigmoid colon and the rectum. The parasympathetic signals intensify the peristaltic waves and augment the effect of the intrinsic neurones to cause increased motility, contraction of the rectum, and relaxation of the internal and external anal sphincters. Thus, the parasympathetic reflex converts the weak intrinsic reflex to a powerful reflex. In Hirschsprung's disease, the innervation of the internal anal sphincter is defective, resulting in loss of reflex inhibition of the sphincter.

The sacral control centre also coordinates the other effects which accompany defecation, including deep inspiration, closure of the glottis and contraction of the abdominal muscles, which forces the faeces downwards and extends the pelvic floor, so that it pulls outward on the anus to expel the faeces. The reflex normally initiates contraction of the external anal sphincter, which temporarily prevents defecation. The conscious

Case 8.2 Chronic constipation

A 35-year-old woman was referred to the gastroenterology clinic with a history of severe chronic constipation. She reported only opening her bowels with frequency of once or twice a week, and that she mainly passes hard pellets of stool. She feels bloated all the time, especially after meals, along with cramping abdominal discomfort. She tried multiple laxatives with little relief. She denied blood in her stools or having lost weight. She has a past medical history of migraines and IBS. She had tried macrogol, senna and lactulose in the past for up to two to three weeks with little improvement in her constipation. She denied any significant family history of medical conditions and works as an office clerk. Her diet is poor with very low fibre. She smokes and drinks alcohol occasionally. Rectal examination identified a good anal sphincter tone with no evidence of rectal prolapse.

Blood tests were performed to rule out hypothyroidism, hypercalcaemia, coeliac disease and anaemia. Her faecal calprotectin (a stool biomarker of inflammation) was normal. An abdominal X-ray confirmed faecal loading throughout her large bowel. Colonic transit studies confirmed slow transit constipation and a defecating proctogram was normal. As her history, examination, and investigations were consistent with the diagnosis of severe chronic constipation, a lower GI endoscopy was not performed as there were no other worrying symptoms.

She was advised to improve lifestyle measures, including increasing her amount of dietary fibre and water as well as getting regular exercise. As a trial of two different classes of laxatives (osmotic and stool bulking) for up to four weeks did not help improve her symptoms, she was given of course of prucalopride, which helped resolve her constipation. She opened her bowels about once every other day with soft stools and had a significant improvement in her abdominal discomfort.

Constipation is a very common complaint in adults that is often variably defined by patients. The Rome 4 criteria define constipation with criteria that include lumpy, hard stools; straining when opening bowels; a sensation of incomplete evacuation; the use of digital techniques to help evacuate; and a decrease in stool frequency (under 3 bowel motions per week). Constipation can be categorised as idiopathic chronic constipation, slow transit constipation, dyssynergic defecation, constipation-predominant IBS and less-frequent secondary causes that include metabolic, neurological and endocrine disorders. Evaluation of patients with constipation should aim to understand the symptoms and rule out secondary causes. Concerning symptoms include rectal bleeding, acute onset of constipation (especially in those over 60 years of age), weight loss and family history of bowel cancer or exemptible disease. A blood test should be performed to rule out anaemia as well as other common secondary causes of constipation, including hypothyroidism, hypercalcaemia and coeliac disease. Lower GI endoscopic evaluation is usually helpful in patients in whom colorectal cancer and IBD is suspected and needs to be ruled out. Occasionally, tests including colonic transit studies, anorectal manometry and a defecating proctogram may need to be performed to help understand the aetiology of constipation and facilitate a more focused management approach.

The first step in the management of chronic functional constipation is dietary and lifestyle modification. Measures including increased fibre in the diet, fluid intake and exercise can be effective, but the evidence for this to date is limited. Following this, a trial of different classes of laxatives such as bulk-forming laxatives (isphagula husk), osmotic (lactulose and macrogol) and stimulants (senna and docusate) can be considered with varying efficacy. In patients in whom these measures have not been successful, other pharmacological agents such as colonic secretagogues (lubiprostone and linaclotide) or a $5HT_4$ receptor agonist (prucalopride) can be used. Finally, biofeedback therapy through retraining the pelvic floor is an important management option for patients with pelvic floor dysfunction and dyssynergic defecation.

mind then takes over, and either it inhibits the external sphincter to cause relaxation and allow defecation to occur, or it keeps it contracted it so that defecation is resisted. Pain inhibits relaxation, and this results in straining. If this becomes chronic, it leads to dilation of the haemorrhoidal veins ('piles') and may even prolapse the rectum through the anal canal. Rectal prolapse is also seen in weightlifters, in whom the process of repeated lifting requires straining against a contracted external sphincter.

The frequency of defecation and the time of day when it is performed is a matter of habit. In two-thirds of healthy individuals, it is between 5 and 7 times a week. In the human adult, approximately 150 g of material are eliminated per day. Of this 150 g, two-thirds are water and one-third are solids. The solids are normally mostly undigested cellulose, bacteria, cell debris, bile pigments and some salts. There is a high content of K^+ ions in the faeces relative to the concentration in the fluid entering the colon because K^+ is secreted by the walls of the colon. The brown colour of faeces is due to the presence of stercobilin and urobilin (see Chapter 4). The odour is caused mainly by traces of other substances, including products of bacterial fermentation.

Ulcerative colitis

Ulcerative colitis is a form of IBD, the incidence of which is rapidly rising in the Western world. Although the exact aetiology of this disease is currently unknown, multiple lines of evidence suggest a dysregulated immune-mediated response to a dysregulated gut microbiota in genetically predisposed individuals.

It affects both men and women and is most common in people aged 20–40 years. Patients typically present with a history of chronic bloody diarrhoea and the diagnosis is made based on endoscopic and histological findings. Unlike Crohn's disease, ulcerative colitis only affects the large intestine with inflammation that starts from the rectum and extends proximally in a continuous manner. The inflammation in ulcerative colitis is limited to the mucosa; therefore, unlike Crohn's disease, patients with ulcerative colitis do not develop fistulas or perianal disease. The damaged mucosa cannot absorb water and ions adequately, and this results in diarrhoea along with bleeding. Frequent bowel movements can result from large volumes of diarrhoea but may also be due to colonic or rectal irritability in this condition.

Case 8.3 Ulcerative colitis

A 22-year-old woman, who had been experiencing intermittent episodes of diarrhoea and rectal bleeding for the past two years, visited her general practitioner. She said each episode lasted for several weeks and more recently these episodes had become more frequent. She would often have to wake up in the middle of the night to use the toilet. Her general practitioner thought the symptoms could be explained by the presence of a few different conditions, including infection, IBS and ulcerative colitis, and she decided to send the patient to see a specialist. Her stool biomarker of inflammation was significantly elevated at 2000 μg/g. The patient was referred to an outpatient clinic followed by a colonoscopy (direct visual examination of the colon). This revealed significant inflammation with confluent ulceration starting from the distal rectum and extending to her descending colon (Fig. 8.11). Stool cultures for microbiological tests were negative. A diagnosis of ulcerative colitis was made based on these findings and biopsies taken from the colon were consistent with this. The patient was prescribed aminosalicylates (mesalazine) given as oral and topical (enema) preparations, which resulted in amelioration of symptoms and normalisation of faecal calprotectin over the course of a month.

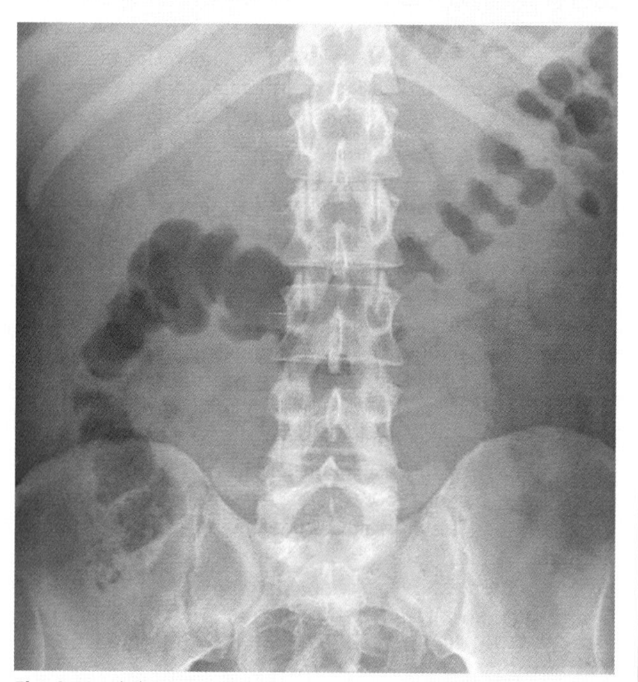

Fig. 8.10 Abdominal X-ray demonstrating thumbprinting of the transverse colon in a patient with severe ulcerative colitis.

Diagnosis

Blood tests may demonstrate signs of a chronic inflammatory process such as anaemia through low albumin, elevated C-reactive protein, erythrocyte sedimentation rate and white blood cell count. It is also important to rule out enteric infections such as *Campylobacter* or *Salmonella* with stool tests. A lower GI endoscopy (colonoscopy or sigmoidoscopy) may reveal erythema, ulceration, mucosal bleeding or loss of vascular pattern. Radiography may show oedema of the colon (thumbprinting or lead-pipe appearance) and some patients with severe disease may show dilatation of the colon (as shown in Fig. 8.10).

Histological findings show that the inflammation is restricted to the mucosa and, to a lesser extent, the submucosa. Near the tips of the crypts are accumulations of polymorphonuclear cells (crypt abscesses). The epithelial cells in the crypts show evidence of degeneration (mucosal atrophy). Ulceration of the mucosa may also be evident.

Treatment

This patient was treated with oral and topical aminosalicylates called mesalazine. This is broken down to 5-aminosalicylate by bacteria in the colon. Its mode of action is through a local anti-inflammatory, and it is usually effective in inducing and maintaining remission. Occasionally, a short, tapered course of corticosteroids (such as prednisolone or budesonide multimatrix) are needed to treat active disease; however, its poor

Case 8.3 Ulcerative colitis—cont'd

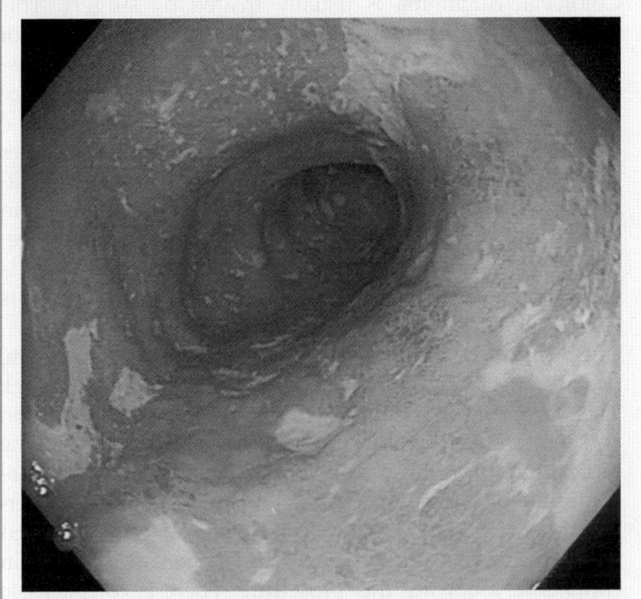

Fig. 8.11 Endoscopic image of a colon showing deep linear ulcers in a patient with severe ulcerative colitis.

side-effect profile and lack of evidence in prevention of relapse limits its long-term use. Other immunosuppressive therapies used as part of escalation of management include thiopurine and biological therapies such as anti-TNFs, anti-integrins and anti-IL12/23 and JAK inhibitors. Faecal microbiota transplantation has shown promise through clinical trials and may have a potential role in the future.

In severe cases or drug-refractory cases, surgery is required to treat ongoing active disease and prevent perforation. This usually involves a colectomy, ileostomy and removal of the colon and rectum. Surgery for ulcerative colitis is curative because, unlike in Crohn's disease, the disease is limited to the large bowel. In most cases, patients will eventually have a part of their small bowel refashioned to form a pouch connected to the anal canal by a procedure called ileal pouch anal anastomosis. This allows restoration of continence; however, in some cases, patients go on to develop complications such as inflammation of their pouch (pouchitis).

Colon cancer

Colorectal cancer is the 4th most common cancer in the UK, accounting for 11% of all new cancer cases with an annual incidence of approximately 42,000. As in most other cancers, it is a disease of the aged, with approximately 44% of all new cases diagnosed in those over 75 years. Colorectal cancer is the 2nd most common cause of cancer death in the UK, accounting for 10% of all cancer deaths (approximately 16,600 per year). Over the last decade, bowel cancer mortality rates have decreased by more than one-tenth and it is projected to fall further over the coming decade. The 5-year survival for what is a very common cancer is approximately 58%. Since it is a very common cancer and the 2nd most common cause of cancer death, the UK government launched the National Bowel Screening programme in 2006. The rationale for this screening programme was to identify asymptomatic individuals with likely early-stage colorectal disease, which is more amenable to curative therapy.

Risk factors

Risk factors for colorectal cancer include the consumption of excess red and processed meat (accounting for 13% of bowel cancer cases) and being overweight or obese (accounting for 11% of bowel cancer cases). There is evidence that 28% of bowel cancer cases in the UK are caused by eating too little fibre. Other risk factors include alcohol, smoking and too little physical activity. Thus, unsurprisingly, over half of all colorectal cancers are thought to be preventable through lifestyle changes. There are also several medical conditions associated with colorectal cancer, including type 2 diabetes (22–30% higher compared to those without diabetes) and IBD (colorectal cancer risk is 70% higher in individuals with IBD compared with the general population). Since colorectal cancer arises through the adenoma-carcinoma sequence, individuals with adenomatous polyps are at greater risk of developing colorectal cancer. Specifically, adenomatous polyps have three histological variants: tubular, tubulovillous and villous adenomas. Tubular adenomas are the most common (approximately 75%) and have <5% chance of harbouring a malignancy whilst villous adenomas constitute 5–10% of total polyps though have a much higher risk of harbouring malignancy (35–40%). Larger polyps and a greater extent of dysplasia are also highly associated with malignant potential. It is largely accepted that if malignant polyps go undiagnosed, they will take approximately 10 years to develop into a carcinoma.

Whilst most colorectal cancers are sporadic in nature, kindred and twin studies estimate that approximately 30% of all colorectal cancer cases are an inherited form of disease. Approximately 5–10% of cases are associated with highly penetrant inherited mutations and clinical presentations that have been well-characterised which include familial adenomatous polyposis (FAP) and hereditary non-polyposis colorectal cancer (HNPCC). It is through the study of these familial conditions that has led to the discovery of the adenoma-carcinoma sequence which describes the development and progression of sporadic colorectal cancers.

Familial adenomatous polyposis

FAP is a familial polyposis syndrome and accounts for approximately 1–2% of all patients diagnosed with colorectal cancer. It is characterised by hundreds to thousands of adenomatous polyps throughout the GI tract with the greatest density in the colon. Without treatment, many of these polyps will progress into cancer and thus patients are offered prophylactic colectomy. Since this condition is attributed to a germline mutation, patients present much earlier in life (average 34 years of age) compared to patients with sporadic cancer. The germline mutation is in *APC*, a tumour suppressor. This gene is involved in several cellular processes, though most notably is crucial in Wnt signalling. In the background of a non-functional APC molecule, β-catenin cannot be degraded within cells and consequently translocates into the nucleus where, in conjunction with transcription factors of the Tcf/LEF family, transcriptionally activates a plethora of genes, many of which are involved in tumourigenesis including c-Myc and cyclin D1. This results in the rapid growth of cells and increases the likelihood of malignant transformation of an adenomatous polyp. There is also a condition known as attenuated familial adenomatous polyposis (AFAP) which is associated with *APC* mutations that predominantly occur outside of the mutation cluster region (MCR) of the gene (mutations in the MCR tend to give rise to a classical FAP phenotype). AFAP is distinct from FAP in that it is characterised by fewer polyps (<100 polyps), later onset (15 years later than FAP) and a lower risk of colorectal cancer.

Hereditary non-polyposis colorectal cancer

HNPCC, also known as Lynch syndrome, is an inherited cancer-susceptibility syndrome that predisposes individuals to colorectal cancer as well as extracolonic cancers. Patients with HNPCC have a very small number of polyps compared to FAP and usually present later in life (mid-forties). It is characterised by germline mutations in one of several DNA mismatch repair (MMR) genes. These genes function by maintaining the fidelity of DNA replication by identifying and excising single-base mismatches and insertion-deletion loops during DNA replication. In brief, these genes survey the DNA and ensure that errors are corrected. Anything that might compromise this process (for example, mutations in MMR genes) will facilitate the accumulation of spontaneous point mutations, deletions and insertions, especially in short repetitive DNA sequences termed microsatellites. These genetic alterations constitute microsatellite instability and are found in most tumours (>90%) from patients with germline mutations in MMR genes. There are six different proteins required for the complete MMR system: MSH2, MLH1, PMS1, PMS2, MSH3, and MSH6. Mutations in MSH2 and MLH1 are thought to account for 90% of HNPCC cases.

Surgical resection

Colorectal carcinoma is usually treated by surgery. This is both to prevent the life-threatening complications of obstruction and perforation and to attempt to cure the disease. Treatment involves a segmental resection of the large bowel along with its arterial blood supply. The arterial blood supply is taken to remove the draining lymph nodes into which tumours commonly spread. This results in little change in GI function unless the rectum is removed, in which case there is loss of storage capacity and more frequent bowel action. The major function of the large bowel is water absorption, and any remaining colon quickly adapts to overcome the loss of function of the resected segment.

Ulcerative colitis, when it requires surgical intervention, usually affects the lining of the whole of the large bowel. Therefore, surgical treatment involves removal of the colon and rectum from the caecum to the anal canal. Despite the radical nature of this resection, it is still possible to restore continuity by joining the terminal ileum to the anus. The terminal ileum is reconstructed to form a new reservoir called a pouch to replace the rectum. Most patients can maintain continence following this procedure. There is considerable adaptation of the small bowel, which reduces its secretions and increases the fluid absorption. Therefore, although patients will not pass formed stools, they will usually only open their bowels three to 4 times a day. Remarkably, the adaptation of the small bowel is such that, even in this extreme situation, salt and water loss is controlled and dietary supplements are rarely required. There may be an increased loss of bile acids because of loss of absorption in the terminal ileum and large bowel. This can lead to persistent diarrhoea but is controllable by oral chelating agents which bind bile salts and so reduce their osmotic potential.

Case 8.4 Colorectal cancer

A 66-year-old man presented to his general practitioner after a positive faecal immunochemical test (part of a bowel cancer screening programme). He reported a history of recent change in bowel habits and had noticed blood in his stool infrequently. He also noticed a sensation of incomplete evacuation of his bowel (tenesmus). He was otherwise well and had a past medical history of high blood pressure. He was referred for an urgent colonoscopy as part of the bowel cancer screening programme. This identified a circumferential cancer in his rectum that was causing partial obstruction of his bowel. He underwent urgent radiological investigations which revealed localised enlarged lymph nodes around his rectum but no distant spread or metastases. Following further evaluation, he was given chemotherapy to downstage the cancer (neo-adjuvant) following surgery to remove his rectal cancer. A stoma was fashioned from the proximal segment of his colon to divert stool into the abdominal wall into a bag. At the annual follow-up, he remained well with no recurrence of cancer.

THE INTESTINAL MICROBIOME

9

Chapter objectives and clinical presentations

After reading this chapter, review your learning by considering the following:

1. Are you able to describe the functions of the intestinal microbiome and how its composition relates to function?
2. Can you list factors that have the potential to alter intestinal microbial composition?
3. Can you explain the term 'dysbiosis'?
4. Are you aware of methods available to study the intestinal microbiome?
5. Can you detail how the microbiome might be involved in disease progression?
6. Do you know the difference between prebiotics, probiotics and faecal microbial transplantation?

In addition, you should be familiar with the following clinical presentations:

- Recurrent *Clostridioides difficile* infection
- Inflammatory bowel disease (in the context of the microbiome)
- Infective diarrhoea

Clinical outlook

The clinical applicability of the intestinal microbiome is rapidly evolving regarding diagnosis and therapy. There is a multitude of studies demonstrating associations between changes in the gut microbiome, and acute and chronic disease. While it is not yet possible to diagnose specific diseases or make decisions around treatment based on an individual's gut microbial profile, this field is likely to advance significantly over the next decade. Modulation of the gut microbiome, however, is currently successfully performed using probiotics and faecal microbiota transplantation for conditions such as *Clostridioides difficile* infection.

Introduction

The importance of the intestinal microbiome is often exemplified by the fact that there are more microbial cells within our body than mammalian cells (around 1.3 times more, with 10^14 microorganisms belonging to over 2000 species and 12 different phyla). However, the full functions and properties of the intestinal microbiome are still largely undetermined. The search term 'microbiome' now surpasses that of 'human genome', further exemplifying its importance in health and disease. This highly complex network of bacteria, viruses (including phages or bacterial viruses), fungi, yeast and archaea (single-celled organisms) reside within the large intestine, synergistically living with their hosts. The healthy gut microbiota is primarily dominated by three to four phyla. Collectively, they act in symbiosis to contain and suppress expansion of pathogenic organisms, facilitate metabolism of dietary substrates and environmental chemicals, and contribute towards intestinal epithelial cell renewal and development of the immune system. The term 'microbiome' refers to all the microorganisms within an environment, whereas 'microbiota' relates to a specific environment, residing within specific niches (such as the intestinal microbiota).

Composition of the microbiome

Initial acquisition of the gut microbiome is still not completely understood. Evidence suggests that the intestinal microbiome is seeded at birth with the most critical and defining contribution from the maternal microbiota. The gut microbial ecosystem and bacterial communities change rapidly in early childhood, stabilise in adults and deteriorate with diversity in old age. The major dominating phyla in the intestinal microbiome are Firmicutes and Bacteroidetes and, to a lesser extent, Proteobacteria and Actinobacteria.

Early development and establishment of the microbiome

In meconium, bacteria are present in low numbers. It is thought that the facultative anaerobic bacteria present in the intestine alter the luminal environment, by decreasing O_2 concentrations and adjusting the pH to facilitate future colonisation by strict anaerobes. The presence of these bacteria in the meconium is suggestive of bacterial colonisation prior to birth. Bacteria have also been found in the blood from umbilical cords of healthy neonates born by caesarean section, and evidence suggests that intestinal microbes could be transported to the placenta and foetus. It has long been considered that the most significant acquisition of the infant microbiome occurs from the mother during passage through the birth canal. Differences in microbial composition are found between infants delivered via caesarean section and those delivered vaginally, and the same bacteria that are found in the mother's vagina or rectum are identified in the infant's faeces after natural delivery. Infants born vaginally are colonised by bacteria such as *Lactobacillus* and *Prevotella*, whereas infants who are born by caesarean section are exposed initially to bacteria found within the skin microbiome. Changes in composition and diversity between infants delivered vaginally and by caesarean section can persist up to 3 years of age. These major microbial differences, and their influence on the differential development of the intestinal immune system (see later) have led to a hypothesis that caesarean-born infants are at a higher risk of developing metabolic disorders later in life. Consequently, interventions are being implemented to ensure caesarean-delivered babies are exposed to vaginal microbes through a process known as vaginal seeding. Early studies have demonstrated such approaches result in successful colonisation of the gut by maternal-derived intestinal microbes.

An increase in lactic acid-producing bacteria appears soon after the onset of milk consumption. Interestingly, a more diverse microbiome is found in formula-fed infants compared to those who are breast-fed. It is possible that mothers transfer their intestinal microbiome via mononuclear cells to breast milk. Upon the introduction of solid foods, which include non-digestible carbohydrates and fibres, there is a further increase in diversity. Diversity and composition changes rapidly over the infant years. Factors that influence the development of the microbiome at this early stage include premature vs. postterm birth, birthweight, hospital vs. home-birth locations, diet, maternal and infant medications, exposure to pets and family size. The microbes to which infants are first exposed are crucial in the subsequent maturation of microbial communities in adulthood.

Factors altering composition throughout life

The gut microbiome is shaped throughout life by numerous factors, including host genetics, age, geographic and socioeconomic factors, diet and disease (Fig. 9.1). Although the microbiome is largely temporally stable and resistant to perturbations in an adult, it does not exist in a single static state, but rather as a dynamic equilibrium. Consequently, the gut microbiota may transiently shift

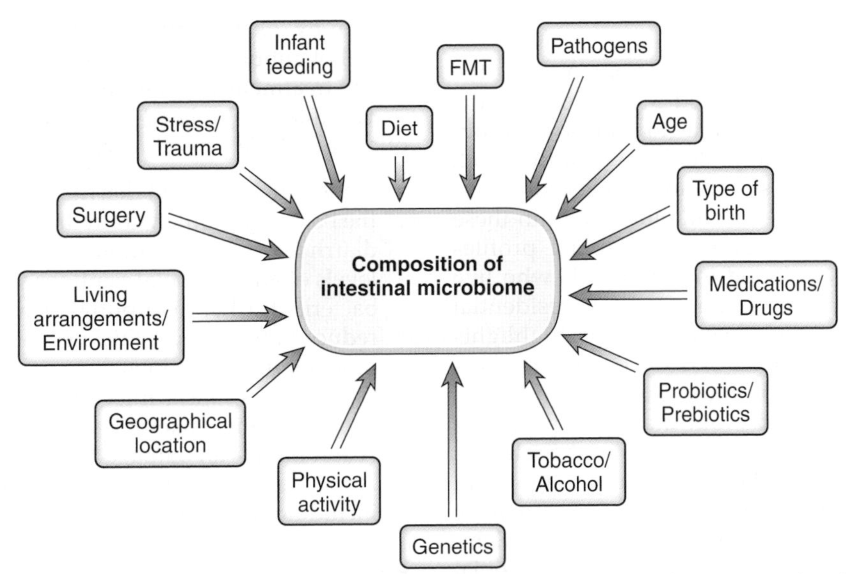

Fig. 9.1 Summary of the many different factors that can alter the composition of the intestinal microbiome. FMT, faecal material transplantation.

following an environmental trigger, such as antibiotics or a gastrointestinal (GI) infection, usually, before recovering to its baseline. These relatively small and transient modulations in the microbiome are commonplace and are not overtly associated with disease.

Diet

Diet is the most influential factor on the composition of the intestinal microbiome – you are what you eat! During and post infancy, the diet is key to shaping the composition of the microbiome. Many components within our diet are non-digestible and inert (such as fibres), yet can be fermented by specific intestinal bacteria. Consequently, diets rich in fibre allow these bacteria to thrive, resulting in changes to microbial composition. Metatranscriptomic studies reveal that microbiome composition is indeed driven by the capacity of the microbial members to metabolise dietary constituents and, specifically, these microbiome-accessible carbohydrates (MACs) that are found in dietary fibres. The abundance of MACs is substantially reduced in the Western diet, which is associated with a reduction in microbial diversity. In addition to dietary fibre, intestinal mucins are also a rich carbohydrate source for bacteria within the colon. Mucus layers are also crucial in mediating the host–microbiota relationship, and the mucus layers found within the colon keep the bacteria distanced from the mucosal lining. The mucus lining (closest to the colonic lumen) is rich in bacteria metabolising the abundant O-glycans present. Reducing MAC intake can result in thinner mucus layers and hence alter the microbial composition. Specialist bacteria within the intestine can alter their substrate utilisation from dietary-derived MACs to host-derived glycans, when dietary availability changes. The fermentation of MACs can lead to the production of short-chain fatty acids (SCFAs). These metabolites have varying roles from regulating immune function to altering intestinal hormone production, having beneficial properties on the host. Butyrate, one type of SCFA, has been shown to have antitumorigenic properties. Diets rich in carbohydrates thus promote butyrate production. Conversely, diets rich in red meat promote the growth of sulphate-reducing bacteria that produce hydrogen sulphide, a toxic metabolite. Consequently, this is one of the many theories of why diets rich in red meat are associated with an increased risk for the development of colon cancer.

The ability to alter the microbiome using an individual's diet in a therapeutic setting is thus being explored. Short-term dietary interventions in healthy humans can lead to significant and rapid alterations in the composition of the intestinal microbiome. However, these changes are not consistent amongst individuals as the starting composition and residence of particular bacterial species will be different. The low fermentable oligo-, di-, monosaccharides and polyols (FODMAP) diet is clinically recommended for the management of irritable bowel syndrome (IBS). This diet requires the reduced consumption of all foods that contain slowly absorbed or indigestible short-chain carbohydrates with a slow re-introduction based on the patient's tolerance to differing foodstuffs. Despite being effective in some patients, there are still controversies over the usefulness of such a change in diet to treat IBS and research continues to address these issues. FODMAP fermentation can lead to the production of gasses and increased luminal water (due to osmosis) which can in turn stimulate mechanoreceptors in response to intestinal distention. The release of SCFAs from fermentation of FODMAPs is also thought to influence intestinal motility and can affect visceral sensitivity. As alteration of FODMAP intake will influence the composition of the intestinal microbiome, it is considered that pathogenic bacteria that flourish on FODMAPs could also be modulating the symptoms found in IBS.

Age

The inception of the intestinal microbiome in the infant is detailed above. At around 3 years of age, the infant microbiome becomes similar to that of an adult. The composition is relatively stable over adulthood, although studies suggest a significant decrease of diversity in the elderly (65–70 years and older). Within these elderly populations, correlations in microbial profiles (including diversity) are found in individuals who live with others (in community settings such as residential care homes) or in isolated dwellings. This highlights how our living arrangements and exposure to others can shape our microbial profiles. Overall, the capacity of the microbiota to carry out metabolic processes such as SCFA production is reduced in the elderly. Consequently, this drop in SCFA concentrations could contribute to intestinal age-associated inflammatory disease incidence. Indeed, many studies have demonstrated that these age-associated shifts in microbial composition can increase the predisposition of developing cardiovascular diseases, cancer, obesity and neurodegenerative diseases.

Antibiotics

Antibiotics and their use in controlling the growth of unwanted pathogenic bacteria can also have non-selective effects and destroy communities of beneficial microbes within the intestinal microbiome. The destruction and compositional changes invoked by antibiotic use can allow the onset of a dysbiosis (see later). These potentially detrimental effects on the intestinal microbiome include reduced species diversity, altered metabolic activity and the selection of antibiotic-resistant organisms, which in turn can lead to antibiotic-associated diarrhoea and recurrent *Clostridioides difficile* infections (CDIs; see Case 9.2). An association between antibiotic exposure during childhood and asthma, allergies and airway illnesses has long been suspected. Continued research has established a link between antibiotic exposure during early ages and the onset of many intestinal and autoimmune-related diseases in later life, including obesity, inflammatory bowel disease (IBD) and colorectal cancer.

Even though antibiotics can reduce bacterial diversity within the colon, bacterial numbers do not change. As bacteria that are susceptible to the antimicrobial agents become depleted, the resistant bacteria are then able to multiply and successfully compete for the space once taken by the other commensals. In some scenarios, these bacteria can be pathogenic and lead to disease. This highlights one of the mechanisms by which the microbiome protects itself from pathogenic growth and invasion. This mechanism, colonisation resistance, ensures that it is difficult for any new and/or pathogenic strains to find a niche within the intestine to thrive. Indeed, antibiotic-resistant strains can thrive in such scenarios, which can be life-threatening when such bacteria are pathogenic. The World Health Organization estimates that the number of antibiotic resistance-related deaths could reach 10 million by 2050. In humans, the gut microbiota contains a pool of antibiotic-resistance genes, acquired by bacteria due to treatment with antimicrobial agents.

The intestinal-related clinical consequences of antibiotic use include the following:

- Antibiotic-associated diarrhoea, where changes in the bacterial profile within the intestine leads to diarrhoea. Such alterations include changes in the levels of antimicrobial peptides secreted by some bacteria (further disrupting microbial patterns), reduced mucus layer thickness and disruption to mucosal tight junctions.
- *Clostridioides difficile* infection. This is a Gram-positive, spore-forming, anaerobic bacteria that produces toxins A and B that can damage the gut mucosa.
- Associated with development of chronic illnesses including IBD, obesity and asthma.

Bile salts

The distribution of bile acids in the small and large intestine can also affect the bacterial composition within the intestine. Primary bile acids can elicit signals to gut bacteria promoting the germination of spores (and hence colonisation of these spore-associated strains) and may also enable the recovery of the microbiome after dysbiosis. Conversely, reduced bile acid concentration in the gut may play an important role in allowing pro-inflammatory microbial species to flourish.

Others

Many other environmental factors have been implicated in shaping the composition of the intestinal microbiome. These include the following:

- geographic location and living conditions/arrangements (rural settings vs. urban towns and cities)
- smoking
- depression
- surgery
- a range of drugs and colon-targeted drugs

Enterotypes

Even though our intestinal microbial composition is shaped by many factors, the microbial profile of faecal samples from American, European and Japanese individuals are similar at the genus level. These similarities are not driven by an individual's age, sex, nationality or body mass index, indicating that there are a limited number of well-balanced symbiotic states. It is unsurprising when you consider that organisms that are phylogenetically related and functionally similar tend to co-exist within the same environmental niches. The three distinct compositions are termed 'enterotypes'. These include enterotype-1 (*Bacteroides*-rich composition), enterotype-2 (mostly *Prevotella* genus bacteria) and enterotype-3

(*Ruminococcus*-rich). Diets rich in animal protein and fat (Western-associated foods) are associated with the *Bacteroides* enterotype, while diets characterised by the predominance of plant carbohydrates are associated with the *Prevotella* enterotype.

There has been considerable controversy about the usefulness of a categorisation system based on bacterial composition which itself is so subject to change. Despite this, there are some clinical relevancies. For example, enterotype-1 has been associated with insulin resistance and the risk of obesity. It is hoped that an enterotype-classification system could help in disease diagnosis, prognosis and understanding pharmacokinetic and drug metabolism profiles of individuals.

Functions of the intestinal microbiome

Digestive functions

The products of fibre and MAC fermentation, namely SCFAs, are an important energy source and maintain epithelial integrity. In addition, SCFAs are ligands for a specific set of G protein-coupled receptors, which are important in the regulation of energy homeostasis. The major SCFAs produced are acetate, propionate and butyrate. Butyrate is the main energy source for colonocytes and can activate intestinal gluconeogenesis. Propionate can have effects in the liver where it regulates gluconeogenesis and satiety signalling. Lastly, acetate is essential for the growth of bacteria and may also regulate appetite. In addition to SCFAs, the intestinal microbiome is responsible for the production of vitamins, namely K and B_{12}. Gut microbial enzymes contribute to bile acid metabolism where primary bile acids are deconjugated to secondary bile acids by enzymes secreted by several bacteria in the colonic microbiome. These secondary bile acids can act as signalling molecules and metabolic regulators of many important pathways. Lastly, it is becoming more evident that non-absorbable and inert dietary chemicals, like polyphenolic compounds, are rendered bioavailable after biotransformation by intestinal bacteria. In the same way, some colon-targeted drugs are delivered as pro-drugs, only having bioactivity once metabolised by bacterial enzymes. The colonic microbiome can also metabolise xenobiotics and drugs which can impact their therapeutic utility in certain diseases and in individuals who have such bacterial species within their intestinal microbiome capable of metabolising drugs.

Host defence and colonisation resistance

As implicated above, the colonic microbiome plays an important defence role to stop the colonisation of invading and pathogenic bacteria and to limit the overgrowth of pathogenic members of the microbiome. The microbiome can effectively compete with pathogens for colonisation and nutrients, in addition to utilising host defence machinery (such as stimulation of host antimicrobial peptides (AMP) and secretions of IgA). This AMP-mediated regulation of bacteria is more predominant in the small intestine where the mucus layer, (which is thick and double-layered in the colon), is diminished. Structural components of bacteria (peptidoglycan, lipopolysaccharide, lipid A, flagella, bacterial RNA/DNA, etc.) and their metabolites can induce the synthesis of AMPs through pattern recognition receptors such as Toll-like receptors, lectin receptors and NOD-like receptors.

Case 9.1 Infective diarrhoea

A 34-year-old man presents to A&E with a 3-day history of abdominal pain, bloody diarrhoea and vomiting. He was previously fit and well with no significant past medical history or drug history. He reported attending a barbecue two days prior to the onset of his symptoms. On examination he had a temperature of 38.9°C with a heart rate of 110 bpm. Palpation of his abdomen revealed generalised tenderness but was otherwise soft with no palpable enlarged organs. His blood tests revealed elevated inflammatory markers with a high white blood cell count and C-reactive protein (CRP). An abdominal X-ray demonstrated a mildly oedematous colon with loss of haustral markings. Stool tests were sent off for microbiology, and this confirmed the presence of *Campylobacter jejuni*. He was treated with fluids and antiemetics. His symptoms started to improve within 24 hours, and he was discharged home. Advice was given to prevent spread of infection that included isolation, hand hygiene and food preparation.

Campylobacter enteritis is one of the most common causes of food poisoning in the Western world resulting in infective diarrhoea. The usual route of transmission is foodborne, through eating undercooked meat and meat products. In addition, in some cases, person-to-person transmission (faecal-oral route) is possible. The incubation period usually varies from 1 to 7 days with symptoms lasting up to a week. Patients often present with acute onset of diarrhoea (often containing blood), abdominal pain and fever. The infection is confirmed on stool testing for microbiology. The mainstay of management is supportive with rehydration and antipyretics. Antibiotics are rarely indicated as most cases are self-limiting.

Host immune development

The gut faces the exceptional challenge of maintaining intestinal immune tolerance and normal homeostasis whilst being tolerant to the beneficial commensals. The microbiome trains and develops major components of the host's innate and adaptive immunity. It is recognised that host immune-microbiome interactions in early life have long-lasting impacts on multiple immune functions that contribute to immune homeostasis and susceptibility to infectious and inflammatory diseases in later life. These mechanisms, however, are still poorly understood.

The capacity to accept the microbiota can also be explained by the relative immaturity of the neonate immune system at birth, and the tolerogenic environment that defines early mammalian life.

The immaturity of the neonate immune system is characterised by blunted inflammatory cytokine production and skewed T- and B-cell development which ensures that the establishment of the microbiota occurs without unwanted inflammation. Early exposure to gut commensal bacteria can also repress cells involved in the induction of inflammatory responses. The neonate immune system recognises bacterial components but responds in a way to promote microbial establishment within the intestine, in contrast to an adult or mature immune system that would produce inflammatory mediators and cytokines. These early responses to microbial ligands condition the gut epithelial cells to become hypo-responsive to subsequent future stimulation. With respect to postnatal immune training, intestinal bacteria also play a critical role in secondary and lymphoid structure development (for example, by dictating the size of Peyer's patches and the number of $CD4^+$ T-cells).

Through these training processes, the establishment of a durable and homeostatic host-commensal relationship is formed. These primary encounters between the host immune system and the microbiota have profound and long-term implications for human health which is detailed for IBD later.

The hygiene hypothesis

Since the 1950s, the incidence of many autoimmune diseases such as multiple sclerosis, Crohn's disease, type 1 diabetes and asthma have soared and similar increases in environmental and food allergies have also been observed. Conversely, there has been an almost mirrored decline in the incidence of infectious diseases thanks to the advent of antibiotics and improved hygiene. This finding has instigated the 'hygiene hypothesis', which correlates the rise in autoimmune and allergic disorders with the decreased exposure to infectious agents and microbes. The hygiene hypothesis is based upon epidemiological data, particularly migration studies, showing that subjects migrating from a low-incidence to a high-incidence country acquire such autoimmune disorders. However, such broad correlations could be irrelevant as many lifestyle and environmental changes have occurred over the past decades as the globe becomes more 'Westernised'. In all these autoimmune disorders, the overactive immune system is the cause of disease and hence the lack of early exposure to microbes and/or the use of antibiotic agents could mis-train or under-educate the immune system in ways described above, leading to this overactivity. Consequently, the intestinal microbiome is implicated. There are increasing data demonstrating that microbiome changes could contribute to the modulation of immune disorders and for IBD.

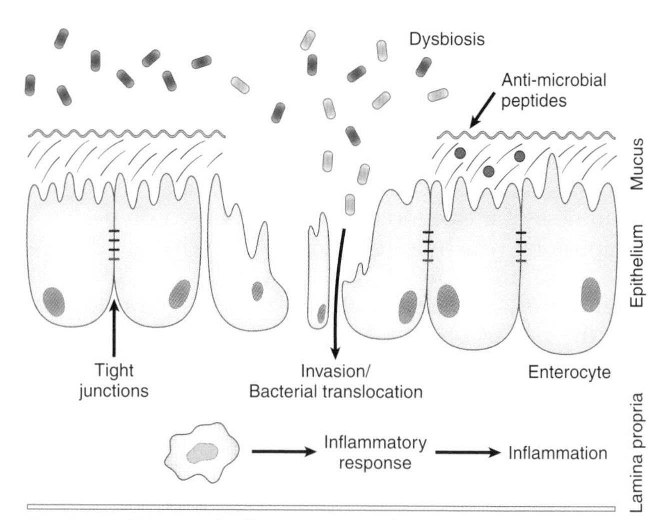

Fig. 9.2 Dysbiosis and inflammation in inflammatory bowel disease. In eubiosis (healthy composition of bacteria), the microbiome plays a vital role in maintaining epithelial integrity through the production of short-chain fatty acids and preventing the expansion of microbial pathogens whilst modulating the immune system. However, the impact of an environmental trigger to cause dysbiosis could result in decreased epithelium integrity and bacterial invasion resulting in the induction of pro-inflammatory cytokines (such as IL-6, IL-7 and TNFα) and inflammation.

Dysbiosis of the intestinal microbiome

A dysbiosis in the intestinal microbiome is a shift or perturbation in the microbial communities that would normally be present. As the composition of communities between individuals is different, the definition of a 'healthy' microbiome and one which is in a dysbiotic state is difficult. One method of characterising a healthy microbiome and a state of dysbiosis is to examine the diversity of richness of communities present. A microbiome associated with health is a rich and diverse microbiome with a high total number of bacterial species and contains less than 10% of the facultative anaerobe phylum, Proteobacteria. This is reversed in a dysbiotic state and specific bacterial species can be identified. For example, in Crohn's disease, a dysbiosis results in fewer bacteria with anti-inflammatory properties and more bacteria with proinflammatory properties.

Dysbiosis in disease

As the intestinal microbiome plays such pivotal role in health, dysbiosis will inevitably impair normal function resulting in both intestinal and extra-intestinal diseases (Fig. 9.2).

IBD

Initial studies implicating the role of bacteria in the pathogenesis of IBD have attempted to identify a single possible culprit as the initiator of the inflammatory cascade seen in IBD. Although specific bacteria have been proposed as direct contributors in the pathogenesis of IBD, no single microorganism has yet reliably been implicated. It is now recognised that the entire gut microbiota is altered in IBD, and this dysbiosis can exacerbate disease progression.

Common compositional profile changes of the intestinal microbiome are found in IBD. These include a decrease in genera of the phyla Bacteroidetes and Firmicutes and an increase in Proteobacteria in patients with IBD when compared to healthy individuals. These alterations appear to be represented by reduced abundance of butyrate-producing and an increase in sulphate-reducing bacteria and other species with pro-inflammatory properties. Collectively, these changes alter the environment of the colon and leads to impaired barrier function, which subsequently increases permeability of the gut and microbes can penetrate the epithelia, exacerbating the immune response.

However, it remains unknown whether this dysbiosis is a cause or consequence of the disease. Recent studies suggest that IBD is a highly multifactorial disease. An environmental trigger (or many) initiates a change in the intestinal microbial composition, yet only in genetically susceptible individuals. This in turn results in the inflammatory response observed in IBD. With the alarming rate at which the incidence of IBD is increasing world-wide, environmental triggers associated with a Western lifestyle are the most likely triggers for this dysbiosis.

Clostridioides difficile infection

Clostridioides difficile is an anaerobic, toxin and spore producing Firmicutes bacterium found within a normal gut microbiome and is largely considered to be a pathobiont. It is believed that other, more dominant gut bacteria confer protection to *C. difficile* infection (CDI) through colonisation resistance. How this is achieved is still unknown, but it is likely through a bile acid-mediated mechanism. Secondary bile acids inhibit the germination of *C. difficile* spores. In a dysbiotic microbiome, less bacteria that produce secondary bile acids are present which provides the opportunity for *C. difficile* to flourish and increase susceptibility toward CDI and increase luminal toxin concentrations. These toxins damage the integrity of the epithelial barrier resulting in an inflammatory response. This initial dysbiosis of the intestinal microbiome provides the opportunity for CDI. The most common reason for the onset of dysbiosis is the use of antibiotics.

Obesity

Sequencing studies have identified microbial composition changes in obese patients in comparison to non-obese cohorts. The changes in composition, and hence the subsequent phenotypic changes include those of increased energy capturing capability, thereby increasing the risk of developing obesity. Murine studies have confirmed that lean mice, inoculated with microbiota from obese mice, demonstrate increased elevations in starch metabolism, body fat and insulin resistance.

Extra-intestinal diseases

It is not only diseases associated with the GI tract and its functions that can be influenced by a dysbiotic microbiome. An ever-increasing list of extra-intestinal diseases is becoming linked with intestinal microbial composition changes. There is a growing appreciation for the role of the gut-brain axis in brain and neurodevelopmental disorders such as autism. Consequently, the role of the intestinal microbiome in the development of neurological diseases is becoming more apparent.

Examining the intestinal microbiome

The ability to characterise and understand the intestinal microbiome is of equal importance for understanding the function of our own genome. The intestinal microbiome has been labelled our 'second genome'. Sequencing methods now enable us to, relatively cheaply, probe and characterise communities within our intestinal microbiome. When assessing the intestinal microbiome, it is well-recognised that differences exist between faecal- and mucosa-associated communities within the same individual. This is an important consideration in sample collection and processing and provides insight into the community niches that bacterial populations within the microbiome prefer. Additionally, two important measures of community diversity are defined with respect to the intestinal microbiome. Alpha diversity refers to the number and richness of species within a population. Beta diversity describes the proportion of specific taxa (for instance, at the phylum, species or strain level).

16S rRNA sequencing

The 16S ribosomal RNA (rRNA) gene is present in all prokaryotes and contains highly conserved genomic regions with other variable regions that are unique to specific bacteria. As such, amplification of this region using polymerase chain reaction (PCR) and subsequent sequencing (for example, next-generation sequencing) can allow the identification of different bacteria within a single sample. This technique is now well-established and allows for high-throughput analysis. However, the DNA sequences identified usually only allow recognition of bacteria at the genus level. Furthermore, as different bacteria have different copy numbers of the 16S rRNA gene, this can skew the interpretation of data when considering relative abundance within a sampled population.

Metagenomics

In a method known as shotgun metagenomics, bacterial DNA is fragmented and randomly sequenced. Once DNA sequences are known, they are subject to bioinformatic analysis and databases to identify the bacteria present in the sample under analysis. In this method, strain-level resolution is possible. Additionally, providing the function of these sequenced genes are known, a sample can be interpreted in terms of how the population of bacteria are functioning and what genes they can express (e.g. to assess metabolism). However, with such a method, databases are required for cross-analysis; these are currently incomplete, making large portions of sequencing data difficult to interpret. They are also currently expensive experiments and require significant bioinformatic interpretation.

Intestinal microbiome as a therapeutic target

The plasticity exhibited by the intestinal microbiota suggests that not only can its composition and function be modified throughout life by extrinsic and intrinsic factors, but also makes it a viable therapeutic target for treatment of gut microbiota-mediated diseases.

Probiotics

Probiotics are formulations that contain microorganisms, and, when taken in appropriate doses and protected in such a way that they reach the colon intact and viable, can engraft, colonise and promote intestinal health. Probiotics compete with pathogenic bacteria for colonisation niches. For example, the probiotic *Escherichia coli* Nissle has been demonstrated to inhibit pathogenic microbes. Interestingly, this strain of *E. coli* has been used in various therapeutic settings for over a century and was one of the first strains isolated for probiotic use. It was isolated from the faeces of a German soldier in the First World War, who, despite his fellow comrades becoming unwell from *Shigella* infection causing gastroenteritis, did not develop any intestinal disease. Other probiotics include *Bifidobacterium*, which has been reported to improve intestinal barrier integrity and exhibits anti-inflammatory effects.

The use of probiotics over the past decades has been largely limited to the self-medication and health supplements, for example, probiotic supplements are readily available from health stores and are found in yoghurt and drinks in supermarkets. This is most likely because the use of probiotics and their efficacy in a clinical setting is highly questioned, and mixed signals in different disease settings have been observed. However, some probiotics are being assessed for the treatment of conditions, such as ulcerative colitis and IBS. Most recently, specific strains of bacteria have also been used in trials to examine their efficacy in the treatment of diabetes and cardiovascular disease, as two examples, but their efficacy remains questionable. This is most likely because studies use different doses, strains and formulations of probiotics, making comparative analysis difficult. In addition, there are concerns around the ability for probiotic bacteria to reach the colon and successfully engraft since the acidic nature of the stomach and colonisation resistance imparted by the microbiome will make this difficult. Consequently, efforts are being made to create formulations that protect probiotic bacteria from any toxic environmental conditions, such as low pH in the stomach. Many probiotics are constituents of fermented foods, as described in Fig. 9.3.

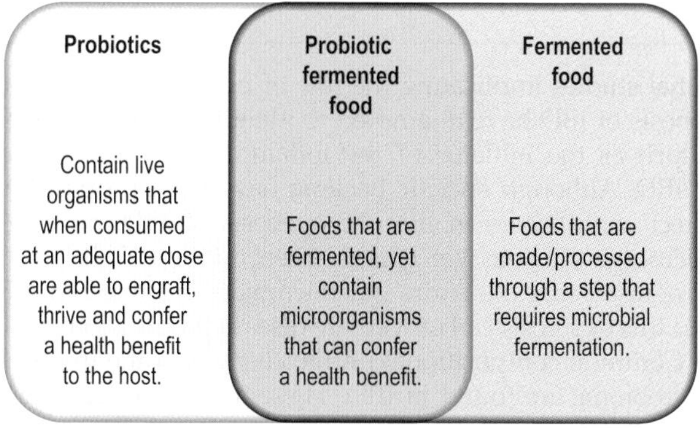

Fig. 9.3 Probiotics can often be contained within fermented food products, but not all fermented foods are probiotics. Probiotics include *Lacticaseibacillus casei or Lactiplantibacillus plantarum*. Probiotic-fermented food examples are yoghurt (which contains live organisms) or cultured/fermented dairy products that contain the fermenting bacterial species. Fermented-only foods are sauerkraut, kombucha and kefir.

Prebiotics

As the microbiome can ferment fibrous substrates that in turn can promote the growth of specific bacterial strains metabolising such nutrients, this can be adopted in a way to support the growth of selective bacteria within the colon. Such an approach, where nutrients are delivered to the colon in a formulation to support the growth of bacteria, is known as prebiotics. Prebiotics do not contain microorganisms, only selective fermentation components. The successful delivery of prebiotic components, such as carbohydrates and oligosaccharides, can promote the growth of *Bifidobacterium* present in the colonic flora which in turn produces SCFAs that are highly beneficial. The efficacy of prebiotics in altering the composition of the intestinal microbiome is more compelling than that of probiotics as it is well-established that a high-fibre diet positively correlates with intestinal health. However, prebiotics in general have limited clinical uses. As we understand how specific prebiotic fibres could be used to selectively enhance bacterial populations, their use may become more established.

Faecal microbiota transplantation

Faecal microbiota transplantation (FMT) is the transfer of a processed stool obtained from a healthy donor into a patient with the aim to correct the underlying dysbiosis by attempting to restore the intestinal microbial community. FMT can be delivered by several routes including colonoscope, nasogastric tube or enema. Fermented faecal suspensions, also known as 'yellow soup', was used as therapy for GI diseases in the 4th century by the Chinese physicians Ge Hong and Li Shizen. In the current medical era, the first reported use of FMT was for the treatment of pseudomembranous colitis in 1958. It now seems likely that these patients were colonised by an overgrowth of toxigenic *C. difficile* as is commonly seen in patients (usually elderly and immunocompromised individuals) who have been treated with broad-spectrum antibiotics. About one third of CDI patients will develop recurrent or persistent disease, refractory to antibiotic treatment. FMT has proved to be highly successful in treating recurrent and antibiotic refractory CDI. In a meta-analysis, FMT was more effective than vancomycin (the common treatment) in resolving recurrent and refractory CDI. Consequently, FMT for recurrent and refractory CDI is now becoming standard practice and is recommended.

Unlike prebiotics or probiotics, FMT delivers a heterogenous mixture of components to the colon of the patient, including bacteria, viruses, partially digested dietary components and intestinal metabolites. It is likely that the high efficacy observed in FMT studies is due to this heterogenous nature. However, this also has potential serious risks as pathogenic bacteria and/or viruses can also be transplanted. This has been observed with reports of possible toxin-producing *E. coli* strains and even SARS-CoV-2 transplanted into patients. Consequently, screening programmes and exclusion criteria are essential when selecting for FMT donors. Despite this, FMT is being examined for a plethora of diseases across the globe, including diabetes, cardiovascular disease and IBD. How FMT is effective in these diseases is unknown but could be attributed to bacterial, SCFA or viral transfer to the patient.

Case 9.2 Antibiotic refractory *Clostrioides difficile* infection

A 74-year-old woman was admitted with a 3-week history of loose stools and fever. She also complained of generalised abdominal discomfort and fatigue. She reports recent use of antibiotics for a lower respiratory tract infection. She had a past medical history of hypertension, type 2 diabetes and asthma. On examination, she was pyrexic with a temperature of 38°C and had mild generalised abdominal tenderness. Her blood tests revealed an elevated white blood cell count and CRP. Stool samples that were sent to the lab for culture were positive for CDI based on PCR and an enzyme-linked immunosorbent assay-based toxin assay. She was isolated in a side room on the ward and strict precautions were taken to prevent spread of the infection. She was commenced on oral vancomycin to treat the infection.

Although there was some initial improvement, her diarrhoea persisted, and her fever reoccurred. She underwent a flexible sigmoidoscopy for further assessment. This showed pseudomembranes in her colon consistent with ongoing CDI. Despite 14 days of oral vancomycin, her diarrhoea persisted. FMT was administered via a nasogastric tube. Her diarrhoea resolved in the next 72 hours, her inflammatory markers improved, and she was successfully discharged home.

Preparation of FMT material

Once potential donors have passed rigorous screening programmes that assess for the history of intestinal diseases or infectious agents that could be present within the stool, stool donations are made. The single best way to prepare FMT material is still under investigation, with questions around storage times and temperature and the importance of preparing material under anaerobic conditions (to preserve the many strains of strict anaerobic bacteria) still unanswered. In general, faeces are processed in less than 6 hours post-defecation. FMT material is prepared by combining the faeces from a single donor (or in some settings, from pooled donors) with saline, which is then homogenised to a slurry. This material is then ready for use or cold storage until ready for transplantation. FMT is predominantly administered via nasogastric tube or colonoscope. The steps taken to prepare FMT are detailed in Fig. 9.4.

FMT in disease

Our understanding of the mechanisms that underpin the success of FMT in certain diseases (and not in others) is currently under investigation. A combination of donor- and patient-centred factors will inevitably determine the

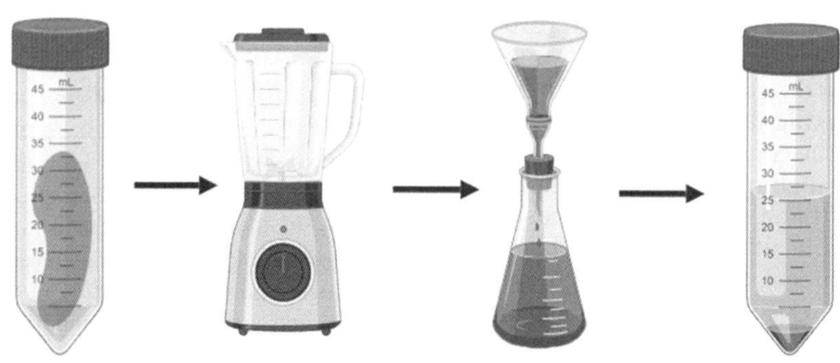

Fig. 9.4 Steps in the preparation of faecal material transplantation (FMT). Stool donations collected from healthy donors are processed within 6 hours of defaecation. Stool weighing at least 50 g is mixed with preservative-free sterile saline and a cryoprotective agent. Stool is then homogenised and filtered. The filtrate is now classified as FMT and can either be used as a fresh infusion or frozen at -80°C for later use.

success of a transplant. For example, the 'super donor' phenomenon has recently been described, where donor material from specific individuals seems to treat disease better than others. This is likely due to the quality of their intestinal microbiome and most probably shaped by their diet and lifestyle. In addition, the patient must also be accepting of the new microbiome, as with any other transplant, which is subject to immune responses and regulation.

With the success of FMT in the treatment of recurrent CDI, many studies are assessing its therapeutic usefulness in a variety of disease settings, including IBD, primary sclerosing cholangitis, obesity, autism and IBS.

abetalipoproteinaemia – a rare autosomal recessive disorder characterised by a low plasma level of betalipoprotein.
achalasia – a motor disorder in which a muscle is unable to relax, particularly the lower oesophagus and the lower oesophageal sphincter (cardiospasm).
achlorhydria – lack of hydrochloric acid secretion in gastric juice.
adenocarcinoma – a malignant tumour of the glandular epithelium (e.g., colonic mucosa).
aetiology – the study of the causes of a disease.
aganglionic – displaying an absence of ganglionic cells.
anaemia – a reduction in total blood haemoglobin.
anastomosis – a connection between two vessels or a surgical joining of two bowel segments to allow flux of the contents from one to the other.
antidiuretic – a substance which diminishes urine production.
ascites – a fluid collection in the peritoneal cavity.
atrophy – wasting or shrinking (of an organ or tissue).
autoimmune – pertaining to the development of an immune response (antibody production) to the body's own tissues.
bacteriostatic – tending to restrain the reproduction of bacteria.
benign – non-malignant (pertaining to tumours).
calculus – an abnormal stone formed in tissues by an accumulation of mineral salts.
cathartic – a (purgative) medicine which increases evacuation of the bowels.
caveolae – invaginations of the cell membrane extending into its cytoplasm.
chloridorrhoea – excessive loss of chloride ions in the faeces.
cholangitis – a bacterial infection of bile in the bile duct.
cholecystectomy – removal of the gall bladder.
cholecystitis – infection (of bile) in the gall bladder.
cholelithiasis – the presence of gall stones.
cholephilic – attracted to bile; easily dissolved in bile.
cholestasis – interruption of bile flow.
cirrhosis – a progressive inflammatory disease in the liver where there is an increase in non-functioning tissue and disruption of the architecture.
colectomy – removal of part of the large bowel (colon).
colic – cyclical intra-abdominal pain owing to dysfunctional peristalsis of the intestine.
colitis – inflammatory disease of the colon.
colostomy – a surgically created opening of the colon in the wall of the abdomen.
computed tomography (CT) – a radiographic scanning procedure where the detailed structure of a tissue is revealed by densitometry. The body is imaged in cross-sectional slices and the computer quantifies the X-ray absorption by the tissues.
constipation – difficulty in passage of stools or infrequent passage of stools.
deglutition – swallowing.
diarrhoea – an abnormal increase in stool liquidity and in daily stool volume.
diuresis – increased production of urine.
diverticulitis – infection in one or more diverticula, usually of the sigmoid colon.
diverticulosis – the presence of pouch-like herniations (diverticula) in the muscular layer of the colon, especially the sigmoid colon.
dysaesthesia – altered perception of oral sensation.
dysbiosis – a change or alternation in the composition in microbial communities.
dysphagia – difficulty in swallowing.
ectasia – dilatation of a duct, vessel, or hollow viscus, usually resulting from obstruction to flow or degenerative changes of the wall.
ectopic – present in an abnormal location (e.g., in pregnancy).
emetic – a substance which causes vomiting.
emollients – substances which alter the consistency (of the faeces).
encephalopathy – any disease or degenerative condition of the brain.
endocytosis – process whereby a molecule or particle becomes surrounded by the cell membrane and engulfed into the cell in a vesicle.
endogenous – originating within the tissues.
endoscopic retrograde pancreatography (ERCP) – a procedure employing a combination of fibre-optic endoscopy and radiography to investigate the presence of biliary and pancreatic disease.
endoscopy – visual examination of a hollow organ (e.g., the gastrointestinal tract) by insertion of an endoscope (an illuminated optical instrument).
enteritis – inflammation of the intestines.
enterotype – classification system based on the bacteriological composition of the gut microbiota.
epigastric – in the upper central abdominal region.
exocytosis – the process by which vesicles release their contents by fusing with the cell's plasma membrane.
exogenous – originating from outside the tissues.
extrinsic – originating (usually situated) outside the tissue.
exudate – a fluid that has oozed out of a tissue and so has a high protein content.
fenestrae – pores.
fibrosis – proliferation of fibrous connective tissue.
fistula – an abnormal passage from an internal organ to the body surface or between two organs.
gastrectomy – surgical removal of the stomach.
gastrinoma – hypersecreting gastrin tumour derived from neuroendocrine cells.
glycosuria – glucose in the urine.
granuloma – a chronic inflammatory lesion characterised by accumulation of macrophages.
haemodynamics – the study of the physical aspects of the blood circulation.
haemolytic – causing the red blood cells to break down and release haemoglobin.
haemorrhoid – a submucosal swelling in the anal canal caused by congestion of the veins of the haemorrhoidal plexus.

hemicolectomy – surgical removal of part of the large bowel with restoration of continuity.
hepatitis – an inflammation of the liver.
hepatoma – a primary tumour of the liver.
homeostasis – constancy of the internal environment of the body.
hydrophilic – attracted to, and easily dissolved in, water.
hydrophobic – not attracted to, and insoluble in, water.
hyperaemia – increased (regional) blood flow.
hyperbilirubinaemia – an abnormally high concentration of bilirubin in the plasma.
hyperglycaemia – increased plasma glucose.
hyperinsulinaemia – increased plasma insulin.
hyperkeratosis – overgrowth of the cornified epithelium layer of the skin (e.g., a wart).
hyperketonaemia – an abnormally high level of ketone bodies in the plasma.
hyperplasia – abnormal growth of a tissue owing to an increased rate of cell division.
hypertension – chronically increased arterial blood pressure.
hypertonic – containing a higher concentration of effectively membrane-impermeable solute particles than normal (isotonic) extracellular fluid.
hypertrophy – enlargement of a tissue or organ because of increased cell size rather than increased cell number.
hypocalcaemia – decreased plasma calcium.
hypochromia – a low haemoglobin concentration in the erythrocytes.
hypoglycaemia – low plasma glucose.
hypoinsulinaemia – low plasma insulin.
hypokalaemia – decreased plasma K1 concentration.
hypotension – low blood pressure.
hypotonic – containing a lower concentration of effectively non-penetrating solute particles than normal (isotonic) extracellular fluid.
hypovolaemia – low blood volume.
hypoxia – deficiency of oxygen (in a tissue).
idiopathic – of unknown cause.
ileitis – inflammatory disease of the ileum.
ileus – loss of peristalsis in the small bowel, usually following surgery, that results in a functional obstruction.
insulinoma – a tumour of the insulin-secreting cells of the pancreas.
intrinsic – originating within the tissue.
ischaemia – decreased supply of oxygenated blood to an organ or structure.
isosmotic – having the same total solute concentration as extracellular fluid.
isotonic – containing the same number of effectively non-penetrating solute particles as extracellular fluid.
jaundice – yellowish discolouration of the skin, mucous membranes, and sclerae owing to deposition of bilirubin.
ketoacidosis – acidosis accompanied by an accumulation of ketones in the body.
lipolysis – breakdown of lipids.
lithotripsy – shattering of (gall or kidney) stones by ultrasound waves.
macrocytic – high mean cell volume (usually pertaining to red blood cells).
malignancy – a tumour with the ability to invade and spread to other tissues and organs.
mastication – chewing.
meconium – greenish material which fills the intestines of the foetus and forms the first bowel movement in the newborn.
meconium ileus – obstruction of the small intestine in the newborn by impaction of meconium (usually in cystic fibrosis).
megacolon – a massively enlarged colon.
megaloblast – an abnormally large, nucleated, immature erythrocyte present in large numbers in pernicious anaemia or folate-deficiency anaemia.
metastasis – the process by which tumour cells spread to distant parts of the body.
microcytic – characterised by the presence of cells with low mean cell volume (usually pertaining to red blood cells).
myogenic – pertaining to (cardiac and smooth) muscle that requires nerve impulses to initiate and maintain a contraction.
necrosis – localized tissue death in response to disease or injury.
neoplasm – an abnormal new development of cells (a tumour).
nexus – gap junction; a zone of apposition between two cells where action potentials can be conducted between the cells.
oedema – accumulation of excess fluid in interstitial spaces.
olfaction – smell.
orad – in a direction towards the mouth.
osmolarity – total solute concentration of a solution.
pancreatitis – inflammatory disease of the pancreas.
peptic ulcer – ulceration of the stomach and or small intestine.
paracrine – relates to an agent that exerts its effects on cells near its site of secretion (by convention, excludes neurotransmitters).
parenteral – relating to treatment other than through the digestive system (e.g., by intravenous administration).
parietal cells – acid-secreting cells of the stomach.
periodontal – pertaining to the area around the teeth.
peritonitis – inflammatory disease of the peritoneum, often secondary to perforation of the bowel.
pinocytosis – endocytosis when the vesicle encloses extracellular fluid or specific molecules in the extracellular fluid that have bound to proteins on the extracellular surface of the plasma membrane.
polydipsia – excessive drinking (usually seen in hyperglycaemia).
polyuria – high urine output.
prophylactic – an agent used to prevent the development of a disease.
purgative – a strong medication used to promote evacuation of the bowels.

roughage – non-digestible dietary fibre, important to promote gut motility.
ruga – a fold of mucosa in the stomach.
satiety – cessation of the feeling of hunger.
scintigraphy – a clinical procedure consisting of the administration of a radiolabelled agent with a specific affinity for an organ or tissue of interest, followed by determination, with a detector, of the distribution of the radiolabelled compound.
sclerosis – hardening of a tissue, especially by the overgrowth of fibrous tissue.
sclerotherapy – a technique using sclerosing solutions to cause obliteration of pathological blood vessels (as in the treatment of haemorrhoids).
secretagogue – a substance that regulates the release of a secretion.
sigmoidoscope – a rigid tubular instrument used for direct visualization of the rectal and sigmoid colonic mucosa.
somatic – pertaining to one of two major divisions of the peripheral nervous system, consisting of sensory neurones concerned with sensation from the skin and body surface and motor neurones to the skeletal muscles, the other division being the autonomic nervous system.
splenomegaly – enlargement of the spleen.
steatorrhoea – a condition where the faeces have a high fat content.
stenosis – a narrowing or constriction of a tube (e.g., bowel) or aperture (e.g., ampulla of Vater).
stent – a short plastic tube.
submodality – subclass of a stimulus which evokes a sensory response.
submucosal – beneath the mucosa.
tetany – a maintained contraction.
thrombocytosis – an abnormal increase in the number of thrombocytes (blood platelets).
tonic – undergoing continuous muscular activity.
vagotomy – division of the vagus nerves.
varices – dilated veins, usually of the oesophagus, owing to raised portal vein pressure.
vasoconstriction – constriction of blood vessels.
vasodilator – a substance which causes dilatation of arterioles.
viscera – body organs (e.g., liver, pancreas).
xenobiotic – an organic substance which is foreign to the body (e.g., a drug or an organic poison).
xerophthalmia – a disturbance of epithelial tissues
xerostomia – dry mouth.

Index

Note: Page number followed by 'f' indicate figure, 't' indicate table and 'b' indicate boxes.

A

D

E

F

G

H

I

N

O

P

R

S